T0182064

Rational Suicide in the Elderly

Robert E. McCue · Meera Balasubramaniam
Editors

Rational Suicide in the Elderly

Clinical, Ethical, and Sociocultural Aspects

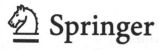 Springer

Editors
Robert E. McCue
Department of Psychiatry
New York University School of Medicine
New York, NY, USA

Meera Balasubramaniam
Department of Psychiatry
New York University School of Medicine
New York, NY, USA

ISBN 978-3-319-81343-1   ISBN 978-3-319-32672-6   (eBook)
DOI 10.1007/978-3-319-32672-6

Printed on acid-free paper

This Springer imprint is published by Springer Nature
The registered company is Springer International Publishing AG
The registered company address is: Gewerbestrasse 11, 6330 Cham, Switzerland

Contents

Contributors

Meera Balasubramaniam, M.D., M.P.H. Department of Psychiatry, New York University School of Medicine, New York, NY, USA

Joshua Briscoe, M.D. Department of Internal Medicine and Department of Psychiatry and Behavioral Sciences, Duke University Medical Center, Durham, NC, USA

Gary Cheung, F.R.A.N.Z.C.P. Department of Psychological Medicine, The University of Auckland, Auckland, New Zealand

Anthony M. Daniels, M.R.C.Psych. Retired Consultant, City Hospital, Birmingham, UK

Simon Dein, F.R.C.Psych., Ph.D. Departments of Anthropology and Medicine, University College, London, UK

Department of Theology and Religion, Durham University, Queen's Campus, Stockton-on-Tees, UK

Darryl Etter, Psy.D. Department of Primary Care—Mental Health Integration, VA Eastern Colorado Health Care System, Denver, CO, USA

Charles S. Grob, M.D. Department of Psychiatry, David Geffen School of Medicine at UCLA, University of California Los Angeles School of Medicine, Los Angeles, CA, USA

Peter S. Hendricks, Ph.D. Department of Health Behavior, School of Public Health, University of Alabama at Birmingham, Birmingham, AL, USA

Warren Kinghorn, M.D. Th.D. Department of Psychiatry and Behavioral Sciences, Duke University Medical Center, Duke Divinity School, Durham, NC, USA

Elissa Kolva, Ph.D. Division of Medical Oncology, Department of Medicine, University of Colorado School of Medicine, South Aurora, CO, USA

Robert E. McCue, M.D. Department of Psychiatry, New York University School of Medicine, New York, NY, USA

Lawrence J. Nelson, Ph.D., J.D. Department of Philosophy, Santa Clara University, Santa Clara, CA, USA

Alan Pope, Ph.D. Department of Psychology, University of West Georgia, Carrollton, GA, USA

Kristin S. Raj, M.D. Department of Psychiatry and Behavioral Sciences, Stanford University School of Medicine, Stanford, CA, USA

Erick Ramirez, Ph.D. Department of Philosophy, Santa Clara University, Santa Clara, CA, USA

Barbara R. Sommer, M.D. Department of Psychiatry and Behavioral Sciences, Stanford University School of Medicine, Stanford, CA, USA

Frederick Sundram, Ph.D., F.R.C.Psych. Department of Psychological Medicine, The University of Auckland, Auckland, New Zealand

Jukka Varelius, Ph.D. Departments of Philosophy, Contemporary History, and Political Science, University of Turku, Turku, Finland

Introduction

Why did we do this book? Both of us are psychiatrists specializing in the treatment of late-life mental disorders and have encountered older patients with no significant mental illness expressing a desire to kill themselves. We were unprepared as to what our clinical response should be. There was little information about this to be found in the psychiatric literature where suicide is considered a sign of a mental disturbance. Our patients did not appear mentally ill, but the threats of suicide were disturbing to us. Were their plans to kill themselves rational, as they insisted? Is there such a thing as rational suicide? How would we know if that is the case? What do we do if it is? What can we do?

The idea of rational suicide in the elderly highlights societal perspectives and stigma at three levels: (a) Is being suicidal a mental illness? (b) Can individuals with mental illness be rational? and (c) How are societal views of the elderly and ageism involved? An older adult expressing a wish to end life understandably evokes many emotions in clinicians. We needed guidance to sort out our cultural beliefs from our personal feelings from our clinical instincts. Therefore, we decided to make sense of what we were experiencing by editing this book.

This book is not about those unfortunate individuals who take their lives as a result of a diagnosable and treatable mental illness. In fact, the odds are that an elderly person who is suicidal has a significant clinical depression. This book is not about these people. Rather, this book is about people at the later stage of life who, without a clearly diagnosable mental illness, have made a well-considered decision to kill themselves. This is rational suicide in the elderly. If the majority of suicides are due to mental illness, why are we addressing the small number who are not mentally ill? As mental health practitioners, we have been trained to consider suicide as a clinical entity within the purview of mental health. However, an increasing number of elderly individuals desire to control the timing and manner of their death and believe that they have a right to determine how they will die. There are organizations such as SOARS (Society for Old Age Rational Suicide), Compassion and Choices, and other right-to-die groups advocating for this. This convinced us that even if the mental health profession is not informed about this topic and ready to confront it, many of our potential patients are.

Our intention is to provide guidance to the clinician in understanding the meaning of death and suicide in old age at a multitude of levels—intrapsychic, interpersonal, philosophical, spiritual, societal, ethical, and legal. We do not espouse a view on whether suicide in the elderly can be rational. However, we have permitted the authors of individual chapters to examine this topic from the lens of their individual beliefs and intellectual points-of-view. We wanted to explore the subject of rational suicide in the elderly from a very broad perspective and allow you, the reader, to draw your own conclusions. The subject of this book concerns death, which has deeply personal and dynamic meanings.

A brief guide to the chapters follows:

Chapter 1, *Can Suicide in the Elderly Be Rational?:* a bio-ethical look at the subject, establishing criteria for determining the rationality of a suicidal wish

Chapter 2, *Would This Be Rational Suicide?:* applying the criteria outlined in Chap. 1 to a real-life case

Chapter 3, *Rational Suicide and the Law:* legal guidelines for clinicians dealing with patients who express a desire to commit rational suicide

Chapter 4, *Refractory Depression and the Right to Terminate Active Treatment:* patients with medical illnesses can be considered as terminally ill and conversations about discontinuing treatment are common; what about patients with psychiatric illness?

Chapter 5, *A Psychological History of Ageism and Its Implications for Elder Suicide:* clinicians cannot isolate themselves from society's norms; older adults have been valued differently throughout history; how is our current view of old age reflected in our beliefs about rational suicide in this population?

Chapter 6, *Rational Suicide in the Elderly: Anthropological Perspectives:* a social anthropological survey of suicide in the elderly and how a culture's beliefs affects its "rationality"

Chapter 7, *Life's Meaning and Late-Life Rational Suicide:* an examination of how understanding our philosophical stance on life's meaning has clinical implications when we are faced with an older patient who has an apparently rational wish to die

Chapter 8, *Baby Boomers and Rational Suicide:* for mental health practitioners treating older adults, it will soon be all about the Baby Boomers; what is there about this cohort that portends a special relationship with rational suicide?

Chapter 9, *Who Are the Elderly Who Want to End Their Lives?:* an examination of the biopsychosocial aspects of those older adults who wish to die

Chapter 10, *Psychological Issues in Late-Life Rational Suicide:* an overview of psychological issues that may play a role in expressions of rational suicide in older adults

Chapter 11, *A Psychodynamic Perspective on Suicidal Desire in the Elderly:* a review of unconscious factors related to suicide and how these must be considered before a determination is made of its rationality

Chapter 12, *The Impact of Psychotherapy on Rational Suicide:* a desire for rational suicide should not lead to therapeutic nihilism; a review of psychotherapeutic measures for these patients

Chapter 13, *Spirituality, Religion, and Rational Suicide:* understanding the spiritual and religious dimensions of suicide and how spiritual interventions may be clinically helpful in older adults who profess a wish to die

Chapter 14, *Classic Psychedelics and Rational Suicide in the Elderly: Exploring the Potential Utility of a Re-emerging Treatment Paradigm:* reviews the evidence that psychedelics may be helpful in restoring the desire to live in older adults who, without being mentally ill, wish to die

Chapter 15, *Epilogue:* an experienced clinician and writer considers the information in this volume about rational suicide in the elderly.

New York, NY   Robert E. McCue
                                                                                    Meera Balasubramaniam

Can Suicide in the Elderly Be Rational?

1

Lawrence J. Nelson and Erick Ramirez

1.1 Introduction

The orthodox view among mental health clinicians is that suicide is an important and largely preventable public health problem that is inextricably intertwined with and usually caused by mental illness [1, 2]. This view holds that because suicide arises out of mental illness, it is irrational, contrary to the interests of the individual, ethically wrong, and ought to be opposed and prevented in all cases. It is undoubtedly true as a general matter that suicide is a serious public health problem and that persons contemplating suicide ought to be discouraged and prevented from doing so. This problem includes many elderly individuals who end their own lives [3]. The elderly perform suicide at higher rates than young people in most countries across the world [4].

This chapter and book explore suicide in the elderly not because only the elderly may have rational grounds for wanting to end their lives and have the mental capacity to make such a choice. Instead, this subject is timely because many mental health clinicians are encountering increasing numbers of elderly persons who express a desire to end their lives and whose symptoms and behavior do not readily constitute mental pathology–and clinicians are questioning how to properly manage these patients. Another important reason for exploring rational suicide in the elderly is that the reasons they offer for wanting to end their lives are very much like those the terminally ill present in support of their right to end their lives. Suicide arising from terminal illness is now quite widely understood as the product of rational processes and has received considerable social and legal approval [5–9].

In contrast to the orthodox view, we do not believe it is true that every elderly person who intentionally takes or desires to take his or her own life is *therefore* mentally

L.J. Nelson, Ph.D., J.D. (✉) • E. Ramirez, Ph.D.
Department of Philosophy, Santa Clara University,
500 El Camino Real, Santa Clara, CA 95053-0310, USA
e-mail: lnelson@scu.edu; ejramirez@scu.edu

© Springer International Publishing Switzerland 2017
R.E. McCue, M. Balasubramaniam (eds.), *Rational Suicide in the Elderly*,
DOI 10.1007/978-3-319-32672-6_1

ill (although we acknowledge many may be, to one extent or another). Nor do we accept the assumption that the diagnosis of a mental illness for a person contemplating suicide necessarily renders the individual irrational, nor would it automatically require that a clinician—and other persons with knowledge of the individual's intentions as well—utilize legal or other forms of intervention to prevent the suicide. In other words, not all suicides among the elderly are irrational, ethically wrong, or should be actively opposed and prevented by others. We acknowledge that determining that a suicide is rational does not by itself mean that it is ethically justifiable although assessing its rationality may be a necessary first step toward reaching this conclusion.

Our primary focus is on how psychiatrists or other mental health professionals (hereafter "therapists") should think about suicide in the elderly in both ethical and professional terms and how they might respond to their elderly patients' disclosure that they are contemplating taking their own lives. We will be primarily addressing elderly patients who disclose a desire to end their own lives and who lack a diagnosis and prognosis that predicts they will very likely die within 6 months. However, this kind of prognostication about when death will occur is inexact [10], and it seems arbitrary to exclude individuals with incurable, but not proximately terminal, conditions such as amyotrophic lateral sclerosis and multiple sclerosis from the population of those who may have a "good" reason to want to die. Consequently, we do not believe the applicability of our analysis and arguments strictly depends on a patient's predicted proximity to the end of her life.

First, this chapter will explore the conventional view that persons who express suicidal desires are invariably mentally ill and that their acting on these desires is irrational and, *as a result*, morally wrong. Desires for suicide can, in many cases, arise without the presence of a mental illness. Furthermore, we will explore the relationship between rationality and mental illness. We argue that the fact that a patient has been diagnosed with a mental illness does not thereby render all desires for suicide automatically irrational. Second, as we do not believe that "suicide" is a concept with a single, widely shared meaning, we will claim that suicides more or less fall into one of three categories and that an analysis of these categories will illuminate the relationship between rationality and suicide. Third, we will examine and question the validity of the common notion that the presence of a terminal illness makes a patient's desire to end her or his life rational. Fourth, we will offer guidelines for assessing the rationality of elderly persons who voice a desire to end their lives. Finally, we will offer some cases that we will use to explain and defend our contention that some suicides in the elderly can be both rational and ethically justifiable.

We will not be addressing the questions of whether it is ethically justifiable for a therapist or other person to assist in someone's suicide at her request or of whether someone may intentionally take the life of another at her request for merciful reasons, i.e., perform voluntary active euthanasia. Likewise, we will not discuss the arguments in favor and against laws that permit physicians to assist in the voluntary suicide of the terminally ill. Furthermore, we will not argue that every rational adult, whether elderly or not, has a right to end his own life voluntarily, a right that would ground an ethical obligation on the part of others never to interfere with any attempt to terminate his life. Respect for the inherent value of human life as well as recognition of the fact that many (perhaps most) suicides are the impulsive, ill-considered acts of mentally unstable individuals should strongly incline the law, general social policy, and common social practice to routinely oppose suicide and encourage persons to prevent others from taking their own lives. Adults who have what they consider to be a rational desire to end their own lives should certainly expect to be called upon to explain and defend their desire, especially to loved ones and to clinicians with whom they have a therapeutic relationship. Whether any persons have an ethical obligation to accept someone's rational case for suicide and leave him or her alone to carry out her desire to die without interference is a question beyond the scope of this chapter.

1.2   Suicide, Mental Illness, and Rationality

The expression of a desire to suicide is often interpreted as symptomatic of underlying mental illness. Statistics often appear to bear this out. Werth, for example, observed that "approximately 80 % of all suicides are related to depression and/or alcoholism… [and] over 90 % of all people who suicided had a psychiatric disorder when they killed themselves" [11]. The relationship between suicidal desire and the presence of a mental illness is thought to be so strong that it is often referred to as the "orthodox psychiatric view" [12].

Although the rationality of a particular desire for suicide is important, it does not yet tell us whether such a desire would be good to act on. We do, however, wish to speak to the view that desires for suicide undermine a person's rationality. On this view, any patient that expresses a desire to suicide is presumed to be irrational because such a desire owes its origin to mental illness. However, this would not automatically render all desires for suicide irrational without the additional supposition that mental illnesses always undermine a person's competence [13]. Although this supposition is common, we will argue that it is false.

The orthodox view assumes that patients who express a desire to suicide are mentally ill and therefore that their desires cannot be the product of a rational process. Such desires require treatment instead of respect on the part of clinicians. Although we will show that these assumptions are common and currently supported by diagnostic assumptions present in the two dominant psychiatric diagnostic manuals (the DSM 5 and ICD 10), we suggest that these assumptions should be rejected. We argue that a desire for suicide can be rational. First, persons without mental illness can have good reasons to end their own lives. We go further, however, and claim that the presence of a mental illness, including depression, does not automatically render desires for suicide irrational.

There is substantial evidence to suggest that most clinicians hold something like the orthodox view. Werth, for example, discovered that health-care practitioners were significantly less accepting and far more likely to take paternalistic preventive action when a nonterminal patient expresses a desire for suicide [11]. He noted that psychological suffering not connected to a terminal illness is seen as impairing a person's rationality, including the rationality of requests for suicide. More recent data suggest that this view remains common in the profession. For example, one study has discovered that clinicians tend to have much less favorable prognostic views about patients with mental illnesses than the general public [14].

Diagnostic categories appear to support the assumptions in the orthodox view. For example, the latest editions of the two dominant diagnostic manuals in psychiatry, the *Diagnostic and Statistical Manual of Mental Disorders* (hereafter "the DSM") [15] and the *International Classification of Disease* ("ICD") [16], both incorporate suicidal desires, ideation, or behavior as a component in the diagnostic criteria for several mental illnesses (e.g., "Suicidal Behavior Disorder" (DSM 5) and "Suicidal Ideation" 2016 ICD-10-CM Diagnosis Code R45.851). Diagnostic classifications like these provide some support for clinicians' assumptions that suicidal desire, behavior, and ideation are products of mental illness. Given the role of the DSM and ICD in clinical contexts, suicidal desire would be seen as an indicator of an underlying mental illness. The DSM makes the link between suicidal desire and rationality-undermining mental illness especially clear. When discussing illnesses comorbid with suicidal behavior disorder, bipolar disorder, schizophrenia disorder, panic disorders, PTSD, alcohol use disorder, antisocial personality disorder, and major depressive disorder are linked to it [15]. Given the stated links between suicidal desire and rationality-undermining mental illnesses, it is not surprising that therapists hold the orthodox view.

Because mental illnesses are conditions that require treatment, desires of patients with these illnesses are typically not viewed as rational. The idea that suicidal behavior, without regard for the context in which the desire arose, can satisfy the diagnostic requirements for a mental disorder is at odds with the acceptance of any form of rational suicide, including assisted suicide in terminal cases. Given the growing acceptance of rational suicide in terminal cases, it is likely that future editions of the DSM and ICD will revise their diagnostic criteria to reflect this change and include rational suicidal desire in at least a limited range of terminal cases.

As currently written, the diagnostic criteria for mental illnesses linked with suicide do not mention their rationality. For example, the criteria for suicidal behavioral disorder do not provide any instruction to clinicians to consider the rationality of their patient's suicidal desire or subsequent behavior in the light of the patient's grounding values and life goals. It also does not ask therapists to consider a patient's subjective well-being or how it would be affected by suicide. Such issues are standard considerations when considering the rationality of suicide in cases of terminal physical illnesses. Additionally, suicidal desires in cases of terminal illness that are seen as rational by many health-care practitioners implies either that these practitioners believe that desires for suicide are not always symptomatic of mental illness *or* that some mental illnesses do not undermine rationality.

However, the diagnosis of suicidal behavioral disorder is not the most commonly invoked illness discussed in connection with suicide, mental health, and rationality. Werth noted that "[o]ne of the primary reasons professionals argue that rational suicide is not possible is because suicidal people are depressed and therefore their cognitive functioning is impaired" [11]. Depression is a serious illness. We do not claim that depression never undermines rationality, nor do we deny that the DSM 5 diagnostic information for major depressive disorder (MDD) [15] properly includes suicidal ideation and suicidal desire as one element for diagnosis. However, it is important to consider how the DSM operationalizes MDD and the role of suicidal ideation within the context of rationality. MDD can be diagnosed if a patient feels, among other symptoms, a:

1. Depressed mood most of the day, nearly every day.
2. Markedly diminished interest in pleasure in all, or almost all, activities most of the day, nearly every day.
3. Recurrent thoughts of death (not just fear of dying), recurrent suicidal ideation without a specific plan, or a suicide attempt or a specific plan for committing suicide [15].

Because many individuals who suicide do so while suffering from MDD and because depression itself is often seen as undermining the rationality of the sufferer, we can again see reason to hold the orthodox view.

There are two related worries that arise about diagnostic criteria and how they link suicidal desires with major depressive episodes. On the one hand, even if it is true that the presence of depression always undermines a patient's rationality, this concern leaves open the possibility that a desire for suicide can arise free from any mental illness. Unless a therapist also believes that desires for suicide are *intrinsically* symptomatic of mental illness, it remains a possibility that some suicides are rational. However, the assumption that suicidal desire is necessarily connected with mental illness runs counter to the belief that at least some forms of self-inflicted deaths are rational and permissible (or, in cases of self-sacrifice, praiseworthy). On the other hand, we argue that depressive episodes do not always undermine the rationality of a person's desires, including desires for suicide. Depressed persons who desire suicide may be expressing a rational desire despite the presence of depression. In order to make headway on whether the "orthodox psychiatric view on suicide" [13] is correct about suicide and rationality, we need to say more about rationality and competence.

To say that a person is rational or competent is to make a claim about her capacities. We agree with Culver and Gert who have argued that "[c]ompetence is task-specific: a person is competent or incompetent to make a will, to perform a neurological examination, or to refuse a suggested medical intervention. It does not follow from the fact that a person is competent to do X that he is competent to do Y" [17]. Philosophers sometimes also discuss rationality in terms of the ability to understand and appreciate the reasons available to a person. Furthermore, rationality and competence require that a person not only demonstrates sensitivity to reasons but that they demonstrate a pattern of responding to reasons that is comprehensible to others. To be sensitive to a reason is to understand the reason. For persons to understand a reason, they must be able to see that a reason applies to their situation and that it calls for some kind of action on their part (to see that my friendship with you is a reason to console you means that I understand what friendship means, that we are friends and that consolation would be good for you). When assessing rationality, we need to be sensitive to how rationality is being discussed and to the particular capacity being assessed.

Rationality is sometimes spoken of in a strongly *objective* sense. An objective sense of rationality sees reason and rationality in a universal way. If rationality is objective in this strong sense, then all rational agents would reach the same conclusions about what to do in a situation because reason pulls in one direction and all truly rational agents would recognize these reasons and act accordingly [18]. We reject this conception of rationality for two reasons. First, we believe that it is *too demanding*. The objective conception of rationality would produce a world without any rational agents in it. This is because of what appear to be irrational features of normal human agency. All of us are subject to heuristics and biases that undermine rationality from the objective point of view. Tversky and Kahneman [19] have documented many of these biases. Though all of us commonly succumb to irrational beliefs due to these heuristics and biases (e.g., by giving in to the sunk-cost fallacy), these forms of irrational beliefs do not render us irrational *as agents*. We still hold each other responsible in light of our choices. For this reason, the purely objective conception of rationality fails to give us the right standard for assessing the rationality of suicidal desires. Second, we reject the objective conception of rationality because we wish to remain pluralistic about the kinds of values that rational agents might have and use when they make decisions. Individuals who value autonomy may rationally come to different conclusions about how to respond to early onset dementia than individuals who believe that life is sacred and should be preserved whenever possible. Value pluralism would allow us to say that these individuals may rationally reach different conclusions about suicide. This would be impossible on a purely objective conception of rationality.

In part to allay concerns like these, rationality is sometimes referred to in a purely *subjective* sense. This sense of rationality assesses beliefs and behaviors by looking at a person's preexisting values and beliefs and judges a person's desires on that basis. For example, the rationality of a decision to forgo reconstructive surgery following a mastectomy is thought to depend entirely on a patient's subjective preference for or against such a surgery. Though a subjective sense of rationality allows for value pluralism, it too should be rejected. In part this is because subjective rationality is *too permissive*: it would count some desires for suicide as rational that, to us at least, are clearly not. For example, suppose that a patient comes to believe that she has a terminal condition that will leave her in great pain and with limited cognitive function. Furthermore, she does not attempt to verify these beliefs and cannot explain how she came to have them. On the basis of these beliefs, she formulates a desire to end her life. Such a desire would be rational in the purely subjective sense because it follows from her preexisting (but mistaken) beliefs in a straightforward way. However, the beliefs that are used to justify her desire for suicide are irrational. She lacks good reason to believe that she has a terminal condition. The same can be said of desires formed on the basis of a schizophrenic hallucination. The purely subjective sense of rationality cannot easily explain why these desires are irrational and is therefore too broad: it would include too many suicidal desires as rational.

For these reasons, we claim that rationality is best understood as a distinctly *intersubjective* concept. Rationality is not something that can be assessed purely by considering only an individual's beliefs and values because those beliefs may be irrational. Similarly, rationality cannot be assessed in a purely detached, objective sense. To say that rationality is intersubjective is to say that it requires third parties to understand a person's reasons in order for those reasons to be rational. For a desire to be understood as rational, it must be *comprehensible* to at least some third-party communities. Comprehensibility does not require that a clinician share a person's beliefs or values in order to make judgments about the rationality of their patient's desires. A pattern of reasons can be comprehensible even if one disagrees with them. Consider the following example from Fischer and Ravizza, "Relative to an agent's preferences, values, and beliefs, reasons are graded in terms of their strength." An agent is rational if she demonstrates an understandable pattern of reasoning. "For example, if a ticket's costing a thousand dollars is a reason not to go to the game, surely (barring unusual circumstances) a ticket's costing two thousand dollars should be a reason not to go to the game…" [20].

If a person claimed that one thousand dollars was too much to pay for tickets but would go to the game if the tickets cost two thousand dollars, we have two possibilities. Either the person is irrational, or we are missing information that makes this pattern of reasoning comprehensible. At face value, the individual in the example is irrational. If one thousand dollars is too much for a ticket to a basketball game, then rationality requires that two thousand dollars is also too much to pay. However, if he were able to provide us with more information, his pattern of response may become comprehensible. For example, suppose it turned out that the agent's company would only reimburse tickets to events if they cost more than one thousand dollars, then the pattern of reasoning suddenly becomes *comprehensible*. It makes sense that he would view one thousand dollars as too high of a cost for him to personally pay but that he would view two thousand dollars as a cost worth (his company) paying for. We can make these assessments of rationality even if we do not share the same values as the person whose rationality we are assessing. For example, one author (E.R.) does not identify as a sports fan. For him, no amount of money is worth paying to attend a game. However, this does not impact his ability to *comprehend* the pattern of reasons above. Intersubjective conceptions of rationality are the only ones that can capture both the objective and subjective aspects of rationality. Others have reached similar conclusions about the nature of rationality: "[a]ny account of irrationality to be incorporated into the concept of competence must be such that no decision is regarded as irrational if any significant number of persons would regard that decision as rational" [17].

What matters from the point of view of assessing the rationality of a desire is that the pattern of reasoning that produces the desire is *comprehensible* not only from the point of view of the individual herself but also from the point of view of at least some third-party groups. If at least some groups comprehend her reasoning, then her desire, whatever other problems it may have, is not irrational. Take, for example, religiously inspired martyrdom. Suicide-bombing may be based on beliefs that many see as false. However, given the existence of religious communities that accept and comprehend martyrdom, such acts are not *irrational*. We may believe that martyrdom is immoral, but it would be a mistake to see it as irrational. These are two different assessments of the behavior.

How does this account translate to desires for suicide and to a therapist's task of assessing whether or not a patient's desire is rational, or whether the presence of a mental illness undermines the rationality of their patient's desire? There are several consequences of adopting the intersubjective view of rationality and competence. Therapists increasingly tend to view suicidal desires as rational when patients are suffering from a terminal illness. The intersubjective view helps to explain why such desires are rational. Even if we personally believe that life is sacred and should not be ended prematurely, we can understand (i.e., we can *comprehend*) how the prospect of a painful terminal illness could produce a desire for suicide. Contrast this with the common but tragic cases of adolescent suicide resulting from the end of a relationship. Although we may see why an adolescent could believe that suicide is the right response to a bad breakup, we also understand that such desires are usually based on irrational beliefs that they will never love or be loved again. Because their desires are grounded not merely on false beliefs but on false beliefs that are irrationally produced, the intersubjective view can explain why these sorts of suicidal desires are *irrational*.

Desires for suicide accompanied by depressive symptoms or even desires that are causally connected with depression are only problematic if they undermine a patient's rationality and competence. It is clear that this is not always the case. Depression is consistent with a desire that is the product of a comprehensible pattern of reasoning and this remains true even if a therapist disagrees with her patient about what a patient *should* decide. Although it should be clear why at least some suicidal desires are rational, our intersubjective conception of rationality can also show that depression need not always undermine the rationality suicidal desires. In 2013, the bereavement exclusion was removed from the DSM 5's MDD criteria. This was a mistake. Bereavement following the death of a loved one is not merely *normal* but *rational*. Many psychiatrists have argued that the removal continues a push to render normal forms of unhappiness as rationality-undermining mental illness. They claim that such a move is a way of "medicalizing and trivializing our expectable and necessary emotional reactions to the loss of a loved one and substituting pills and superficial medical rituals for the deep consolations of family, friends, religion, and the resiliency that comes with time and the acceptance of the limitations of life" [21]. Because it is (widely) comprehensible why someone would feel "[m]arkedly diminished interest in pleasure in all, or almost all, activities most of the day, nearly every day" and a "depressed mood" following the loss of a loved one, on our account, bereavement is a rational expression of the love that a person has for the recently deceased [15]. Although the removal of the bereavement exclusion was an error, it is instructive that a diagnosis of MDD following the loss of a loved one shows us that depression need not always undermine rationality even from the point of view of psychiatry.

For our purposes, the upshot of this discussion is that suicidal desires that result from at least some forms of mental illness can be *rational*. It is comprehensible that a person diagnosed with terminal cancer, neurocognitive disorder stemming from

Huntington's disease, or locked-in syndrome may satisfy the criteria for MDD. Furthermore, it seems comprehensible that rational people would, on the basis of these diagnoses, desire to end their lives [22].

Although we have argued that suicidal desires can be rational in many cases, including cases where a person is suffering from mental illness, we acknowledge that the opposite is also true. MDD, schizophrenia, manic-depression, and bipolar disorder can so affect a person's mental state as to render them irrational. Nevertheless, the presence of illnesses like these should not automatically be seen as undermining the rationality and autonomy of a patient's desires to end her life. In order to clarify our position further, we must now turn to the question of suicide and its many meanings.

1.3   The Meanings of Suicide

What is "suicide"? A common definition is simply "one who dies by his own hand" [23]. However, we decline to use the second definition from this source, "one who commits self-murder," as it begs the moral question. Individuals engage in self-destructive behavior for a variety of reasons and in varied circumstances. There is no such thing as a generic suicide or a suicide without surrounding facts and circumstances. We have already argued that some suicides do not arise out of mental illness or irrationality.

We propose to divide suicide into three categories to sort out significant conceptual and ethical differences in instances of dying by one's own hand. First, suicide can be understood as an expression of ultimate personal responsibility or of radical autonomy ("per se suicides"). Second, suicide can be understood as instrumental to the agent's conception of personal well-being ("remedial suicides"). Third, suicide can be understood as instrumental to an agent directly affecting other persons, i.e., to inflict harm on someone else or to prevent another from being harmed ("other-directed suicides").

Although most suicides are instrumental, what can be interpreted as per se suicides do happen. 19-year-old Kipp Rusty Walker repeatedly plunged a 6-in. blade into his chest on stage at an open mic night after playing a song called "Sorry For All the Mess" and died shortly afterward. The audience clapped and cheered believing it was piece of theater. A friend of his tried to explain: "It was almost like he wanted to prove a point, like there's no point in being scared of death because it's going to happen to us anyway" [24]. Whether possibly rational in some attenuated sense, per se suicides ought presumptively to be prevented and strongly discouraged because, on their face, they appear irrational and incomprehensible.

Remedial suicides include instances of self-destruction in which persons seek to avoid future harm or indignity, to escape intolerable circumstances in their own lives. Perhaps most common, individuals end their own lives to stop their pain and suffering arising out of physical illness (e.g., disseminated bone cancer), depression, psychosis, hopelessness, loneliness, financial ruin, scandal, and so on. However, other motives drive remedial suicides as well.

Reports exist of an indeterminate number of African-American slaves who committed suicide in the antebellum South rather than live under the horrors of slavery such as vicious beatings, flogging, rape, and forced separation from family. A contemporaneous account of one slave's suicide observed "it was said she started to lose her mind and preferred death to that" [25]. A 2014 report by Amnesty International documents that a number of women captured by the so-called Islamic State operating in the Middle East have killed themselves to escape the torture, rape, and other forms of sexual violence inflicted by their captors [26]. Furthermore, even though those who refuse medical treatment needed to save or maintain their own lives are not usually thought of as suicides, the fact remains that they purposefully failed to do something that would have allowed their lives to continue, and they almost always do so because they find their present lives unsatisfactory or unbearable due to pain, loss of function, suffering, great fatigue, or general misery. The late Justice Scalia has argued that there are many ways to commit suicide and refusing life-saving medical treatment is one of them.

> For insofar as balancing the relative interests of the State [in preventing suicide] and the individual is concerned, there is nothing distinctive about accepting death through the refusal of "medical treatment," as opposed to accepting it through the refusal of food, or through the failure to shut off the engine and get out of the car after parking in one's garage after work [27].

Other jurists disagree with this characterization of refusing treatment as suicide [28]. Who may be right in this particular debate, if anyone actually is, depends on what they understand suicide to be and what they believe constitutes an acceptable reason to die.

No single ethical evaluation can properly be made of all remedial suicides. While slave "owners" or Islamic State terrorists should of course be condemned for their inhumane treatment of others, those who end their own lives to escape the pain and indignity of inhumane captivity cannot reasonably be seen as acting irrationally or wrongly, especially if they lack any reasonable prospect of rescue. Competent individuals who refuse life-saving medical treatment can be understood as lacking a specific intent to die, as valuing bodily integrity about length of life, and as not setting the death-producing force in motion and therefore dying of "natural causes." Those who die by their own hand to avoid the ravages of perhaps long-standing mental illness, painful physical disease, or other sources of debilitating and presumably unrelenting suffering may or may not be doing wrong to themselves and to others close to them. We would want to know much more about the specifics of their particular situation to make a judgment about whether their reasons would be comprehensible to overcome the ethical presumption that persons should not intentionally end their own lives.

Other-directed suicides typically involve someone intentionally killing himself or putting himself at very great risk of dying in order to save another from death or harm or to uphold a deeply held religious, ethical, or political value. The most familiar examples of other-directed suicides would be a soldier who falls on a grenade or intentionally draws enemy fire to save his comrades, or the mother who pushes her child out of the path of a speeding car. Some individuals go on hunger strikes in protest of what they deem unjust or oppressive behavior on the part of a government or another social group. For example, dissidents in Cuba who were politically opposed to the Castro regime have died as a result of hunger strikes [29]. Yet there are those who end their lives in order to punish or wreak revenge on others. Still other individuals voluntarily risk—and suffer—death responding to situations dangerous to themselves and others. Three workers at the Chernobyl nuclear plant died after knowingly exposing themselves to massive doses of radiation in order to prevent an explosion that would have released huge quantities of radioactive material into the air that might have killed or injured millions [30]. After a deranged student opened fire at random people at Virginia Tech University, a professor held the door to his classroom shut to keep the shooter out; he succeeded but took five bullets as he did so, including a fatal one to the head. All but one of his students survived [31].

People also end their lives to remain faithful to their religious convictions. In the early Christian era, soldiers captured Domnina and her two daughters, and these women "knew the things terrible to speak of that men would do to them, and the most terrible of all terrible things, the threatened violation of their chastity." Domnina believed that "to surrender their souls to the slavery of demons was worse than all deaths and destruction" and offered "the only deliverance from all these things-escape to Christ," i.e., death. She and her daughters deliberately plunged into a river and drowned [32]. The Catholic Church made Domnina a saint, an exemplar of religious virtue. Although the Church has for many centuries condemned suicide, one of the most important Church Fathers, Augustine, recognized an exception for "those who acted on God's direct order" [33]. "By this means Augustine could accept as martyrs those whom he and his community admired, while pagans like the Stoic Cato he could label as self-murderers" [33]. Given their wide variation, it is impossible to ethically evaluate all other-directed suicides in the same manner.

In short, "suicide" is not a simple descriptive term; it has ethical, religious, and emotional import. Some of the instances of self-killing we have discussed are rational, i.e., the individuals involved have reasons for their acts that others can more or less readily understand and be hard-pressed to flatly object to, even though they would not embrace those reasons themselves. We do not want this discussion to be construed as making the case that many suicides are both rational and ethically unobjectionable. Similarly, our rejection of an invariable connection between mental illness and suicidal wishes does not demonstrate that the two are unconnected. Our position is more modest: some elderly individuals exist who are rational, have good, comprehensible reasons to want to end their lives, deserve to have their wishes taken seriously, and should receive help from their therapists in scrutinizing their very serious decision to engage in suicide.

1.4 The Paradigm of Terminal Illness Making Suicide Rational

Bascom and Tolle have documented that "it is not uncommon for patients with terminally illness to consider PAS [physician-assisted suicide]. Many physicians will receive a specific request for PAS from a patient" [34]. Our concern in this chapter is not primarily with the terminally ill elderly who express a desire to end their lives but with any elderly patient who does so. Nevertheless, the reasons the terminally ill give for wanting physician assistance in ending their lives are worthy of attention. If these reasons are largely the same ones nonterminal elderly cite to support wishes to end their lives, then the ethical and conceptual issue arises of whether a diagnosis of terminal illness is the decisive factor in determining whether a patient's desire to end her life is rational and deserving of respect. The reasons the non-terminally ill—and possibly rational—elderly have to end their lives are for most part the same ones expressed by the terminally ill. We do not, however, believe that the presence of a terminal diagnosis, with its inherent inexactness, is *necessary* for a desire to die to be rational.

The following is the list of reported reasons that Bascom and Tolle found in a wide range of studies as to why the terminally ill request PAS. We omit pain and physical suffering from this list to emphasize other sorts of reasons persons may have for wanting to die:

> Being a burden; being dependent on others for personal care; loss of autonomy; loss of control; loss of control over bodily functions; loss of dignity; loss of independence; loss of meaning in their lives; poor quality of life; ready to die; saw continued existence as point-less; tired of life; unable to pursue pleasurable activities; "unworthy dying"; wanted to control circumstances of death [34].

To see that these are at bottom the same reasons mentioned by many elderly persons desiring to die, we refer the reader to other chapters in this volume. We also note that these reasons can roughly be mapped onto our division of suicidal motivations: most are associated with remedial suicides (loss of dignity, control independence, poor quality of life, unable to pursue pleasurable activities), others with other-directed suicides (being a burden, dependent on others for personal care), and a few possibly with per se suicide (tired of life, ready to die). This mapping indicates that individuals often not only have a variety of reasons for suicide but also reasons of fundamentally different types.

Do all requests for PAS from the terminally ill come from persons with mental illness? We have already argued that this claim is implausible. It is true that the terminally ill are facing death sooner than those who lack that diagnosis, but the mere predicted proximity of death does not, indeed cannot, eliminate or alleviate the distressing or intolerable symptoms and life circumstances, such as loss of functions and loss of control over their lives, which lead an elderly person to consider suicide. It is extremely likely that the circumstances or symptoms which appear on Bascom and Tolle's list are not experienced and disvalued only by the terminally ill. Physician-assisted suicide for the terminally ill has a considerable amount of social support and more may be forthcoming. Four states have legally approved physician-assisted suicide for the terminally ill [5–8]. Between January and September 2015, more than 25 state legislatures considered bills to authorize PAS [35]. The medical literature contains approval of physician-assisted suicide [10, 36], although, to be fair, it contains condemnation as well [37]. This support at least suggests that when other elderly persons consider suicide and rely upon the very same experiences the terminally ill do, their desire ought not be dismissed out of hand as irrational and unfounded by anyone, especially their therapists.

Bascom and Tolle wisely advise that although "physicians should remain mindful of their own personal concerns [about dealing with requests for assistance in suicide], these concerns should not override their willingness to explore the motivation behind the patient's request. When a physician responds to requests for PAS with avoidance or rejection, opportunities to alleviate suffering may be missed" [34]. The same is true for therapists whose elderly patient expresses a desire to end his life. They should invite further discussion about the patient's reasons and situation. Implicit in this approach is the rejection of an automatic assumption that the patient is mentally ill and is in immediate need of treatment or of being involuntarily civilly committed to prevent suicide. Additionally, even if the patient can be or has been diagnosed with a mental illness, therapists should not automatically assume that their patient's illness renders their desires for suicide irrational. The patient may be exploring options as he perceives his life nearing its end, looking for information and advice about how to manage the future, or seeking help in managing his existential situation. Interestingly, Bascom and Tolle offered evidence that in general "physical symptoms rarely serve as the primary or sole motivation behind the request [for PAS]. Instead, individual values appear to have primacy" [34]. Surely the same will be true for elderly individuals disclosing to therapists a desire to die by their own hand.

1.5 Assessing Rationality in the Elderly

Not all elderly patients who express a desire to end their lives will be rational when doing so, but some surely will. The question then arises how to determine which desires are rational, *comprehensible*, and which are not. We offer four indicia that can be used to determine whether a decision of an elderly person to end her or his life may be considered rational. These broadly overlap with the criteria for rational suicide offered by Battin [38]. The application of these indicia to any given case requires practical wisdom and the exercise of reasoned judgment; they do not provide some sort of algorithm.

1. *The ability to demonstrate rationality.* The individual must have the mental capacity to follow valid logical form when reasoning from premises to conclusion and understand the consequences of what she intends to do—and what is likely to happen if she acted differently. Though we make reference to logical validity, we do not mean to imply that an individual must be able to do this inerrantly. We may well not agree with, share, or even *personally* understand an individual's values or attitudes that lead them to the conclusion that continuing to live is not worth it, but these by themselves do not render someone else's choice irrational as long as their pattern of reasoning connects reasons together in a way that some groups comprehend. Both ending one's own life without

being able to reason logically about such a final act and allowing someone to end his life when he lacks this ability is wrong.

2. *Realistic information and judgment about the life-world.* Any rational choice to act on a matter of great significance must be grounded in a realistic reckoning of the state of the agent's life-world. A psychotic person who attempts to kill himself by setting himself on fire at the order of a demon has a bizarre take on the world that cannot possibly support a rational choice to commit suicide. Less dramatic perceptions and beliefs about the world can unduly influence a choice to end life: very low self-esteem, exaggerated or false conceptions of one's disabilities, or the perceived denial of love from family members or friends that is readily apparent to other observers. Suicides based on religious convictions may seem out of touch with reality or bizarre, but then suicides for sincere political or moral values would seem to be equally out of touch with reality to someone who does not accept those values.

For a person's suicide to possibly be considered rational, he must make a careful and largely accurate assessment of his situation as it exists in the shared life-world. An individual should have adequate information about his present situation and future, although uncertainty clouds the latter to some extent. An individual needs to know her health problems and medical condition, her prognosis, and the alternatives realistically available to address whatever health or social difficulties exist. She should correctly acknowledge the material circumstances of her existence and find them seriously wanting such that living on is worse than death.

The rationality of an individual and the intelligibility of her or his reasons for behavior are intersubjectively determined. Beliefs that motivate an action are not irrational only because they are false but also because they are incomprehensible to others. A politically motivated suicide should be comprehensible even to those who do not share political convictions or who believe that they lack the will to starve themselves to death. It should be comprehensible to others that a 95-year-old person who suffers daily from arthritis, general weakness, and the inability to walk more than a few steps and has outlived her entire family—but does not have a terminal illness—would consider ending his life because he is stuck with a quality of life he cannot bear any longer.

3. *Lucid state of mind, intelligible emotion, and authentic will.* Depression or other forms of mental illness are likely to be present among elderly inclined to take their lives. Studies of suicide among the elderly have demonstrated that "bipolar disorder, major depression, and severe pain were associated with the largest increases in suicide risk" among 11 illnesses known to be linked to a significantly increased risk of suicide [3]. Yet the on-the-ground clinical picture of the elderly and suicide appears more complicated. In one study of suicide in the elderly, "the coexistence of multiple illnesses confers marked increase in the risk of suicide" [3]. Among those who visited a physician shortly before suicide, the five most common diagnoses were "anxiety, unspecified gastrointestinal symptoms, depression, unspecified cardiac symptoms, and hypertension" [3]. Non-depressive factors, such as uncontrolled pain, other distressing medical

symptoms, and serious decrease in overall quality of life, are also operative in these patients' lives.

If depression or other forms of mental illness are present, therapists should, of course, intervene and attempt to treat these problems or refer the patient to other clinicians who can help. The same is true for distressing medical symptoms. However, other reasons already identified for why patients may seek death—loss of autonomy and control, loss of independence, and meaning in life—are likely present as well and contribute to, even primarily cause, the patient's dissatisfaction with life or depressed mood. In many patients with terminal illness, "depressed moods will represent normal reactive sadness, rather than clinical depression," that is, their moods are intelligible given their existential situation [21]. The same is true for the non-terminally ill. Elderly people who are experiencing the disintegration of their former selves because of physical limitations, unwanted and unavoidable dependence on others, and the inability to engage in satisfying activities may have comprehensible reason not to value their future.

An elderly person, whether terminally ill or not, who expresses a desire to end her life must do so clearly, repeatedly, and voluntarily if it is to possibly be rational and ethically respectable. As a suicidal act must be presumed fatal (in fact generally elderly persons attempt suicide with much higher lethality than younger persons [3]), it has irreversible consequences for the suicidee and likely has serious consequences for those close to them as well. For the same reasons, suicide should not be the product of impulse rather than deliberation over time. Of course the decision to end life must be voluntary and not the result of undue influence, duress, or fraud; it must be an individual's authentic choice to die rather than continue in his or her present state.

4. *Congruence with fundamental values and critical interests.* Individuals typically embrace some fundamental values that matter to them and that guide their lives over a long period of time, often their entire adult life span. Dworkin described "critical interests" as those personal goals and desires that make life worth living and reflect one's true identity [39]. The rationality of an individual's act then depends on its consistency with these fundamental values and critical interests. We have already mentioned several categories of people who preferred to end their own lives than continue living under certain circumstances: a person starves himself to death to advance a political or moral cause; a sex slave kills herself rather than endure further rape and beatings; and a patient refuses what he knows to be life-sustaining medical treatment because he cannot abide his quality of life. Asserting that the hunger striker or the person who sacrifices his life to save others from harm is not a "suicide" because one endorses the "good" reasons that support their acts while rejecting all other possible reasons does not adequately solve the problem of identifying objectionable acts of self-destruction from those that are not. None of this is to claim that self-destruction is or should be a common means of honoring one's fundamental values, especially since one cannot pursue their interests when dead. Most of the time individuals must be alive to enjoy or at least have the possibility of satisfying their cherished values and interests. Suicide permanently ends the existence of the valuing self.

Persons do not have to be protesting momentous events in history in order to choose to die rather than to live "in this kind of world." Someone's world can become uninhabitable for a variety of reasons and circumstances including serious medical problems that impair the person's functioning in addition to personal or social difficulties that cause him harm and damage his sense of self. Dying enables the individual to avoid future harms and indignities, what we have previously called remedial suicide. Some individuals can conclude they would be better off dead, although we acknowledge some paradox inhabits this claim.

We have already noted that loss of dignity, loss of independence, loss of meaning to life, and poor quality of life can lead some to suicide. These concepts, vague as they seem, matter to many people. They point to fundamental values and critical interests that should be carefully considered by a therapist confronted with elderly patients who are considering ending their lives. In addition, some elderly individuals may have other-directed reasons for suicide, and these could be vitally connected to their fundamental values. However, we think it odd that an elderly person would have *only* other-directed reasons to end her or his life.

Finally, a fundamental value everyone ought to have to some degree is avoiding harm to oneself and others with whom one is connected by family relation, friendship, and community. Suicide can be understood as the ultimate harm to the self. Yet individuals whose self-destruction is rational attempt to avoid causing themselves harm and suffering and perhaps others close to them by doing so. In other words, they find their lives full of relentless suffering that cannot be alleviated, and they consider *that* to be their worst fate, not death. Seeking death is a rational means to avoid enduring inescapable suffering. This idea is one of the cornerstones of the Dutch acceptance of euthanasia and PAS [40]. Like the Dutch medical association, we believe unacceptable suffering is not limited to somatic pain caused by disease [40]. To be rationally consistent with what ought to be one of her fundamental values, an individual contemplating suicide should demonstrate awareness and consideration of the potential harmful effects of her self-inflicted death on others, especially family members and close friends. Furthermore, a decision to end one's life should typically not be made without the involvement of others close to him or her, not only to gain their counsel but also to avoid the shock a self-inflicted death can cause them.

1.6   Cases and Commentary

In this section, we offer several cases of elderly persons contemplating suicide and provide some commentary regarding their rationality and moral permissibility. The first is taken almost verbatim from her own account of her struggle with dementia and decision to end her own life which she made public on the internet.

Gillian Bennett was an 85-year-old former psychotherapist with dementia who decided to "end my own life by taking adequate barbiturates...before my mind has totally gone. Ethically, this seems to me the right thing to do." She knew that she had dementia for three years before coming to this decision and noted "Ever so gradually at first, much faster now, I am turning into a vegetable." She can't remember that her granddaughter will be visiting in three days time; she can't find the coffee. "Every day I lose bits of myself, and it's obvious that I am heading towards the state that all dementia patients eventually get to: not knowing who I am and requiring full-time care.... I, Gillian, will no longer be here."

She understood that a time would come when "one is no longer competent to guide one's own affairs." She considered her options: "I have choices which I have reviewed, and either adopted or discarded. I think I have hit upon the right choice for me." Here are her options as she perceived them. First, "have a minder care for my mindless body." She saw this as involving financial hardship for her family or entangling them "in a seemingly endless round of chores that could erode even their fondest memories of me." Second, "Request whatever care [in a facility] the government is willing to provide." She did not want her family to be expected to visit her often and "thank the caretakers for how well they are looking after the carcass." Third, "end my own life...." She did not believe that ending her life was a loss. "Understand that I give up nothing that I want by committing suicide. All I lose is an indefinite number of years of being a vegetable...having not the faintest idea of who I am." She did not come to her decision in isolation from her family. "All [my immediate family] know that it matters to me not to become a burden to them, or to Canada. I have discussed my situation with them all." She also made sure no one in her family could be accused of assisting her suicide and risking criminal prosecution for doing so.

As far as we can tell from her account (which may be incomplete), Ms. Bennett had the ability to reason, despite her dementia, about her situation and understood the consequences of her decision to end her life. She was also able to imagine—and reject—what she believed the future held for her: a need for institutionalization as her dementia would progress, and her biographical life, her personality, would be gone. Her stated pattern of reasons are comprehensible and demonstrate how her suicide relates to the problems she sees in her life. She does not tell us, however, whether her physician provided her with the scenario of her worsening dementia, although one could infer this was the case as no one in her family apparently challenged her assessment. She seems to be in touch with the reality of her present condition, her likely future, and her options. She is aware of what she does not want: being bodily alive but lacking a self and living in such a condition in an institution at the expense of her family or her country. She reaches the conclusion that continued "mindless" living is worse than death [41]. Her account strikes us much more as a reasonable and fair reaction to being in the bad state of progressive dementia ("bad" as judged by her own values) than the product of clinical depression or other forms of mental illness. Although she may satisfy the diagnostic criteria for clinical depression, it is not clear that this depression, if present, would be fatal to her rationality. Ms. Bennett's decision also appears congruent with her fundamental values. She does not believe she is harming herself ("Understand that I give up nothing that I want by committing suicide."), and she consulted her family and encountered support rather than objection. In addition, she was careful to have her relatives not violate the law by assisting her.

In sum, we would conclude that Gillian Bennett made a rational and ethically justifiable decision to end her own life, with the understanding that others in a similar situation could (and some definitely would) choose differently. On August 18, 2014, she dragged a mattress to a favorite place near her home on an island in British Columbia, downed the lethal dose of drugs she had gathered, chased it with a shot of whiskey, and died [42].

A second case comes from a brief article by Rita Marker, an opponent of assisted suicide.

Georgia, a 68-year-old widow, is a retired psychologist. For several years, she has considered her life situation and has expressed a wish to die before reaching what she considers an unacceptable old age. She has lived a full life. Although she is mildly depressed, her judgment is not impaired. She has discussed her decisions with persons whose opinions she values highly. After careful deliberation, she comes to the conclusion that she will end her life [43]. Ms. Marker's purpose in offering and briefly discussing this case is to demonstrate the difference between a rational and a morally correct decision to die by suicide. We agree: "a decision may well be both rational and wrong." She also wants to persuade us that a rational decision for an individual to die does not provide the justification for a public policy that permits that individual to obtain assistance in ending his life, a matter this chapter will not address.

In any event, Georgia's decision has little to commend it—except it follows valid logical form: (1) she should die before an unacceptable old age; (2) she has nearly reached an unacceptable old age; (3) therefore, she should bring about her own death. However, we know nothing of what makes old age "unacceptable" to her or why her future appears so bad that she prefers death to it. No mention is made of whether she is suffering or has good reasons to believe she will be suffering in the future, nor do we know what good things exist in her current life. Moreover, we are given no idea of the reactions to her plan from those "persons whose opinions she values highly." Did they explore ways to manage whatever it is about old age that bothers her? Consequently, without a more detailed explanation, we cannot judge the rationality of her conclusion that "old age" is "unacceptable" to the point of making her intent to seek death understandable and worthy of respect. We have approached rationality as carrying some objective features, although we also attempt to acknowledge and work with the notion that reasons can be subjective. Charitably speaking, it may be possible to fill in the reasons for Georgia's decision in such a manner that it becomes comprehensible (rational), although we would need to learn a great deal more about Georgia to do this.

The Netherlands Right to Die organization (NVVE) contends that such persons who desire to die have "completed life;" they are:

> People who suffer from a complex constellation of factors connected with old age. These are non-life threatening conditions and physical deterioration (poor eyesight, deafness, difficulty walking, fatigue, apathy, incontinence), resulting in a loss of independence and personal dignity, dependence on care, loss of status and control, a shrinking social network, loss of a sense of purpose and meaning, disengagement from society, fear of the future and the absence of future prospects. [40]

A Dutch citizens group calling themselves Uit Vrije Wil (By Free Choice) have lobbied (unsuccessfully so far) for an amendment to existing Dutch law which permits physicians to perform euthanasia and assist in the suicide of a patient if certain conditions are satisfied. The amendment would "make it possible for people aged 70 and older who feel they have completed life and wish to die in a dignified manner to [legally] receive assistance in doing so if they expressly request it" [40]. While the legislative proposal of By Free Choice is very far from what any American state would even consider, its description of a "completed life" may help us understand what might underlie the elderly's preference to die by suicide rather than wait for a "natural death."

The judgment of an elderly person that his life simply is no longer worth living or that his life is "complete" and therefore he wishes to end it himself could well be too subjective and free-floating to merit respect. That person's standards could be seriously irrational ("I can't do everything I did when I was 30, and nothing else will do") and his values very strange ("I must win at chess every time I play or life isn't worth living"). On the other hand, there may be much more behind the statement that "my life is complete and I wish to die in a dignified manner." Any elderly person's expression of a desire to die calls for an individualized response out of respect for the worth of human life and respect for that particular person. The therapist who encounters someone like Georgia should make a serious effort to explore the individual's *specific* reasons and concerns that have led him to want to die. We suggest that the four indicia of a rational decision be applied to this end.

Of course, the mental status and mental health of any elderly person who wishes to end her life must be assessed, but an automatic assumption that the patient must be clinically depressed and needs hospitalization seems unwarranted to us. From a conservative risk management point of view, one could argue that any patient, regardless of age or situation, who expresses a desire to end his life must be prevented from doing so, and involuntary civil commitment is the most reliable method for doing so. Yet is this reaction the only one that comes within the standard of care for a therapist confronted by such a patient? It is not clear to us that it is, especially when it is at least questionable what involuntary commitment will achieve. Once the patient is hospitalized—if she is indeed rational, in firm touch with reality, and serious about what is wrong in her life—she will very likely first stop talking about her wish to end her life and then cooperate with "treatment." Then she would probably have to be released and will surely be reluctant to talk with that therapist again.

According to the third indication of a rational decision, the patient must be making a voluntary decision about his life, one that has been well-considered and expressed over time rather than impulsive or grounded in what others might think of his quality of life. Elderly persons who are considering ending their lives likely have some sort of disability (restricted mobility, hearing or visual deficits, weakness, mental processing) that leads them to be unsatisfied with their present lives and future prospects. Also, the elderly may feel their lives lack dignity due to their dependence on others and inability to function. In this regard, it is likely worth reflecting on whether patients have suffered from forms of discrimination against the elderly or the disabled. If they have, their decision to end their lives may be unduly influenced by the discriminatory acts and attitudes of others.

While prejudice against the disabled and the elderly certain exists, it is not clear that the effects of such prejudice infects their desire to end their lives in all cases to the extent that their decisions cannot possibly be properly respected. It is true that the simple fact of being dependent on others should not be a source of guilt or shame or make someone feel that he no longer deserves to live. Almost everyone at every age is dependent on others in one manner or another, just as nearly everyone who lives long enough will have more need of help from others to live safely and well. On the other hand, individuals are entitled to cherish their independence and to strongly disfavor being totally dependent on others, particularly when they may have lost their sense of self as Gillian Bennett feared so much.

References

1. Swanson J, Bonnie R, Appelbaum P. Getting serious about reducing suicide: more "how" and less "why". JAMA. 2015;314:2229–30.
2. Moscicki E. Opportunities of life: preventing suicide in elderly patients. Arch Intern Med. 2004;164:1171–2.
3. Juurlink D, Herrmann N, Szalai J, Kopp A, Redlmeier D. Medical illness and the risk of suicide in the elderly. Arch Intern Med. 2004;164:1179–84.
4. Sachs-Ericsson N, Van Orden K, Zarit S. Suicide and ageing. Aging Ment Health. 2016;20(2):110–2.
5. Oregon Revised Statutes. Sections 127.800-127.995. 2015.
6. Revised Code of Washington. Sections 70.245.010-70.245.904. 2015.
7. Vermont Statutes Annotated. Sections 5281-5292. 2015.
8. California Health & Safety Code. Sections 443-433.217. 2016.
9. Dugan A. In U.S., support up for doctor-assisted suicide. Washington DC: Gallup; 2015 [cited 2016 Jan 13]. http://www.gallup.com/poll/183425/support-doctor-assisted-suicide.aspx.
10. Quill T, Cassel C, Meier D. Proposed criteria for physician-assisted suicide. N Engl J Med. 1992;327:1380–4.
11. Werth JL. Rational suicide? Implications for mental health professionals. Washington, DC: Taylor and Francis; 1996.
12. Varelius J. On the moral acceptability of physician-assisted dying for non-autonomous psychiatric patients. Bioethics. 2016;30(4):227–33. doi:10.1111/bioe.12182.
13. Hewitt J. Why are people with mental illnesses excluded from the rational suicide debate? Int J Law Psychiat. 2012;36:358–65.
14. Hugo M. Mental health professionals' attitudes towards people who have experienced a mental health disorder. J Psychiatr Ment Health Nurs. 2001;8:419–25.
15. American Psychiatric Association. Diagnostic and statistical manual of mental disorders: DSM-5. Washington, DC: American Psychiatric Association; 2013.
16. World Health Organization. The ICD-10 classification of mental and behavioural disorders: clinical descriptions and diagnostic guidelines. Geneva: World Health Organization; 1992.
17. Culver C, Gert B. Competence. In: Radden J, editor. The philosophy of psychiatry: a companion. New York: Oxford University Press; 2004. p. 258–71.
18. Kant, I. Groundwork for the metaphysics of morals. Gregor M, Timmermann J, translators. Cambridge: Cambridge University Press; 2012/1785.
19. Tversky A, Kahneman D. Decision making under uncertainty: Heuristics and biases. Science. 1972;185:1124–31.
20. Fischer J, Ravizza M. Responsibility and control: a theory of moral responsibility. New York: Cambridge University Press; 1998.

21. Frances A. DSM 5 Is guide not bible—ignore its ten worst changes. APA approval of DSM-5 is a sad day for psychiatry. Psych Today. https://www.psychologytoday.com/blog/dsm5-in-distress/201212/dsm-5-is-guide-not-bible-ignore-its-ten-worst-changes.
22. Cholbi M. Suicide: the philosophical dimensions. Peterborough: Broadview Press; 2011.
23. Oxford English Dictionary. [cited 2016 Jan 13]. http://www.oed.com.libproxy.scu.edu/view/Entry/193691?rskey=GAUMDb&result=1#eid.
24. Suicide as performance art. [cited 2016 Jan 13]. http://abbey-roads.blogspot.com/2011/04/suicide-as-performance-art.html.
25. National Humanities Center. The Making of African American Identity: Vol. 1, 1500–1865, Suicide among slaves: a 'very last resort,' pp. 1–4.
26. Amnesty International. Escape from hell: torture and sexual slavery in Islamic state captivity in Iraq. London: Amnesty International; 2014. p. 4–8.
27. U.S. Supreme Court. Cruzan v. Superintendent, 497 U.S. 261-351. 1990.
28. California Court of Appeal. Bartling v. Superior Court, 163 Cal. App. 3d 189-98. 1984.
29. Cuban hunger striker Wilmar Villa dies in jail. [cited 2016 Jan 13]. http://www.bbc.com/news/world-latin-america-16644899.
30. McGinty S. Lead coffins and a nation's thanks for the chernobyl suicide squad. The Scotsman [Internet]. 2011[cited2016Jan13].http://www.scotsman.com/news/stephen-mcginty-lead-coffins-and-a-nation-s-thanks-for-the-chernobyl-suicide-squad-1-1532289#axzz3qUsceh85.
31. Moynihan C. Professor's violent death came where he sought peace. New York Times [Internet]. 2007 [cited 2016 Jan 13]. http://www.nytimes.com/2007/04/19/us/19professor.html?rref=collection%2Ftimestopic%2FLibrescu%2C%20Liviu&action=click&contentCollectio n=timestopics&region=stream&module=stream_unit&version=latest&contentPlacement=2& pgtype=collection&_r=0.
32. Eusebius. The martyrdom of st. domnina and her two daughters. [Internet]. New York: Fordham University; 1996 [cited 2016 Jan 13]. http://legacy.fordham.edu/halsall/source/euseb-domnina.asp
33. Stivala J. Death before dishonour! Suicide of Christian victims of rape. Eras. 2011;13(1):1–23.
34. Bascom PB, Tolle SW. Responding to requests for physician-assisted suicide. JAMA. 2002;288:91–8.
35. Orentlicher D, Pope T, Rich B. Clinical criteria for physician aid in dying. J Palliat Med. 2015;18:1–4.
36. Brody H. Assisted death—a compassionate response to a medical failure. N Engl J Med. 1992;327:1384–8.
37. Callahan D. When self-determination runs amok. Hast Cent Rep. 1992;22(2):52–5.
38. Battin MP. Can suicide be rational? Yes, sometimes. In: Werth JL, editor. Contemporary perspectives on rational suicide. Philadelphia: Brunner/Mazel; 1999. p. 13–21.
39. Dworkin R. Life's dominion: an argument about abortion, euthanasia, and individual freedom. New York: Vintage; 1996.
40. Royal Dutch Medical Association. The role of the physician in the voluntary termination of life [Internet]. Utrecht: KNMG; 2011 [cited 2015 Nov 10]. http://knmg.artsennet.nl/Publicaties/KNMGpublicatie-levenseinde/100696/Position-paper-The-role-of-the-physician-in-the-voluntary-termination-of-life-2011.htm.
41. Gillian Bennett [Internet]. Bowen Island, British Columbia: personal site; 2014 [cited 2015 Nov 10]. www.deadatnoon.com.
42. Mason G. A suicide note that should be read by everyone. The Globe and Mail. 2014; [cited 2015 Nov 11]. http://www.theglobeandmail.com/globe-debate/a-suicide-note-that-should-be-read-by-everyone/article20161330/.
43. Marker RL. Foreword 2. In: Werth JL, editor. Contemporary perspectives on rational suicide. Philadelphia: Brunner/Mazel; 1999. p. xxi–xxii.

Would This Be Rational Suicide?

2

Robert E. McCue

2.1 Introduction to Mr. D

Mr. D has it figured out. Twenty years earlier, he decided that when the time came, he would kill himself by jumping off the steep cliffs of the Hudson Palisades at Fort Lee Historic Park. This New Jersey park has spectacular views of the Hudson River and upper Manhattan. He has visited the park throughout the years and has always been struck by the grand juxtaposition of natural and man-made beauty. It would be a beautiful place to die when it was time.

Mr. D is now in a locked psychiatric unit in New York City. He is a 78-year-old divorced man who lives alone in his one-bedroom apartment. His health has been deteriorating over the past year, and his medical problems include severe coronary artery disease, congestive heart failure, implanted pacemaker, Barrett's esophagitis, prostatic carcinoma (treated with radiation), and lower extremity weakness (of unknown etiology which requires him to use a walker). Mr. D has seen a close friend deteriorate and end up in a nursing home, helpless and dependent. He is determined that this will not be his fate. He selected a Tuesday in October to kill himself. On the Monday before, he mailed letters to 12 neighbors, friends, and professionals informing them of his plan, explaining his reasons and bidding them good-bye. On the appointed Tuesday, he dressed in a suit, hailed a taxi, and went to the park. However, the day was rainy and overcast. The park was muddy and gloomy, and the view of Manhattan obscured by mist. The setting was more miserable than grand. He decided to go home and return the next day, when better weather was predicted. However, a neighbor who received his letter called emergency services. When Mr. D returned to his apartment, he was met by the police and brought to a local hospital where he was admitted involuntarily to the psychiatric unit.

R.E. McCue, M.D. (✉)
Department of Psychiatry, New York University School of Medicine,
1 Park Avenue, New York, NY 10016, USA
e-mail: Robert.mccue@nyumc.org

© Springer International Publishing Switzerland 2017   23
R.E. McCue, M. Balasubramaniam (eds.), *Rational Suicide in the Elderly*,
DOI 10.1007/978-3-319-32672-6_2

Mr. D was born in Wyoming and raised by his mother and a stepfather. He has no siblings. He reports that both biological parents were alcoholics. From the age of 9 until 17, he was sexually abused by his stepfather. He describes his childhood as horrible. At 18, he left and joined the armed forces. After discharge from the service, he moved to Georgia, went to college, and married. The marriage did not work out, and they divorced after 7 years. There were no children. He then moved to New York City and began experimenting with homosexual relationships. After some failed attempts, he decided that he did not want a committed relationship with either a man or woman. He never had a problem with drugs or alcohol. He has never had mental health treatment. He had been gainfully employed as an administrative assistant for a large corporation until he retired at age 65. He has had friends and an active social life, but in recent years, this has been less so as his friends are ill or have died. He enjoys writing music and graphic design, but is aware that his skills are deteriorating with age. For many years, Mr. D has told friends, acquaintances, his attorney, and his internist that he was going to kill himself when he thought the time was right. "It is my life and I should be able to dictate its course." Over the past 6 months, as his medical problems worsened, he began to wind down his life in anticipation of the planned suicide in October. He wants an "organized, clean, and proper death."

When assessed in the emergency department before being admitted, Mr. D denied feeling depressed and was described as euthymic. However, because of his intention to kill himself, he was admitted with the diagnosis of depressive disorder NOS (unspecified depressive disorder in DSM 5 [1]). In the hospital, Mr. D has variably been described as personable, pleasant, euthymic, or "somewhat depressed." He relates in a cooperative and courteous manner. His speech is articulate and coherent; his thought processes are logical. There is no evidence of psychosis. He continues to deny feeling depressed, but is angry at wasting resources because of the unnecessary hospitalization. He insists that it is his right to kill himself, that he is not mentally ill, and that he knows his life's value better than anyone else. He becomes irritable when anyone questions this. He promises that he will not commit suicide in the hospital as this is not his plan. He scored 27/30 on the Montreal Cognitive Assessment [2] and 5/15 on the Geriatric Depression Scale [3]. The positive scores on the latter were from low energy and decreased participation in activities, which he plausibly attributed to his medical problems, as well as not feeling wonderful to be alive, not feeling happy most of the time, and feeling bored. Mr. D denies any major problems with sleep, appetite, or concentration. Aside from the suicidality, there is little about Mr. D to suggest a mental illness, let alone requiring him to be involuntarily hospitalized. Now what?

Mr. D is based on an actual patient. His story may be similar to those of other older patients who present themselves to us, voluntarily or involuntarily, with a clear intention to suicide, but without much else to suggest a serious psychiatric disorder. These patients present a challenge for those of us in clinical care. Someone threatening suicide is an alarm that a therapeutic intervention is urgently needed. But how do we approach someone with few signs and symptoms of a mental illness? Would considering this a case of rational suicide be of clinical value?

Formal psychiatric diagnostic criteria (DSM 5) do not recognize the entity of rational suicide. However, there have been discussions of it in the health-care field, particularly about providing assistance or aid in dying for terminally ill patients. Several sets of criteria have been developed [4–9] to determine whether a request to die or an intention to kill oneself is rational. Most require that the intention is voluntary and well considered and stems from a terminal or irreversibly debilitated condition. We will use the four criteria presented by Nelson and Ramirez in Chapter 1 of this book to examine Mr. D's case in the hope of better understanding how to help him.

2.2 Criterion 1: The Ability to Demonstrate Rationality

Mr. D's position: He has a consistent and coherent reason for wanting to kill himself. He believes that physical deterioration, disability, and dependency lie ahead. At 78, he feels that he has done everything he wants to do. At this age and with these medical problems, death is not far off, so he prefers to die on his own terms and in the manner of his choosing. In other matters, Mr. D is thoughtful and logical, so there is little evidence to question his ability to think rationally.

Affirmative: Beliefs such as Mr. D's are not rare among older adults. Lloyd-Williams et al. [10] interviewed 40 older English adults, between the ages of 80 and 89, who were living alone in the community. Most were happy about the lives they led. The prevalent fear was about how they would die, not of death itself. They were frightened of becoming a burden to others and of developing a chronic, debilitating illness (e.g., stroke). It was important for them to have a choice about when and where to die. Most did not think the medical profession wished to engage in a discussion with them about these issues Kjølseth et al. [11] performed psychological autopsies on 23 suicides of older adults (average age = 78) in Norway to understand the experience of life before the suicide. While some were depressed, it was not prevalent. The stronger themes were life had been lived, they were now becoming a burden, their functional decline was leading to a perception of losing oneself, and life had entered a final stage where death was close and was to be accepted. Philosophy has examined the rationality of suicide. In Prado's view [12], it can be neither irrational nor immoral to want to die in order to shorten a condition that lessens the self and carries unacceptable debility, dependency, and futile suffering. For Schramme [13], suicide can be a rational act if life has lost its meaning. These issues are further discussed in Chapters 1 and 7.

Negative: Can the wish to die be a purely rational decision? Siegel [4] wrote that suicidal intent stems from emotions and that, therefore, it is impossible for it to result from pure logic. It is also difficult to be rational when in pain, either physical or psychological, as Mr. D may be even if it cannot be classified by formal diagnostic criteria. Farsides and Dunlop [14] noted that the will to live and the belief that life is not worth living fluctuates over time, so that an apparent rational stance is not fixed. There is evidence for that. A review of cases of physician-assisted suicide in the Netherlands [15] found that when a request for euthanasia or assisted suicide was denied, a substantial number of people changed their minds about wanting it. Likewise, in the latest review of Oregon's Death with Dignity Act [16], since 1997, 1545 people have met the criteria for assisted suicide and were given lethal prescriptions, but only 991 (64 %) died from ingesting them.

2.3   Criterion 2: Realistic Information and Judgment About the Lifeworld

Mr. D's position: He has multiple medical problems and requires a walker to ambulate. He has been living alone and finds it more difficult to do routine household chores. At some point in the not-too-distant future, he will require assistance to remain in the community or will have to move to an institutional setting. He believes that this would jeopardize the freedom that he values. He is more alone as friends have died or moved away. Medical illness and aging have made it difficult to do the activities that have given him satisfaction. He believes that he has accomplished all that he has wanted to in his life. While his current state may be tolerable, he sees his condition deteriorating soon to a point where continuing to live would just be prolonging dying.

Affirmative: At 78 years of age, Mr. D has a life expectancy of 10 additional years by the calculations of the Social Security Administration [17]. However, he is not a healthy man. From their study of Medicare enrollees, DuGoff et al. [18] estimated that for every chronic condition, there is an average of a 1.8-year reduction in life expectancy. So, Mr. D may really expect to live another 4–5 years. The average American man has a period of 5 years of debility before dying [19]. Mr. D's fears of imminent physical decline and dependency are realistic. He has always valued his independence, so that its diminution will seriously impair the quality of his life. In their review of physician-assisted suicide, Zaubler and Sullivan [20] found that when it was requested, issues of quality of life were more important than depressive symptoms, particularly for people with strong needs for control and independence. Pearlman et al. [21] similarly found that people who have requested physician-assisted suicide were motivated by debilitation from illness, a loss of control leading to a loss of sense of self, and fears about the future. Just as Mr. D. witnessed his close friend deteriorate in a nursing home, many of those who requested physician-assisted suicide in this study had had negative past experiences with how someone close to them has died.

Negative: Mr. D and others who fear a prolonged dying process with impaired quality of life are reacting to a structure of health care that does not address the needs of people at the end of these lives and barely acknowledges their existence. There is evidence [22, 23] that suicide is related to sociocultural factors and that a desire for suicide may reflect a lack of integration with family, religion, or economic life. As professionals, we may know of resources that Mr. D is unaware of. There may be interventions to integrate Mr. D into a social network so that he will no longer wish to kill himself. There are supportive or palliative programs that could make Mr. D's final years tolerable and pleasant.

2.4 Criterion 3: Lucid State of Mind, Intelligible Emotion, and Authentic Will

Mr. D's position: He denies being depressed and reports, "I am not unhappy." From clinical observations, he is not in a persistent state of sadness. His admitting diagnosis of depressive disorder NOS is a noncommittal diagnosis not indicative of a serious mood disorder. Mr. D's negative response to the question on the Geriatric Depression Scale asking if he is "happy most of the time" seems appropriate for the current state of his life. Mr. D does not have cognitive impairment or a thought disorder. His plan to kill himself is clearly his own decision.

Affirmative: As discussed in Chapter 1, the orthodox view of psychiatry is that suicidal ideation is always a sign of a mental disturbance. In Hardwig's view [19], during the late stages of life, death (and suicide) has a different significance than at younger ages. At the end of life when death is near, dying, whether by suicide or not, does not mean a curtailment of expectations and hope to the extent it does for younger people. It is part of life's trajectory. Some older adults do have a mental illness that makes them suicidal and requires treatment, but the evidence suggests that not all do. In Cattell's review of late-life suicide [24], he found that although depressive illness was an important predictor, it was not present in 20–30% of the suicides. Linden and Barnow [25] studied 516 elderly people in (West) Berlin looking for those with a desire to die who were free of psychopathology. One hundred fifteen (21%) had thoughts about wanting to die and life not being worth living. In the majority of cases, a psychiatric disorder was present per DSM criteria; however, in 13 cases it was not. Jorm et al. [26] studied 923 elderly Australians. Twenty-one (2%) had a persistent wish to die. Depression was a significant factor associated with this wish, but there were others *independent of depression*: unmarried status, poor health and disability, hearing impairment, visual impairment, and living in a nursing home. Harwood et al. [27] looked at the rates of psychiatric disorders in elderly English suicides. About 20% had no psychiatric diagnosis at the time of death. As mentioned above, Kjølseth et al. [11] performed psychological autopsies on elderly suicides in Norway and did not find premorbid depression to be prevalent. Similar findings occur with terminally ill patients who request physician-assisted suicide [21, 28, 29]. Schneidman, considered the father of suicidology, believed that suicide stemmed from psychological pain and should not be thought of in terms of a psychiatric disorder [30]. In her recent review of suicide and ethics from the perspective of a psychiatrist, Ho [31] also emphasized that suicide cannot always be equated with having a diagnosable mental illness.

It would be fatuous to describe Mr. D as happy or expect him to be. His childhood was miserable, intimate relationships have been a challenge, friends have gone, and his health is deteriorating. The diagnosis of depressive disorder NOS was as much to justify an admission as indicative of a true mental illness. Horwitz and Wakefield [32] have argued that states of normal sadness are now being claimed by the medical establishment and classified as mental disorders. Parker [33] also cautioned against medicalizing unpleasant parts of human existence. Mr. D has reasons to have a dark view of the rest of his life. His not being "happy most of the time" seems more reality-based than otherwise.

Negative: The diagnostic criteria of DSM are assuredly far from perfect, but we should not be limited by these imperfections. Suicide in the elderly is a serious problem strongly associated with depression. Mr. D is not a happy man and is intent on killing himself, not because his present condition is intolerable but because of fears of what may happen in the future. From the palliative care field, there is an entity called "demoralization syndrome." It denotes someone with severe existential distress, hopelessness, and loss of meaning to life [34]. A patient with demoralization syndrome is unable to think clearly about the rest of life. While not part of DSM nosology, clinicians are encouraged to consider its validity when making decisions about a patient's capacity to make a decision regarding physician-assisted suicide. Mr. D may have a demoralization syndrome that distorts his view of life. There are also recommendations for treating this syndrome in palliative care patients [35].

Mr. D arrived at the place where he was to die, but changed his mind because of the weather. His desire to die was clearly not absolute. This presence of ambivalence is striking in studies of people requesting physician-assisted suicide [14, 36, 37]. People change their minds. Schneidman [38] considered ambivalence to be the common cognitive state in suicide. Boloş et al. [39] explored ethical aspects of depression and suicide and emphasized that ambivalence almost always precedes suicidal acts. The act may not be an end in itself but an attempt to communicate with others. According to Leenaars [40], "the prototypical psychological picture of a person on the brink of suicide is one who wants to and does not want to. He makes a plan for self-destruction and at the same time entertains fantasies of rescue and intervention." This underlying ambivalence must be recognized and explored to better understand the significance of a patient's suicidal wishes.

Muskin [41] stressed the importance of using a psychodynamic perspective to understand the underlying thoughts and emotions of those requested physician-assisted suicide. In their earlier criteria of how to assess competency, Appelbaum and Roth [42] even included the understanding of psychodynamic factors. Writing about the legalization of physician-assisted suicide in the Netherlands, Schoevers et al. [15] doubted whether it was possible to make an objective decision about death without taking into account unconscious feelings and that this was not easily done. What was the underlying motivation for Mr. D's plan to kill himself by jumping off a cliff? Are there things that he wishes to communicate that can be expressed in ways other than jumping off a cliff?

2.5 Criterion 4: Congruence with Fundamental Values and Critical Interests

Mr. D's position: He values his independence, self-reliance, and ability to make decisions about his life. For him, losing these would significantly impair the quality of his life and diminish his personhood. He is not religious so he does not consider his suicide as immoral. Most friends are gone, and he feels alone in the world. He believes that his suicide will not seriously harm others, but will spare the community the unnecessary expense of sustaining a life that has lost its value. Killing himself at the time is consonant with his values.

Affirmative: In the medical field, sustaining life and avoiding death is of utmost importance and a goal of many medical interventions. However, to some people, including Mr. D, there are things worse than death. These include being in a coma, being demented, severe suffering, complete dependence on other people or life-sustaining interventions, and facing a condition with an extremely poor prognosis [29]. As noted above [10], for many older people, it is the manner of death that is feared rather than death itself. Being independent is important to Mr. D, but as a result of improvements in medical technology, he will soon survive longer than he can care for himself.

Will his suicide negatively affect others? Mr. D cannot be considered in isolation, as he does have some acquaintances and friends who may be deeply hurt by his suicide. In writing about preemptive suicide and dementia, Davis [43] contrasted two views of rational suicide: the more conventional one of it being a selfish and individualistic act dismissive of others versus it being an act out of concern for family and the community with the aim to not waste resources and avoid exposing loved ones to a long, agonizing dying process. Mr. D does acknowledge his individualism, but thinks that illness and age have limited his ability to contribute to society. Moreover, he considers the cost of caring for him in a deteriorating state while awaiting death to be a complete waste of resources that could be more beneficially deployed. He does not believe that he has any close relationships who will deeply mourn him, and those friendly relationships that he does have will benefit from his estate, if it is not used up by needlessly prolonging his dying process.

Negative: Mr. D wants to remain independent and self-reliant. We can acknowledge the value of these qualities. However, while there are some restrictions to his mobility, he has been living alone and making his own decisions. Is he not still independent? His fears about the future are based on what happened to his friend, but there is no certainty that the same will happen to him. Spoletini et al. [44] reported that the fear of anticipated suffering leads to more suicide in cancer patients than the actual suffering itself. While his life will change in the future, it is only his guess (and fear) that there will be significant insults to his self-reliance that will radically diminish the quality of his life. Mr. D may minimize the impact that his death would have on others. His remaining friends and acquaintances may be deeply hurt by his killing himself and value his company more than he realizes. Lastly, his suicide will probably be viewed by others as a lonely act of a distraught man rather than a brave attempt by him to maintain control of the essence of his humanity.

2.6   Conclusion

Since the middle of the twentieth century, medical science and technology have led to a remarkable increase in longevity. At a certain point, though, prolonging life becomes prolonging death. For many people, dying has become a drawn-out process to which the medical profession and our culture have not adjusted. Some people may want to eek the last second out of life, but many, including Mr. D, do not. Hardwig [19, 45] wrote about how we aim to defeat and delay death, as it once came too early and unexpectedly. However, that is no longer the case. We now find ourselves in a situation of dying too late. We too slowly approach an end that is in sight. How do we manage this relatively new phenomenon? Well, Mr. D found a solution for himself.

From Mr. D's perspective, his suicide would be rational. He has thought about this plan for many years; it is not a result of impaired thinking from a major mental illness or cognitive disorder it is based on a realistic view of his future; and it is congruent with the high value he places on control and independence. If we limit ourselves to that which is overt and understandable, we would have to agree with him that his suicide would be rational. The criteria for rational suicide may be clearly stated and easily understood, but people are not so easily comprehended. Human behavior cannot be understood only in terms of what is observable and describable. We cannot make definitive statements about Mr. D's desire to kill himself without exploring his ambivalence, internal conflicts, and changing motivations and moods.

Under different set of circumstances, Mr. D may have committed suicide according to his plan. From a distance, it would have been considered a case of rational suicide. It was only by chance (or was it?) that he entered the mental health system and has now become a patient. We are now involved and his desire, rational or not, has become a clinical issue. As clinicians, our instinct is to help him. But how? What do we do for someone who does not have a diagnosable mental illness but who is in an understandably difficult situation? Set aside DSM and the medical model, and do not treat Mr. D as a patient with an illness. As Schneidman suggested [30], we address this situation "directly, phenomenologically, without the intervention of the often obfuscating variable of psychiatric disorder." Mr. D has made a seemingly understandable decision based on what he knows of his life and current situation. However, there may be things, external and internal, that he does not know. Our goal will be to help him find this information. We must empathically acknowledge the hard facts of Mr. D's life and his fears that if he does not kill himself, he will enter a prolonged deteriorated state devoid of purpose. These fears are not from a mental illness but the unfortunate product of Mr. D's personality traits colliding with a culture unprepared for a prolonged period of late life. To Mr. D, his life may have lost meaning, but it may be possible for us to restore meaning and become healers of a frightened, lonely man. How do we do that? You will not find the solution in the treatment guidelines that abound in psychiatry. There are no easy answers to a situation that barely existed 30 years ago. However, guidance can be found in Chapters 12–14. These explore spiritual, psychological, and psychopharmacological interventions for people, like Mr. D, who are facing the fear of dying too late.

References

1. American Psychiatric Association. Diagnostic and statistical manual of mental disorders. 5th ed. Arlington: American Psychiatric Publishing; 2013.
2. Nasreddine ZS, Phillips NA, Bédirian V, et al. The Montreal Cognitive Assessment, MoCA: a brief screening tool for mild cognitive impairment. J Am Geriatr Soc. 2005;53(4):695–9. doi:10.1111/j.1532-5415.2005.53221.x.
3. Yesavage JA, Sheikh JI. Geriatric Depression Scale (GDS): recent evidence and development of a shorter version. Clin Gerontol. 1986;5(1–2):165–73. doi:10.1300/J018v05n01_09.
4. Siegel K. Psychosocial aspects of rational suicide. Am J Psychother. 1986;40(3):405–18.
5. Quill TE, Cassel CK, Meier DE. Care of the hopelessly ill. Proposed clinical criteria for physician-assisted suicide. N Engl J Med. 1992;327(19):1380–4. doi:10.1056/NEJM199211053271911.
6. Werth JL, Cobia DC. Empirically based criteria for rational suicide: a survey of psychotherapists. Suicide Life Threat Behav. 1995;25(2):231–40.
7. Battin MP. Can suicide be rational? Yes, sometimes. In: Werth JL, editor. Contemporary perspectives on rational suicide. Philadelphia: Brunner/Mazel; 1999. p. 13–21.
8. Werth JL, Holdwick DJ. A primer on rational suicide and other forms of hastened death. Couns Psychol. 2000;28(4):511–39.
9. Hewitt J. Why are people with mental illness excluded from the rational suicide debate? Int J Law Psychiatry. 2013;36(5–6):358–65. doi:10.1016/j.ijlp.2013.06.006.
10. Lloyd-Williams M, Kennedy V, Sixsmith A, Sixsmith J. The end of life: a qualitative study of the perceptions of people over the age of 80 on issues surrounding death and dying. J Pain Symptom Manage. 2007;34(1):60–6.
11. Kjølseth I, Ekeberg Ø, Steihaug S. Why suicide? Elderly people who committed suicide and their experience of life in the period before their death. Int Psychogeriatr. 2010;22(2):209–18. doi:10.1017/S1041610209990949.
12. Prado CG. Moral individualism and elective death. Int J Law Psychiatry. 2013;36(5–6):471–6. doi:10.1016/j.ijlp.2013.06.003.
13. Schramme T. Rational suicide, assisted suicide, and indirect legal paternalism. Int J Law Psychiatry. 2013;36(5–6):477–84. doi:10.1016/j.ijlp.2013.06.008.
14. Farsides B, Dunlop RJ. Is there such a thing as a life not worth living? BMJ. 2001;322(7300):1481–3. doi:10.1136/bmj.322.7300.1481.
15. Schoevers RA, Asmus FP, Van Tilburg W. Physician-assisted suicide in psychiatry: developments in The Netherlands. Psychiatr Serv. 1998;49(11):1475–80. doi:10.1176/ps.49.11.1475.
16. Oregon Death with Dignity Act: 2015 data summary. Oregon Public Health Division. http://public.health.oregon.gov/ProviderPartnerResources/EvaluationResearch/DeathwithDignityAct/Documents/year18.pdf. Accessed 12 Feb 2016.
17. Life Expectancy Calculator. Social Security Administration. https://www.ssa.gov/OACT/population/longevity.html. Accessed 6 Feb 2016.
18. DuGoff EH, Canudas-Romo V, Buttorff C, Leff B, Anderson GF. Multiple chronic conditions and life expectancy: a life table analysis. Med Care. 2014;52(8):688–94. doi:10.1097/MLR.0000000000000166.
19. Hardwig J. Going to meet death: the art of dying in the early part of the twenty-first century. Hastings Cent Rep. 2009;39(4):37–45. doi:10.1353/hcr.0.0151.
20. Zaubler TS, Sullivan MD. Psychiatry and physician-assisted suicide. Psychiatr Clin North Am. 1996;19(3):413–27. doi:10.1016/S0193-953X(05)70298-7.
21. Pearlman RA, Hsu C, Starks H, et al. Motivations for physician-assisted suicide. J Gen Intern Med. 2005;20(3):234–9. doi:10.1111/j.1525-1497.2005.40225.x.
22. Clarke DM. Autonomy, rationality and the wish to die. J Med Ethics. 1999;25(6):457–62.
23. Van Orden KA, Witte TK, Cukrowicz KC, Braithwaite SR, Selby EA, Joiner Jr TE. The interpersonal theory of suicide. Psychol Rev. 2010;117(2):575–600. doi:10.1037/a0018697.

24. Cattell H. Suicide in the elderly. Adv Psychiatr Treat. 2000;6(2):102–8. doi:10.1192/apt.6.2.102.
25. Linden M, Barnow S. 1997 IPA/Bayer Research Awards in Psychogeriatrics. The wish to die in very old persons near the end of life: a psychiatric problem? Results from the Berlin Aging Study. Int Psychogeriatr. 1997;9(3):291–307. doi:10.1017/S1041610297004456.
26. Jorm AF, Henderson AS, Scott R, Korten AE, Christensen H, Mackinnon AJ. Factors associated with the wish to die in elderly people. Age Ageing. 1995;24(5):389–92. doi:10.1093/ageing/24.5.389.
27. Harwood D, Hawton K, Hope T, Jacoby R. Psychiatric disorder and personality factors associated with suicide in older people: a descriptive and case–control study. Int J Geriatr Psychiatry. 2001;16(2):155–65.
28. Chochinov HM, Wilson KG, Enns M, Lander S. Depression, hopelessness, and suicidal ideation in the terminally ill. Psychosomatics. 1998;39(4):366–70.
29. Rich BA. Pathologizing suffering and the pursuit of a peaceful death. Camb Q Healthc Ethics. 2014;23(4):403–16. doi:10.1017/S0963180114000085.
30. Shneidman ES. Rational suicide and psychiatric disorders[letter]. N Engl J Med. 1992;326(13):889–90.
31. Ho AO. Suicide: rationality and responsibility for life. Can J Psychiatry. 2014;59(3):141–7.
32. Horwitz AV, Wakefield JC. The loss of sadness: how psychiatry transformed normal sorrow into depressive disorder. New York: Oxford University Press; 2007.
33. Parker M. Medicalizing meaning: demoralization syndrome and the desire to die. Aust N Z J Psychiatry. 2004;38(10):765–73. doi:10.1111/j.1440-1614.2004.01460.x.
34. Kissane DW, Clarke DM, Street AF. Demoralization syndrome—a relevant psychiatric diagnosis for palliative care. J Palliat Care. 2001;17(1):12–21.
35. Kissane DW. The contribution of demoralization to end of life decisionmaking. Hastings Cent Rep. 2004;34(4):21–31. doi:10.2307/3528690.
36. Chin AE, Hedberg K, Higginson GK, Fleming DW. Legalized physician-assisted suicide in Oregon—the first year's experience. N Engl J Med. 1999;340(7):577–83. doi:10.1056/NEJM199902183400724.
37. Mishara BL, Weisstub DN. Premises and evidence in the rhetoric of assisted suicide and euthanasia. Int J Law Psychiatry. 2013;36(5–6):427–35. doi:10.1016/j.ijlp.2013.09.003.
38. Shneidman ES. A conspectus for conceptualizing the suicidal scenario. In: Maris RW, Berman AL, Maltsberger JT, Yufit RI, editors. Assessment and prediction of suicide. New York: Guilford; 1992. p. 50–65.
39. Boloş A, Ciubară AM, ChiriYă R. Moral and ethical aspects of the relationship between depression and suicide. Rom J Bioeth. 2013;10(3):71–9.
40. Leenaars AA, Edwin S. Shneidman on suicide. Suicidol Online. 2010;1:5–18.
41. Muskin PR. The request to die: role for a psychodynamic perspective on physician-assisted suicide. JAMA. 1998;279(4):323–8.
42. Appelbaum PS, Roth LH. Clinical issues in the assessment of competency. Am J Psychiatry. 1981;138(11):1462–7. doi:10.1176/ajp.138.11.1462.
43. Davis DS. Alzheimer disease and pre-emptive suicide. J Med Ethics. 2013;40:543–9. doi:10.1136/medethics-2012-101022.
44. Spoletini I, Gianni W, Caltagirone C, Madaio R, Repetto L, Spalletta G. Suicide and cancer: where do we go from here? Crit Rev Oncol Hematol. 2011;78(3):206–19. doi:10.1016/j.critrevonc.2010.05.005.
45. Hardwig J. Medicalization and death. APA News. 2006;6(1):2–14.

Rational Suicide and the Law

3

Lawrence J. Nelson

3.1 Introduction

Given the assumption that some suicides in the elderly can be rational and ethically permissible (the arguments for and against which are made elsewhere in this volume), this chapter explores the legal aspects of such cases with special attention to the concerns that the clinicians who treat such patients may have. First, some general legal background on suicide will be provided. Second, the criminal law regarding assisting a suicide will be discussed. Third, as five states now have legalized physician-assisted suicide for the terminally ill, some in our society have concluded that under certain conditions, suicide can be rational and ethically acceptable to the point that the law will permit it to occur without sanction to the participants. This section will examine these laws as they can inform our understanding of rational suicide. Finally, I will examine the potential civil liability for clinicians who treat competent elderly persons who have expressed a desire to end their lives.

3.2 Legal Background

No jurisdiction within the United States currently has a statute that makes successful suicide a crime, nor does any state make it a crime to attempt suicide. Rather than being considered criminal, the law considers suicide to be a manifestation of mental illness that should be addressed by mental health-care professionals. Minnesota, for example, repealed its statute criminalizing suicide in 1911 [1]. Several reasons support this conclusion. Criminal sanctions will not deter attempts to commit suicide. If suicide is truly caused (most often, if not exclusively, it is

L.J. Nelson, Ph.D., J.D. (✉)
Department of Philosophy, Santa Clara University,
300 El Camino Real, Santa Clara, CA 95053-0310, USA
e-mail: lnelson@scu.edu

© Springer International Publishing Switzerland 2017   33
R.E. McCue, M. Balasubramaniam (eds.), *Rational Suicide in the Elderly*,
DOI 10.1007/978-3-319-32672-6_3

assumed) by mental illness, then the moral responsibility of the self-destructive individual for his behavior is at least in serious doubt. "The current psychiatric view is that attempted suicide is a symptom of mental illness and, as such, it makes no more sense to affix criminal liability to it than to any other symptom of illness" [2]. Put differently, the failed suicide does not morally deserve to be punished for what she has done. Finally, the typical self-destructive individual is very unlikely to be rehabilitated in prison and quite likely to either kill himself there or suffer more from his illness.

However, English common law found both suicide and attempted suicide to be a crime. Self-killing was a felony in England for well over 700 years and was decriminalized in that country only in 1961 [3]. The reaction of the common law was influenced by the moral views of the Catholic Church which considered suicide "a mortal sin instigated by Satan" which led to "excommunication, punishment of the body of the deceased (exhibition of the dead body on the gallows), and burial in unconsecrated ground…, such as at a cross-roads, pinioning the body by driving it through with a stake, and a preclusion on attendance by a minister…" [3]. Burial at a crossroads was highly undesirable as the soul of the evil departed could not "rest in peace." Furthermore, the successful suicide forfeited his property to the crown because he had deprived the king of his property. It would be a serious understatement to think the stigma that currently attaches to suicide lacks historical depth.

3.3   Assisting a Suicide

The great majority of states (40) have statutes that expressly make assisting a suicide a crime, even though the suicidal individual herself commits no crime. As American common law also condemned assisting a suicide [2], it is not at all unlikely that a person who assisted in a suicide would be prosecuted in the remaining states that lack a statute expressly prohibiting such assistance. In addition, 48 states expressly disapprove of suicide and assisting a suicide either in statutes dealing with durable powers of attorney for health care or with advanced directives for medical care [4]. Consequently, it should be assumed for all practical purposes that assisting a suicide in any American jurisdiction is criminal.

The state has a variety of reasons for prohibiting persons from assisting a suicide. First, such a law manifests the state's interest in preserving human life, although a closer analysis shows that the state's efforts to preserve human life are inconsistent. For example, the government has no constitutional duty to feed or house its citizens, or to protect them from the violent or homicidal acts of private individuals [5]. Second, the state has a moral obligation to protect vulnerable groups—the poor, elderly, and disabled—from the abuse of those who might improperly induce or force them into ending their lives. Third, as physicians would likely be approached to help people end their lives by means of prescription medications, these laws preserve the ethical integrity of physicians and other clinicians as healers who are fundamentally obligated always to preserve life and so be opposed to participating in a suicide. Finally, states may fear that accepting assisted suicide will start society down a path toward voluntary or even involuntary euthanasia [6].

Although statutes prohibiting assisting a suicide are worded in various ways, it is clear that "assisting" primarily means that the accused actively participated in the events prior to the commission of the lethal act by the suicidal person, almost always by furnishing the practical means for causing death—the poison, the rope, the firearm, the knife—for the use of that person, knowing what he intended to do with it. Any person who unwittingly provides the means of self-killing to someone cannot be held criminally or ethically responsible for involvement in that death.

In contrast, if a person actually performs the fatal act, e.g., holds the pillow over the face of another or administers the poison with his consent, then he or she has committed murder, "and it is wholly immaterial whether this act is committed pursuant to an agreement with the victim, such as a mutual suicide pact" [2]. In other words, the legal distinction between murder and assisting (it could also be called "aiding" or "aiding and abetting") a suicide rests on the difference between the active and passive role of the second party in the actual death of the suicide. If she knowingly provided the actual means for accomplishing the suicide, she has assisted or aided a suicide. If she actively participates in performing the lethal act (pulling the gun's trigger), she is guilty of murder.

Earlier I noted that "assisting a suicide" *almost* always means knowingly furnishing the physical means of producing death. The qualifier is there for a reason. A number of states prohibit not only assisting or aiding a suicide but also "advising" or "encouraging" another to commit suicide. A recent decision by the Minnesota Supreme Court has held that a person cannot be criminally prosecuted for providing another with advice or encouragement to commit suicide because the statutory terms "advising" and "encouraging" violated the First Amendment's free speech guaranty by their breadth. In this case, William Melchert-Dinkel contacted two different people online and feigned understanding their situation while posing as a young nurse to win their trust, falsely claimed that he too would kill himself, and attempted to persuade both to hang themselves and to let him watch the hangings on a webcam. Both killed themselves, the former by hanging and the latter by drowning. One of them was 32 years old and had suffered from significant mental and physical health problems for many years, including a condition that was "like having [the] flu all the time." The other was a 19-year-old college student [1].

Despite ruling that informing someone about suicide or providing verbal support or courage to do so cannot be made criminal, the court also decided that some speech by itself can rise to the level of "assisting" a suicide because it enables a suicide and has a direct, causal connection to it. The court found that this constitutes conduct not protected by the First Amendment [1]. Unfortunately, the court never explains how speech alone can have a direct, causal connection to suicide, and this lacuna in its analysis renders its conclusion of dubious validity.

No therapist treating a suicidal patient, elderly or not, should be concerned that their therapeutic conversations could amount to "assisting" a suicide in violation of the criminal law, unless the therapist engaged in outrageous and bizarre conduct similar to that of Mr. Melcher-Dinkle—which is hard to imagine unless the therapist was in serious need of therapy himself. The same is true for therapists who express sympathy for or understanding of an elderly patient's rational conclusion that she finds her current life burdensome and her future bleak to the point where she is contemplating ending her life. Assisting a suicide requires "a level of involvement beyond merely expressing a moral viewpoint or providing general comfort or support" [1]. Furthermore, I am aware of no criminal prosecution of a therapist for failing to prevent a patient's suicide and thereby "assisting" a suicide (civil liability for negligently failing to prevent a suicide will be discussed below).

Could someone who gave another a book (or referred them to it) like Derek Humphrey's *Final Exit* which contains information about "the practicalities of self-deliverance" be successfully criminally prosecuted for assisting a suicide? The First Amendment free speech guaranty protects the publishing of such a book, giving it to someone, discussion of it, or telling someone of its existence. "The constitutional guaranties of free speech protect the freedom of individuals to speak, write, print or otherwise communicate information or opinion" [7]. On the other hand, while the Constitution prevents the state from punishing those who write, publish, discuss, or use a book, this does not mean that it is ethical, professionally proper, or wise to do so. The clinician's first or primary ethical obligation to a patient is not, as commonly thought, "to do no harm." Rather it is to benefit, be useful or helpful, to the patient and then not to harm [8]. Whether a patient could ever be benefited by being directed to such a book by a clinician is of course ethically controversial and surely not a matter that can be decided by the law.

From a legal point of view, the most prudent position for a therapist to adopt in relation to an elderly patient's arguably rational desire to end her life is either opposition if that is what, after careful investigation and reflection, the clinician believes is in the patient's best interests or neutrality if, after the same process, the clinician believes that the patient's desire is not unreasonable or the product of seriously disordered thinking. As indicated in chapter one of this volume to which I contributed, Gillian Bennett's suicide cannot fairly be called irrational or thought to be generated by a serious mental illness. If she had disclosed her intentions to her own therapist and the latter made professionally proper inquiries into the patient's reasoning, mental state, and personal values, the therapist very likely would be in a legally defensible position if she were neutral toward Ms. Bennett's plans.

3.4   Legalized Physician-Assisted Suicide

Four states (Oregon, Washington, Vermont, and California) have statutes that permit physician-assisted suicide for competent, adult, terminally ill patients, and one allows the practice by court ruling (Montana) [9–13]. The laws in Oregon and Washington were enacted by citizen ballot initiatives, while those in Vermont and California were enacted by the legislature. The four sets of statutes are basically quite similar: only adults with the mental capacity to understand what they are doing can make a request for a prescription from a physician that they must personally use to end their lives; the patients must be properly informed of their medical situation and alternatives by their attending physician; two physicians must confirm that the patient is terminally ill (i.e., have an incurable and irreversible disease that reasonable medical judgment determines will produce death within 6 months) to qualify for receiving the prescription; the physician must determine the patient has mental capacity to make an informed choice and refer the patient to a mental health clinician if he suspects the patient's judgment is impaired by a psychiatric disorder; the patient must make repeated requests for the prescription, including a written request properly witnessed. The Baxter decision states that if a terminally ill, competent adult patient receives a lethal medication from a physician and takes the medication herself, the physician who prescribed the drug has a defense to any legal charges of wrongdoing.

No physician or other clinician is required to participate in an assisted suicide. Physicians who do participate are immune from all legal and professional sanction, although a health facility or organization can prohibit activities related to assistance on their premises. Only assistance in suicide is permitted; active euthanasia and all other forms of mercy killing remain criminal. Coercion, undue influence, or fraud directed to those choosing assisted suicide are prohibited.

The approval of regulated physician-assisted suicide in these states demonstrates that their citizens and legislators (a majority of one or the other, although by no means all of either) believe that some suicides are rational and not generated by impaired judgment due to a mental disorder. It is implausible to contend that decisions to end life become rational only because the individuals are terminally ill. Furthermore, the choice of having less than 6 *months* to live is neither talismanic, nor the only reasonable conception of "terminal illness," nor the only possible qualification in addition to informed consent needed for the ethical and legal permissibility of assisted suicide. It is very likely that 6 months was chosen by those who drafted these laws for strategic political purposes and not because it is the "true" definition of the term.

Likewise, it is implausible that terminally ill persons lose their right to life, have less personal stake or interest in remaining alive, or that the state has less interest in protecting their lives. The law treats the lives of all persons as having equal worth:

> The lives of all are equally under the protection of the law, and under that protection to their last moment. The life of those to whom life has become a burden—of those who are hopelessly diseased or fatally wounded—nay, even the lives of criminals condemned to death, are under the protection of the law, equally as the lives of those who are in the full tide of life's enjoyment, and anxious to continue to live. [14]

Yet many conclude that terminally ill persons can rationally and ethically waive their right to life when done voluntarily, can have good reasons not to remain alive for whatever time they may have left, and do not want the state's protection to prevent them from voluntarily taking their own lives. In short, the presence of terminal illness by itself is not the only factor that can make someone's desire to end her life understandable, rational, or ethically justifiable. States could, if enough citizens and or legislators chose to, broaden the criteria for qualification for physician-assisted suicide, although the wisdom of any such law would surely be hotly contested.

The states that have permitted PAS for the longest periods of time are Oregon and Washington. A review of what those individuals in Oregon (1998–2013) [15] and Washington (2012–2014) [16] who have obtained a lethal prescription are concerned about at the end of their lives can help us understand why some elderly persons who are *not* terminally ill might wish to rationally end their lives as well. The most commonly mentioned concerns for those seeking physician-assisted suicide were loss of autonomy (OR 92 %, WA 91 %), loss of ability to engage in activities that made life enjoyable (OR 89 %, WA 91 %), loss of dignity (OR 81 %, WA 81 %), burden on family, friends/caregivers (OR 50 %, WA 61 %), losing control of bodily functions (OR 40 %, WA 53 %), and inadequate pain control or concerns about it (OR 24 %, WA 37 %) [15, 16].

These appear to be fundamentally the same factors as those that motivate many elderly, but not terminally ill, individuals to express to therapists and others a desire to end their lives. However, this is not intended to be an argument for expanding "death with dignity" laws to include the nonterminally ill elderly. That is a discussion beyond the scope of this chapter. Nevertheless, I am suggesting that the presence of these same concerns in the elderly—or reasons why continuing to live is no longer a felt necessity—tells us that their experiences of what life presently has and will likely hold for them in the future can reasonably lead them to consider suicide.

It seems unlikely that psychiatrists, who would be able to write the lethal prescriptions permitted by these laws if they can competently diagnose the terminal illness and fulfill the other requirements under the law, will actually be the ones approached by patients seeking physician-assisted suicide. Oregon officials do not keep track of the areas of practice of physicians who write these prescriptions, although we do know that in 2014, 83 different physicians wrote 155 such scripts, in number ranging from 1 to 12 [15]. Given that 91 % of those citizens who used the Oregon Death with Dignity law between 1998 and 2013 had cancer (79 %), amyotrophic lateral sclerosis (7 %), or chronic lower respiratory disease (5 %), they would much more likely seek assistance from their primary attending internist than their psychiatrist [15].

3.5   Civil Liability and Treating the Suicidal

Therapists who encounter elderly patients expressing what appears to be a rational desire to end their lives have the same basic legal obligations toward them as they do toward all patients under the civil law: to provide them with professional service that conforms to the standard of care. Any claim that a professional has been negligent in treating a patient rests on the plaintiff proving the four elements of negligence by the preponderance of the evidence: (1) a duty of care existed between the therapist and the individual who was allegedly harmed, i.e., a therapist-patient relationship existed at the time of the alleged wrongdoing; (2) the therapist breached her duty by failing to meet the standard of care applicable under the circumstances; (3) the patient suffered harm; and (4) the therapist's conduct in question was the legal cause of this harm, i.e., the alleged breach of the standard of care was the actual cause of the harm (but for the breach, the patient would not have been harmed) and the proximate cause of the harm (the harm was foreseeable to the therapist as a consequence of his actions) [17].

It is not uncommon for professional negligence (malpractice) lawsuits to be brought against therapists after a patient attempts suicide or succeeds in killing himself [18], which could well be due to the emotionally damaging aftermath of guilt, bewilderment, and anger experienced by remaining family members. A study of malpractice claims from the 1980s showed that post-suicide lawsuits accounted for the largest number of malpractice lawsuits and largest settlement amounts against psychiatrists [19]. Another study demonstrated that among psychologists insured by the American Psychological Association, claims related to patient suicide were the sixth most common type but accounted for the second highest total costs [20]. However, lawsuits against mental health professionals remain relatively rare, only a small portion of claims go to trial (6 to 10 %), and clinicians win up to 80 % of those that do go to trial [21]. No study focusing only on lawsuits over suicide among the elderly could be located.

Although the risk of a civil lawsuit related to an attempted or completed suicide cannot be eliminated, legal risk is inherent in all professional practice and, in the last analysis, also inherent in virtually all of life's activities. After all, anyone with the court filing fee and a little legal knowledge on how to draft a complaint can file a lawsuit. Free-floating anxiety over and excessive reaction to the possibility of litigation can damage the quality of professional service to patients as well as the professional integrity of the mental health practitioner. Baerger has argued that:

> Clinicians must resist resorting to defensive clinical practices in an attempt to shield themselves from potential lawsuits. In other words, clinicians must resist relying on excessively restrictive treatments (e.g., involuntary hospitalization, unnecessary medication, unwarranted physical restraint) in an effort to protect themselves from criticism or censure.... [T]he best protection against potential liability for suicide is for the clinician to have followed acceptable standards of practice throughout treatment. [21]

Baerger has proposed five recommendations for minimizing a clinician's exposure to liability in the treatment of suicidal patients. The following is a discussion of each of these recommendations in light of the focus of this volume on the elderly patient who expresses a rational desire for suicide:

1. "The clinician must conduct a comprehensive examination of the patient at intake" [21]. A patient who evinces a desire to end his life should, of course, receive a standard of care clinical assessment. I leave the details of that to mental health experts, but note that Baerger believes there is "no need to follow a standardized interview schedule for such an assessment. Intake formats will vary greatly depending upon the patient's presenting problem and the reason for referral" [21]. Whatever the form and content of the examination, maintaining positive therapeutic relationships with patients provides clinicians with protection from lawsuits even if particular outcomes are not positive.

In the chapter of this volume "Can Suicide in the Elderly Be Rational?," Professor Ramirez and I proposed a set of indicia for determining whether a decision to end one's life could be considered rational. I suggest that a therapist utilize this set (or similar criteria [22, 23]) as part of a comprehensive mental evaluation of an elderly patient, especially because the patient's reasons for wanting to die will likely be more subjective and existential. Given that an elderly patient contemplating a rational suicide is not necessarily likely to meet the criteria for mental conditions that are strongly associated with suicide (such as major depression, other mood disorders, schizophrenia, post-traumatic stress disorder, substance abuse disorders, and borderline or antisocial personality disorders), a careful review of the individual's reasons for wanting to die and the circumstances of his lifeworld, as well as what can possibly be done to change those reasons and circumstances, is strongly indicated. Some commentators have observed that therapists will not be found negligent if a patient's suicide is judged to be voluntary [23]. If therapists are unfamiliar with elderly patients who appear competent, rational, and are contemplating suicide, they should consult with a colleague who has experience with these patients.

2. "If the patient is at risk (e.g., likely to attempt to harm him- or herself in the near future, hospitalization should be seriously considered and only rejected in the event of a comprehensive safety plan" [21]. This recommendation may be difficult to apply to elderly persons who want to die primarily for reasons having to do with functional disabilities, loss of independence and control, and loss of life's meaning and purpose and who often have a justified negative reaction to their situation rather than manifest mental illness. In any event, it should be noted that "as long as documentation is adequate, cases arising from a failure to hospitalize have typically been favorable to clinicians" [21]. In addition, if rational suicides do exist, then we must reject the simple equation of a desire to kill oneself with the presence of a mental illness that eliminates the individual's mental capacity to make decisions which others should respect.

    The threshold question is whether the elderly person meets the legal criteria for involuntary civil commitment: the patient must suffer from a mental illness and pose an imminent threat to his own safety, a threat likely to be carried out in the near future [24]. Then the question of the purpose or goal of hospitalization arises. While a period of involuntary commitment might allow for deeper clinical evaluation, exploration of alternative solutions to the patient's negative feelings about her situation, and some treatment, a truly rational person will, once detained, refrain from expressing any desire to die and cooperate with whatever therapy is offered. In all likelihood then, the patient will no longer legally qualify for commitment and have to be released, particularly once judicial review of the detention occurs. Consequently, if a competent elderly patient presents with a desire to die supported by understandable reasons and involuntary commitment is not appropriate, therapists should carefully explain and justify their conclusion in the patient's medical record. Finally, it bears mention that clinicians treating outpatients should not be found liable for failing to assume physical custody over suicidal patients [21].

3. "The clinician should review the level of risk a patient presents at particularly stressful times in the patient's life" [21]. This recommendation is intended to avoid the situation in which the clinician adopts an initial treatment plan for a patient and then does not adjust it to conform to changed circumstances in the

patient's life as this can increase the risk of litigation. The elderly patient who considers himself at the end of his life, lacks a desirable future, and has a rational desire not to continue living may have already encountered enough stressful events of sufficient magnitude so that one more stressful event will not alter his situation significantly. Nevertheless, from a risk management point of view, a therapist is advised to keep in touch with a patient's current situation and to adapt their therapeutic assessment and intervention to it.

4. "The clinician should maintain accurate records that explain significant treatment decisions and that clearly delineate the reasons for rejecting hospitalization for at-risk outpatients and the reasons for choosing discharge for at-risk inpatients" [21]. Every lawyer advising any health-care professionals will tell them in no uncertain terms that if litigation ever arises over what they did or failed to do in their practice (and either can be the source of a negligence claim), "if you didn't document it, it didn't happen" or, alternatively, "if you didn't write it down, you are inviting the inference by opposing counsel, the judge, and the jury that you're not telling the straight story from memory." Careful and thorough documentation in the patient's record is not only the best evidence of what actually happened between the therapist and the patient but also the best way to refresh the therapist's memory of what occurred when he or she is called upon to testify at a deposition or trial.

Baerger has rightly pointed out that many clinicians embrace "the erroneous belief that not maintaining comprehensive treatment records will protect them in the event of a lawsuit. In fact, nothing could be further from the truth" [21]. Probably even worse is the idea that it is wise to alter the record. "Clinicians who attempt to alter the clinical record after the fact are making a fatal mistake. Tampering or inserting new material after the fact can insure that the psychologist [or other therapist] will lose the case regardless of the reasonableness of the treatment decisions made by the clinician" [18]. Actually, therapists who make a bad or suspect decision but whose reasoning and justification for that decision are clearly articulated and well documented are in a more legally defensible position that colleagues make reasonable decisions but fail to document them or do so poorly. For example, the law does not hold clinicians liable for mistakes in judgment, but it is much harder to explain and justify a judgment as made in good faith and in accord with the standard of care, even if wrong in hindsight, if the circumstances and reasons for that judgment are badly—or not at all—documented.

Thorough documentation is particularly important in the case of the elderly patient with a rational desire to die. This is the case not only because of the tension and ambiguity in the term "rational suicide" as conventionally understood but also because justification for concluding that the desire is rational requires explication of personal values, treatment options that exist but are unacceptable to the patient, and the evidence that demonstrates the patient's mental capacity and grasp of reality. The following is an example of a hypothetical outpatient note that helpfully explains the clinician's action.

I considered hospitalizing the patient but rejected it for several reasons. The patient did not meet the commitment criteria and did not want to enter the hospital. He had never tried suicide before. I was concerned that, given his declining self-esteem, if I hospitalized him at this point, I would be making it much more likely that he would kill himself. So, even though I knew there was an elevated risk of not hospitalizing this patient, I determined that it was outweighed by the clinical risks of hospitalizing him [25].

In short, any therapist treating an elderly patient who is considering rational suicide is well advised to carefully and thoroughly document all of the clinical, personal, and existential factors that are operative in the case at hand. Accurate documentation "is a sine qua non of demonstrating professional competence" [18]. Furthermore, the stronger a therapist's documentation is of the evidence for finding the patient able to act truly voluntarily, "the more remote the prospect for malpractice liability for suicide may be, since it is thus more likely that the [patient's] independent and competent action is the proximate cause of the outcome" [23].

5. "The clinician must take special precautions against suicide when treating the at-risk patient, including–where appropriate–involving the patient's family or friends in safety or discharge plans" [21]. The involvement of an elderly patient's family and friends may not be so important for implementing an adequate safety or discharge plan as it is for ensuring that the patient's desire to die is well thought out, persistent, and in accordance with the patient's fundamental values. If the family and friends do not oppose the patient's plan and may even endorse it (e.g., the Bennett case in Chapter 1 of this volume), the clinician has learned something very important. The same is true if they oppose the patient's desire and want to intervene. The latter situation rightly puts the onus on the family to take affirmative steps to make the patient's life more bearable.

Of course therapists have an ethical and legal obligation to maintain their patients' confidentiality; the failure to do so can destroy or damage a strong working therapeutic alliance between therapist and patient. However, "it is important to note that confidentiality is not absolute and that there are circumstances under which breaking confidentiality is both legally and ethically required" [21]. Preventing an impending suicide by informing family members of the patient's intent, for example, is generally a valid reason for breaching confidentiality as doing so is in the patient's own interests. It should be an unusual "rational" suicide when the patient's loved ones are unaware of her desire to die and have not had an opportunity to take action that might change the patient's mind. On the other hand, as dysfunctional and abusive families exist, good reasons might exist for their exclusion from the patient's plans. In any event, when an elderly person expresses an intent to take her own life, a clinician's suspicions should be aroused if her family is not involved in the patient's deliberation about a choice of last resort.

In conclusion, while undoubtedly the existence and meaning of rational suicide is contested among mental health professionals and others, the contents of this volume and the work of a variety of commentators demonstrate that it is not a bizarre or fringe concept [22, 23]. Studies show that significant numbers of mental health professionals believe the concept is meaningful and report that they have worked with clients they considered to be rational when contemplating suicide [23]. The fact that clinicians respond in different ways to patients who are considering suicide for reasons they find compelling does not necessarily mean that any particular clinical response is *the* standard of care. Courts have held that if there are several professionally acceptable approaches to a situation, then a clinician may choose among them, even if that is not the dominant approach, provided that it is endorsed by a significant or respectable minority of clinicians with similar training and experience [23].

Laws pertaining to a professional's legal responsibilities vary from state to state. For example, in some jurisdictions, psychiatrists and psychologists may be held to differing standards of care, with the former facing stricter requirements [21]. Moreover, the application of law to a particular situation is fact sensitive. Consequently, it is advisable for clinicians to consult with a lawyer who represents them personally (and not an institution for which they work) to better understand what legal risks they might face in managing a competent elderly patient who no longer wishes to live.

References

1. Supreme Court of Minnesota. State v. Melchert-Dinkel, 844 N.W.2d 13–25. 2014.
2. Supreme Court of California. In re Joseph G., 34 Cal.3d 429–40. 1983.
3. Mendelson D, Freckelton I. The interface of the civil and criminal law of suicide at common law (1194–1845). Int J Law Psychiatry. 2013;36:343–9.
4. Supreme Court of the United States. Vacco v. Quill, 521 U.S. 793–810. 1997.
5. Supreme Court of the United States. DeShaney v. Winnebago County Department of Social Services, 489 U.S. 189–213. 1989
6. Supreme Court of the United States. Washington v. Glucksberg, 521 U.S. 702–92. 1997.
7. California Court of Appeal. Donaldson v. Lungren, 2 Cal.App.4th 1614–25. 1992.
8. Nelson LJ. Primum utilis esse: the primacy of usefulness in medicine. Yale J Biol Med. 1978;51:655–66.
9. Oregon Revised Statutes. Sections 127.800-127.995. 2015.
10. Revised Code of Washington. Sections 70.245.010-70.245.904. 2015.
11. Vermont Statutes Annotated. Sections 5281–5292. 2015.
12. California Health & Safety Code. Sections 443–433.217. 2015.
13. Supreme Court of Montana. Baxter v, Montana, 224 P.3d 1211–40. 2009.
14. Supreme Court of Ohio. Blackburn v. State, 23 Ohio St. 146, 163. 1872.
15. Oregon.gov [Internet]. Salem: Oregon Health Authority; 2015 [cited 2015 Nov 23]. https://public.health.oregon.gov/ProviderPartnerResources/EvaluationResearch/DeathwithDignityAct/Pages/ar-index.aspx.
16. Death with Dignity [Internet]. Tumwater: Washington Department of Health; 2012–2014 [cited 2015 Nov 24]. http://www.doh.wa.gov/YouandYourFamily/IllnessandDisease/DeathwithDignityAct.
17. Griffin M. Working with suicidal patients. The Therapist 2011; July–August:1–8.
18. Bongar B, Stolberg R. Risk management with the suicidal patient. Washington DC: National Register of Health Service Psychologists; 2009 [cited 2015 Nov 23]. http://www.e-psychologist.org/index.iml?mdl=exam/show_article.mdl&Material_ID=100.
19. Robertson JD. Psychiatric malpractice: liability of mental health professionals. New York: Wiley; 1988.

20. Bongar B, Maris RW, Berman AL, Litman RE. Outpatient standards of care and the suicidal patient. In: Bongar B, Berman AL, Maris RW, Silverman MM, Harris EA, Packman WL, editors. Risk management with suicidal patients. New York: Guilford; 1998. p. 4–33.
21. Baerger DR. Risk management with the suicidal patient: lessons from case law. Prof Psychol Res Pr. 2001;32:359–66.
22. Battin MP. Can suicide be rational? Yes, sometimes. In: Werth JL, editor. Contemporary perspectives on rational suicide. Philadelphia: Brunner/Mazel; 1999. p. 13–21.
23. Werth JL. Rational suicide? Implications for mental health professionals. London: Taylor and Francis; 1996.
24. Testa M, West SG. Civil commitment in the united states. Psychiatry (Edgemont). 2010;7:30–9.
25. Packman WL, Harris EL. Legal issues and risk management in suicidal patients. In: Bongar B, Berman AL, Maris RW, Silverman MM, Harris EA, Packman WL, editors. Risk management with suicidal patients. New York: Guilford; 1998. p. 150–86.

Refractory Depression and the Right to Terminate Active Treatment

Barbara R. Sommer and Kristin S. Raj

4.1   Introduction

This chapter discusses whether patients with treatment-refractory depression have the same right as patients with other refractory illnesses to control when to terminate active treatment of their depression. The chapter questions the rationale for compelling such patients, refractory to many trials of ever more complicated medication regimens, to continue with treatment, even when doing so would be unlikely to help.

Before discussing this ethical issue, it is important to describe the patients to whom it applies. We begin by defining treatment-refractory depression (TRD), with some of its possible biological underpinnings, and then we discuss some newer strategies for treatment, some now established and others that remain investigational. Then we will discuss the concept of "terminal depression," in which the refractory patient has become so disabled that their very life is shortened by the psychiatric disorder. To draw parallels with other treatment-refractory disorders, we will discuss the concept of capacity in patients with refractory medical disorders and the influence of depression on their decisions. Such comparisons between medical and psychiatric patients are not common in the United States but are made in some other countries, and we will discuss the potential ramifications of such comparisons.

The chapter aims to discuss only the rights of patients who want to terminate active treatment. Many patients and their families want to pursue all options, even if prior treatments have been ineffective, and we are not addressing this group. Likewise, we will not discuss the group of patients who may wish to terminate care specifically with the intent to commit suicide.

B.R. Sommer, M.D. (✉) • K.S. Raj, M.D.
Department of Psychiatry and Behavioral Sciences, Stanford University School of Medicine,
401 Quarry Road-2337, Stanford, CA 94305-5723, USA
e-mail: brsommer@stanford.edu

© Springer International Publishing Switzerland 2017   45
R.E. McCue, M. Balasubramaniam (eds.), *Rational Suicide in the Elderly*,
DOI 10.1007/978-3-319-32672-6_4

In the USA, the legal concept of a medical patient's autonomy over end-of-life care has been discussed at least since 1969, when attorney Luis Kutner discussed the living will and the right to terminate care in the event of an incurable condition [1]. In 1976, after the case of Karen Ann Quinlan, which discussed the physician's obligations in the termination of life support, the moral burden of a patient's death was placed on the disease, rather than on the physician [2]. While TRD is not generally considered a terminal illness, directly causing death if untreated, the issue of when to terminate active medical treatment is similar. The advocacy for a terminally or incurably ill person to refuse life-sustaining measures intended to prolong life artificially [3] is to be differentiated from physician-assisted suicide.

4.2   Treatment-Resistant Depression (TRD)

Despite the availability of modalities to treat depression such as antidepressants with differing biochemistries, augmentation strategies (anticonvulsants, antipsychotic drugs, lithium, thyroid hormone), psychotherapy, and interventional neuromodulatory treatments (electroconvulsive therapy (ECT), repetitive transcranial magnetic stimulation (rTMS), and vagus nerve stimulation), a minority of patients does not improve with therapy. Overall, 50 % of patients with major depression fail to reach full remission despite adequate treatment, and 30–50 % of responders do not respond in the long term (greater than 50 % reduction of symptoms on the Hamilton Rating Scale for Depression) [4–7]. In the comprehensive STAR*D study of treatment outcomes, evaluating an outpatient cohort of over 4000 patients with nonpsychotic depression, remission was best for the first two treatment steps, with over 50 % responding if they stayed in treatment. The participants who required additional treatment steps were found to have poorer treatment outcomes, and while the overall remission rate was 67 %, patients requiring multiple trials with augmentation experienced only 13.0 % remission rates. Furthermore, the patients requiring more treatment steps had a higher relapse rate [8].

In the longer term, follow-up studies have found that up to 12 % of patients suffering from major depression have a poor outcome even after 5 years of treatment [9, 10] and the likelihood of recovery seems to decrease over time [11]. One meta-analysis found that the risk of relapse increased after each successive trial and that the all-cause mortality rate from natural causes was 32 % after 7 years [11]. The result for treatment-refractory patients is a lower quality of life than treatment-remitted patients, with more work missed and more frequent medical visits, which may account for the $29–45 billion thought to be the ultimate cost of such depressions [7].

Although TRD has many definitions in the literature, with attempts to stage the entity [10, 12, 13], most outcome studies describe the phenomenon as a failure to achieve remission despite two different antidepressant trials of adequate duration (at least 1 month) [10, 14–16]. Other outcome studies of therapies specific to TRD give alternative, more stringent definitions of the disorder. For example, studies of the effectiveness of deep brain stimulation (DBS) define refractory depression as a major depressive episode of at least 1 year, with failure to respond to a minimum of four different antidepressant treatments, psychotherapy, and ECT [17, 18]. Another study used the following criteria: at least 4 episodes of MDD, or chronicity of an episode over 2 years, more than 5 years after the first episode of MDD, failure to respond to more than 5 weeks of maximum doses of antidepressants from at least 3 different classes, and at least 2 different augmenting strategies, such as thyroid hormone (T3), lithium, stimulants, antipsychotic medication, anticonvulsants, buspirone, or a second antidepressant. ECT consisting of greater than 6 bilateral treatments and at least 20 psychotherapy sessions must also have been administered [19].

Requirements to meet a diagnosis of TRD include verification both of the diagnosis and of adequate treatment trials. Specifically, patient adherence to each medication regimen must be documented, with assessment of symptoms over time, either with depression instruments or with diary or self-report [10]. Community-based surveys have shown that fewer than 50 % of patients receive either an adequate dose or duration of antidepressant treatment [20]. The diagnosis of treatment refractory should not be made unless adequate psychotherapy also has been tried. The effects of cognitive behavioral psychotherapy (CBT) recently have been shown to be as effective in treating severe depressions as in treating mild or moderate depression, and many patients with severe depression have not been found to need concomitant medication therapy [21]. Thus, while lack of CBT historically has not been used in defining TRD, current evidence suggests that it should be included. Likewise, the importance of spirituality has been evaluated in an observational study of 160 medical patients at the end of their lives. Greater spiritual well-being, assessed with a scale measuring the extent to which one derives support through spirituality, was seen as conferring relative protection from end-of-life despair and from asking for a hastened death [22]. This was an observational study unable to account for the possibly overlapping factors of spiritual well-being and depression. Nevertheless, prior to the designation of TRD or terminal depression, chaplaincy contributions may be important in many cases.

4.3   Terminal Depression and the Case of Mr. A

These alternative definitions, all describing "treatment resistance," lend support to the concept of a spectrum ranging from treatment responsive, resistant, refractory, and then terminal. In this range, a partial response is defined as less than a 50 % reduction in Hamilton Depression Rating Scale, as mentioned above. Refractory patients either suffer from nonresponse or worsening of symptoms over time [4]. Along the continuum of nonresponse to treatment, terminal depression implies a rational belief that a patient will ultimately die of natural causes without his/her depression improving, despite multiple reasonable adequate trials of medications, interventional treatments such as rTMS or ECT, psychotherapy, and intervention by clergy as appropriate [23]. It may be considered in patients with the increased medical morbidity that often accompanies depression and that cannot be adequately treated in the face of the depression [24]. For example, a study of primary care patients found that treatment resistance was associated with both overweight and frank obesity, with higher rates of disability and comorbidity [25]. Although one cannot infer causality, it is likely that the health problems and depression exacerbate each other.

In particular, the geriatric population may suffer from depressive signs and symptoms that are complicated by additional factors that may lead to the diagnosis of terminal depression [25]. Older patients may experience a decline in physical health, with decreased food consumption and ambulation. Frail older patients may be at risk for falls and, after staying in bed for protracted periods also may run the risk of deep vein thrombosis. Complicating this picture is the risk of delirium posed when older patients are given multiple medications [26]. While treating such patients with all available regimens is the standard of care, there are instances when such patients do not improve or even decline because of the medications, and remission becomes a frank impossibility. We describe here a case of such a patient whose case gave rise to our definition of terminal depression. This case has been described in detail elsewhere by the authors of this chapter [23]:

Mr. A first experienced a profound depression at age 59. There were no confounding medical illnesses, medications, or family stresses, and he did not present with concurrent psychosis or dementia. His prominent difficulties were with poor sleep and appetite and lack of energy, and he was treated with citalopram and psychotherapy. This led to a remission for 5 years after a psychiatric hospitalization, and Mr. A was able to resume his job. However, his depression recurred 5 years later when Mr. A's wife found him to be irritable, isolative, and psychotic. He no longer was able to function as the professor he had been. When his outpatient psychiatrist prescribed an increase in citalopram, he refused, having lost confidence in the medication on which he again became symptomatic. Suffering from anergy and paranoia that others were poisoning his food, he stopped eating. He had intrusive thoughts and auditory hallucinations. A CT scan of his brain was normal. Mr. A remained alert, oriented, and fluent in his speech. Neurological examinations were unrevealing.

Soon Mr. A stopped eating altogether and lost 45 lb. With extreme poverty of thought and slowness of speech, he was voluntarily admitted for his third psychiatric hospitalization. At times he refused to get out of bed to perform activities of daily living, and despite his lack of the classic waxy flexibility on physical examination, the staff considered the diagnosis of catatonia. He described a somatic delusion about esophageal and intestinal blockage, causing him to refuse to eat or drink. An MRI of the brain was consistent only with nonspecific chronic small vessel ischemic disease. Also noted was mild global prominence of the ventricles and sulci consistent with mild cerebral tissue loss, specifying that the loss was slightly greater than expected for individual his age. A Mini Mental State Exam (MMSE) was 29/30, missing one point for "serial 7s," and a diagnosis of dementia was ruled out.

Mr. A received a course of 16 bilateral ECT treatments during this hospitalization, with scores on the Montgomery-Åsberg Depression Rating Scale (MADRS) decreasing only from 53 to 34, reflective of continuing very severe depression. However, he became less paranoid and began oral intake again, gaining 20 lb. The

ECT did not result in demonstrable cognitive impairment, save for some loss of autobiographical memory.

Five months after discharge, the patient relapsed and required another psychiatric hospitalization. Another medication regimen was prescribed, and while the neurovegetative symptoms improved, he continued to complain of depressed mood. Given the magnitude of his functional decline from his baseline, a course of 16 ECTs was again administered. Unfortunately, his MADRS score only decreased from 45 to 33. At the time of final discharge, he was able to participate in some ward groups and activities and was able to leave his room for short escorted walks with his wife or with staff. He continued to exhibit constricted affect and to appear dysphoric, and he stated he felt "frustrated" for lack of overall improvement in his mood. He did not appear psychotic.

Mr. A's wife stated that about 6 months later, he became "tired of seeing the psychologist and of taking medications," telling her, "Enough is enough." His refusal to take medications was again followed by refusal to eat, and another psychiatric hospitalization ensued. His primary care provider felt that Mr. A had capacity to make his own decisions and after consulting with an ethicist, informed Mr. A's wife that it was "ok to let him go." Medication adherence became an issue, as Mr. A was at this point refusing to abide by a daily regimen. His ability to assess the advantages and disadvantages of another course of ECT were intact. He remembered these risks and benefits based on recall from his prior ECT experience. In hospital, the patient did allow pharmacological treatment, and his anxiety improved, enabling him to get out of bed with aid from physical therapy once or twice a day.

It was at this point that that the patient decided that he was no longer interested in any treatment for depression. He was able to recall that he had had several psychiatric hospitalizations and ECT with little effect. Feeling a burden to his wife, he felt that there was nothing left to ameliorate his low level of functioning. He no longer wanted his wife to visit. When she did see him, she often cried at his deterioration and entered counseling herself. He acknowledged to one of the authors that he felt he had lost his dignity. A palliative care consultation was called, but he refused to see the team.

While he appeared to have capacity to refuse treatment, given his severe depression with somatic delusions, an ethics consultation was sought to determine if the team could abide by his wish. It was determined that the patient did indeed have capacity and he was transferred to a skilled nursing facility, nasogastric tube (NGT) in place. He continued to demonstrate paucity of speech, with long latency of response. After 3 weeks at the skilled nursing facility, the patient pulled the NGT and said "goodbye" to his wife. He died several days later. A complete list of his medication regimen is listed in the paper cited above.

We propose that Mr. A may be thought of as having suffered from the psychiatric equivalent of a terminal illness. Like other patients suffering from medical disorders who do not respond even to the most up-to-date strategies and who are considered "nonresponders," his prognosis became increasingly grave. As it became progressively more difficult for him to experience a sustained remission, he began to spend increasing amounts of time in hospitals. His treatments were aggressive, and while one may argue over the details of some combinations of treatments, there is no argument that he received adequate trials of several antidepressants in adequate doses, with evidence-based augmentation strategies. Furthermore, he was administered ECT twice. Nonetheless, no treatment, save citalopram at the onset of his symptoms, was helpful for a sustained period.

Mr. A was competent in his understanding that after having had many available psychiatric treatments, one viable option was to continue with enteral (tube) feeding and even more medications in an assisted living environment. Alternatively, he could have accepted ECT, which had not caused sustained remission in the past and which gave rise to autobiographical memory loss. In addition to his psychiatric diagnosis of major depression with psychosis, he may have also been suffering from the depression and demoralization often superimposed on patients in the terminal phases of medical illnesses and which may increase the desire to die [27, 28]. Mr. A also likely suffered from a mild vascular neurocognitive disorder, which was not felt to decrease his capacity to make decisions regarding his health care. Mr. A was a voluntarily admitted patient who, while depressed, was never suicidal during any of his admissions and who clearly understood the ramifications of the different courses that could be taken on his behalf. His capability was in line with most research findings that even patients with very severe depression maintain their competence to make health care decisions [29].

This case differs from the landmark Chabot case in the Netherlands in 1994, in which the Supreme Court ruled that to assess capacity, it is the seriousness of the suffering that is important, rather than whether the patient suffers from a psychiatric versus medical disorder. In this case, the Court found the physician guilty because he had not obtained a face-to-face evaluation by an independent medical expert. Our case also differs from a case described from the Netherlands in 2013, when a patient with what we would call terminal depression requested and was granted physician-assisted suicide. In this latter case, the patient had wanted to end her life of suffering after years of intermittent suicidal feelings and plans. In our case, while the patient knew that withdrawal of nasogastric feeding would hasten his death, he was not suicidal per se [30].

4.4 Biological Substrates of TRD

There may be several ways to understand the biological mechanisms of treatment-refractory or terminal depression. Research suggests that some late-onset depressions are associated with abnormalities in the anterior cingulate and dorsolateral prefrontal cortex, thought to be central pathways in depression [31, 32]. Such abnormal changes are thought to diminish the possibility of a full response to medications or to electroconvulsive therapy (ECT), which make use of such pathways [31]. Vascular pathology, particularly common in the elderly, may play an important role in the refractoriness of depression by virtue of such limbic area disruptions.

It is thought that up to three-quarters of patients with depression who present to psychiatrists in older age (over 50 years old) have a late-onset form, associated with such cerebrovascular disease and decreased responsiveness to antidepressant treatment [33]. In 1994, Hickie et al. described TRD in patients who had not responded to the following regimens: imipramine in doses of at least 150 mg, tranylcypromine 40 mg, phenelzine 60 mg for at least 4 weeks, at least 8 treatments in a course of ECT, and chlorpromazine in doses of at least 300 mg equivalents in the case of psychosis. In the study group of 39 patients treated on inpatient units for periods up to 15 weeks, the authors found that there was a strong correlation between poor treatment response to either pharmacologic treatment or ECT and the extent of subcortical white matter lesions on MRI. The findings were independent of the presence of concurrent essential hypertension. While this correlational study examined only a small sample of inpatients with very severe depression, the authors were able to conclude that white matter hyperintensities were associated with older age of first psychiatric episode, lack of family history of depression, with neuropsychological deficits, and a poorer response to treatment [34]. The concept of vascular depression was developed in the 1990s, differentiating early-onset from late-onset depression [24, 32, 35–37]. Whether depression increases the likelihood of acquiring vascular disease [38, 39], whether vascular disease increases the likelihood of acquiring depression [34], or whether these two disorders co-occur in a group with predisposition to both is unclear, but the result is a difference in outcome between depressed patients with and without cerebrovascular disease [40, 41].

Smaller frontal lobes, indicating neuronal atrophy, may be another risk factor for late life depression, thus suggesting either that there may be at least two anatomical pathways to the disorder or that the magnitude of vascular ischemia is the basis for such atrophy [42]. This frontal lobe impairment, clinically manifested by executive dysfunction, also has been demonstrated as a predictor of poor response to antidepressants.

There is ongoing research on the complicated interplay between genetic expression differences and risk for depression. For example, effectiveness of escitalopram, sertraline, or extended release venlafaxine, along with risk of side effects from these medications, has been associated with variants of the ABCB1 gene, which encodes P-glycoprotein. Genetic variants of this gene have been thought to account for differing brain concentrations of these medications in an 18–65-year-old population [43]. In patients whose first depression occurred in older age (60–75 years old), variants of certain regions of the SLC6A4 gene, impacting serotonergic function, have been found to give rise to a more robust response to serotonin reuptake inhibitor (SSRI) antidepressants such as citalopram [44].

4.5   Novel Antidepressant Approaches to TRD

Recently, new techniques have emerged that attempt to treat TRD with greater effectiveness, often with greater site specificity than pharmacological agents can offer. The changes in limbic microcircuitry associated with ensuing high incidence of partial or nonresponse may require such novel treatments, which we believe may give hope in the treatment of TRD, both in young adults and in the elderly.

A. *Deep brain stimulation (DBS)*

Several studies have shown that deep brain stimulation (DBS) gives rise to significant changes in motivation and depressed mood in young adult patients with TRD [17–19, 45], but older patients have not been studied with this technique. Future studies of DBS for the treatment of TRD may give rise to more optimism, particularly in young adults who do not have the cortical striatal abnormalities seen in late life depression but whose circuitry is likely variable in different individuals [46].

B. *Ketamine*

Another novel antidepressant approach has used the *N*-methyl-D-aspartate (NMDA) antagonist anesthetic ketamine, which many open trials have suggested induces a decrease in symptoms by from 25 to 78 %. Although the effects were far more rapid than are seen from traditional antidepressants, in general these effects were short lived, and only the young adult age group has been studied [47, 48]. Two recent meta-analyses evaluated its effects, one using data from seven trials and 147 participants [49] and the other using data from a total of 1242 subjects receiving either ketamine or other NMDA antagonists [50]. Ketamine was found to positively augment the treatment effects of ECT after an initial treatment, but these effects waned by the end of the series [49]. Many of the ketamine studies included a small number of patients, and some were seen as biased. The authors called for more rigorous trials before concluding efficacy versus nonefficacy [50]. Because other NMDA antagonists such as D-cycloserine and rapastinel only slightly affected depressive symptoms, the authors concluded that other mechanisms of action besides NMDA antagonism for ketamine must be found [50].

C. *Repetitive transcranial magnetic stimulation (rTMS)*

DBS and ketamine trials have studied the younger adult population, with age cut-offs of 65 years old, but the use of repetitive transcranial magnetic stimulation (rTMS) has been used and studied in a small number of late-onset vascular depression patients as well [51], and another more comprehensive open trial of 257 patients found that in this treatment-refractory group, whose ages ranged from 18 to 90 years old, 205 patients were able to complete the 1-year trial. Of them, around two-thirds experienced a sustained positive response to treatment with minimal adverse effects [52].

D. *Vagus nerve stimulation (VNS)*

Vagus nerve stimulation (VNS) is another recent intervention and FDA approval was obtained in 2005 for the treatment of severe depression. This technique uses a pacemaker-like device implanted to generate electric pulses and to stimulate the vagus nerve. In a 2-year open naturalistic follow-up study of adult outpatients with chronic or recurrent depressive episode, but not necessarily TRD, there was a response rate of 42 %. Remission rates were 22 % at 2 years [53]. To investigate the effects of VNS on patients with TRD in particular, Rush et al. performed an open trial of 30 patients with a mean age 47.5. They found 12 responders with improved social functioning after 4–9 months of follow-up [54]. The effects of VNS, while modest in the treatment of TRD, are significant in this hard-to-treat group. The effects in elderly patients with TRD, evaluating both primary and side effects, have not comprehensively been studied.

These novel treatment modalities show great promise, but most are investigational, require hospitalization with infusions or surgery, and are not readily available to the general population. Furthermore, the newest potential treatments often have not been studied in the older population, who may have different response rates because of the associated vascular changes or frontal atrophy.

4.6   Decision-Making Capacity

While depressive disorders in general are not considered terminal, older patients, in particular the "oldest old," over 85, fare poorly with TRD [55, 56]. In a large cohort study of 5751 individuals over 65, the 496 depressed subjects without disability at the start of the study were found to be at increased risk of disability (by 67%) and immobility (by 73%), after 6 years, compared to their nondepressed counterparts. These findings were independent of medical disorders [57]. Moreover, medical comorbidities are common in this population, and patients with depression accompanying a medical illness may suffer from significantly greater impairment than patients without such disorders [55]. After a patient has undergone several courses of antidepressant treatment without therapeutic effect, the malnourished, frail, older, depressed individual may be seen as suffering from the psychiatric equivalent of a medical illness, culminating in a terminal disorder if untreated. The question then arises as to whether such a severely depressed patient has the capacity to choose to terminate pharmacological care after multiple failed attempts at treatment, knowing that the outcome may even hasten death [23].

Applebaum has described four major components in decision-making capacity. The patient must be able to clearly communicate a treatment choice, understand the relevant information about the condition and treatment options, appreciate the choices and their consequences, and engage in rational discussion of these options. A patient must be able to make a choice about treatment without frequent vacillation about the decision and must understand the risks, benefits, and alternatives of all choices, including the choice to withdraw treatment. In summary, the patient must possess insight into the condition and the ramifications of accepting or withholding treatment [58].

Rudnick argues that while Applebaum's four primary tenets of capacity may be unaltered in depression, "coherence of personal preferences" may be disrupted. A depressed patient's treatment preferences should be compared to what his preferences may have been while well and should be respected if consistent [59]. This raises the issue of psychiatric advance directives, discussed later in this chapter, which are honored in some but not all states in the USA [60, 61].

When a patient suffers from depression, end-of-life issues generally are delayed until the depression has lifted, with the implicit assumption, as above, that passive suicidal thoughts and feelings of hopelessness will abate or disappear [62]. Patients

are most often considered temporarily incapable of making such important decisions when depressed. Studies show that in general they have more optimism after
antidepressant treatment, and this optimism also may apply to decisions about
advanced directives [62, 63]. Indeed, a patient with a chronic medical condition and
an untreated depression should first have their depression treated prior to the possibility of prematurely invoking the right to die. A few studies have examined the
effect of depression on hypothetical preferences for life-sustaining therapy, with
contradictory findings. One found no relationship and the other observed higher
depression scores correlating with more acceptance of limiting life-sustaining ther-.
apies [64, 65].

Ganzini and Lee found that when elderly patients had both mild to moderate
depression and medical illness, the depression exerted little influence on choices
about life-sustaining medical treatment, and there was no significant increase in
choosing medical therapy once their depression remitted [66]. Thus, one might conclude that mild depression would not interfere with judgment in the decision to
terminate psychiatric care. The same group found that treatment of severe depression did increase preferences for life-sustaining medical treatments [66], suggesting
patients suffering from more severe depression will seek more medical care when
treated.

While a sense of grief or disappointment is not uncommon in patients with serious medical illnesses, fewer than half of people with terminal medical illnesses
meet strict criteria for major depression [67]. Nonetheless, depressive cognitive distortions without a formal diagnosis may result in a negatively biased sense of important potential outcomes. Moreover, these subtle depressive cognitive impairments
may not represent the choices that a patient otherwise would have made based on
their previously expressed values [62, 68], findings which seem at odds with those
of Ganzini et al.

There is little in the literature that discusses capacity as it pertains to depression
as the primary medical disorder. As articulated by Appelbaum and Roth, "Of all the
psychopathological processes associated with refusal [of treatment], depression is
the most difficult to recognize, because it masquerades as, 'Just the way I would
think if it happened to me' … The depressed patient is frequently able to offer 'rational' explanations for the choices that are made"[69]. In general, psychiatrists have
been more reluctant than other physicians to accept the right to withhold treatment.
The perspective is that a patient wanting to stop active treatment is surely suicidal,
resulting from psychiatric illness. However, if the depressive disorder is refractory
to treatment, the question becomes moot. Depressive disorders are similar to other
medical disorders, in that the patient's desires would be different if the disorder
were treated, but when in a refractory state, response is unobtainable. This logic
brings into question whether anyone with a desire to end life-sustaining treatment
has capacity to make that decision [62]. But the criteria for capacity and a patient's
assessment of their quality of life continue to apply.

The legal case of Elizabeth Bouvia is an important example that addresses this
issue. Ms. Bouvia was a young woman with severe cerebral palsy and pain, admitted to a psychiatric ward after presenting with what was seen as suicidal ideation.

Being unable to feed herself or swallow, she nonetheless refused tube feeding. The attending psychiatrist opposed her refusal, believing that her views represented the suicidal feelings of a psychiatric disorder, which caused her admission to his service. The appellate court upheld Bouvia's refusal [70]. Legal scholar Alan Meisel described this tube feed refusal not as a desire to commit suicide but rather as resignation to accept a potentially earlier death [71]. Thus, the court moved toward a view that knowledge of a hastened death did not negate one's right to refuse medical treatment. In this case, refusing an invasive and long-term treatment was not seen as the same as the active desire to end life.

4.7   End-of-Life Decisions in Psychiatric Patients in Europe

One way to consider the discussion of capacity in patients with depression without concomitant life threatening illness, is to understand the way other countries have addressed this issue in the more extreme case of physician-assisted suicide. In 1997, the Supreme Court in the Netherlands ruled that in rare cases, unbearable psychological suffering *may* justify physician-assisted suicide. A subsequent study of patients with psychiatric diagnoses found that 30 % of psychiatrists had received such requests and that 2 % were granted. Half of these patients had concomitant medical disease, often terminal. Thus, assisting psychiatric patients in their desire to end their lives has been rare in a country with among the most liberal laws in assisted suicide [72]. In Belgium, euthanasia was given for "unbearable mental suffering due to an irreversible disease" in 3.5 % of total cases [73]. The psychiatric patients requesting such services tended to be young (64 % under 50 years old). Suffering was the major determinant causing requests for physician-assisted suicide or euthanasia. Dependency, loss of autonomy, pain, feeling a burden, but most of all hopelessness about the future contributed to these requests. The psychiatric patients were described as suffering from unbearable suffering most of the time [74].

To ensure the appropriateness of the rationale, the capacity of the patient, and to ensure that no treatable symptoms are present, the authors called for multidisciplinary meetings involving patient and family [73]. Specific recommendations included multiple psychiatric consultations as a part of a comprehensive assessment, thorough written documentation, and assessment of issues of transference and countertransference. Elderly patients complaining of severe bereavement, physical pain, and "fatigue of life" are not considered candidates for physician-assisted suicide with the expansion of palliative care services. For such patients, specific treatment of each symptom is seen as the appropriate course of treatment [75].

While our chapter does not include the discussion of euthanasia or of physician-assisted suicide, it is worthwhile to discuss the ways in which European countries use these laws in thinking of a psychiatric patient's wishes as a part of the above advice on end-of-life decision-making. Some case reports emerging in the lay press may be stimulating this discussion. For example, in June 2015, a 24-year-old Belgian woman with longstanding depression, having had a number of psychiatric hospitalizations was given the right to undergo physician-assisted suicide despite her young age and lack of a terminal medical illness [76]. In the Netherlands, the Termination of Life on Request and Assisted Suicide Act of 2002 was passed. However, the dilemma of requests from patients with psychiatric disorders request for physician-assisted suicide has been debated ever since. So far the outcome of such debates has been the recommendation that these options require more scrutiny than those given to patients with medical disorders. Nonetheless, decisions on end-of-life care of psychiatric patients have not been *a priori* be ruled out [75].

4.8 Discussion

This discussion was intended to explore the autonomy of capable patients with non-suicidal TRD to make decisions about their regimens in a fashion similar to patients with other medical disorders. Conversations about the potential cessation of active pharmacological care should be considered for patients who do not respond to treatment and who seek treatment discontinuation. Such patients would then be free of side effects of ineffective medications, which have even been reported to exacerbate cognitive impairment in some cases [77]. Clinicians should encourage patients with TRD to continue to receive active non-pharmacological treatments such as psychotherapy, spiritual care, and caregiver support, all integral components to treating geriatric medical and psychiatric patients in general [55].

Instilling and fostering hope in treating a patient with TRD remains an important part of the work of psychiatrists and has been considered a crucial component in the treatment of any patient [78]. While discussing the consideration of a patient to terminate active treatments, it thus remains key to balance a sense of hopefulness regarding other life potentials for the patient, even if remission of the depression is unlikely.

Termination of active medical treatments in this population is not entirely analogous to patients with other medical disorders. Compared with refractory medical disorders, psychiatric disorders are not life threatening in the same way, and patients may be destined to live potentially long lives, albeit with untreatable morbidity. We suggest that despite these differences, patients have the same rights to stop treatments if they are without significant therapeutic value. As is the case in other medical disorders, such decisions should be based on stricter criteria for capacity than the criteria used for less potentially risky decisions [79].

Current investigations of neuromodulatory treatments are exciting and hold hope for future treatment of patients with TRD. At this time, not all patients have access to these new treatments, which have not been studied extensively in geriatric patients. Novel techniques to improve symptoms are being developed so rapidly that response and remission rates are likely to improve in the future. Even now, the Fava criteria [13] that often define TRD may need to be updated to include the novel trials listed above and also CBT.

In the future, patients with TRD will be unlikely to want to discontinue biological care as advances in treatments improve outcome. At this time, however, when patients refuse continued pharmacological intervention, we question the usual response of psychiatrists to give medications involuntarily, in the face of the side effects and cost, when there is little to no expectation of improvement. In such cases, however, providers should inform patients that future techniques may well be of greater value, and indeed patients need a great deal of education about newer techniques on the horizon.

A meta-analysis describing end-of-life decision-making has been studied in six Western European countries, the Netherlands, Switzerland, Denmark, Sweden, Belgium, and Italy [80]. In this naturalistic study performed in 2003 of over 20,000 deaths, the authors found that one-third of patients had died unexpectedly, such that end-of-life decisions could not be made. In the other two-thirds, end-of-life decisions were made from 23 % of the time (Italy) to 51 % (Switzerland). Medications were explicitly given to hasten death from 1 % (Belgium) to 3.4 % (Netherlands) of the time. While end-of-life decisions were often made in all the countries studied, there was variability in the types of decisions. The authors called for regarding end-of-life care as having the same importance as the more traditional goals of physicians of curing disease and avoiding premature death [80]. These decisions are rarely discussed in the field of psychiatry.

As is the case with medically ill patients, advance directives may at times be a way in which to address decision-making in treatment-refractory psychiatric illness. While not accepted in much of the United States, these directives allow an individual during a symptom-free time to state preferences about treatment should they become incapable. Directives may have the potential to minimize coercion and hospitalization as individuals are able to make their wishes known in advance [61]. However, it has been argued that a patient's views on treatment may change with illness and that even patients with severe depression are usually competent, as discussed above. Thus, if a patient were to decide to terminate medical treatment during the course of a depression, after having requested aggressive treatment in the advance directive, treatment decisions may become even more difficult [60]. We believe, though, that the idea of advance directives should be considered for all patients, including psychiatric patients. The issue of a patient changing his mind during an exacerbation is similar in both psychiatric and medical patients, and most often these directives are more helpful than not.

In viewing psychiatric disorders as similar to medical ones, some have called for the psychiatric profession itself to do likewise, considering the illnesses they treat as potentially refractory. Parker et al. specifically call for psychiatrists to discuss the acceptance of end-of-life decisions in the context of accepting that psychiatric disorders are analogous to medical disorders as patients fail to respond to treatment [81]. With the above cautions in mind, this chapter attempts to do just that while also describing the factors that differentiate psychiatric and medical patients.

References

1. Kutner L. Due process of euthanasia: the living will, a proposal. Indian Law J, 1969;44(4), Article 2.
2. Truog RD. End-of-life decision-making in the United States. Eur J Anaesthesiol. 2008;25 Suppl 42:43–50.

3. Company HM. The American Heritage medical dictionary. Boston: Houghton Mifflin Company; 2007.
4. O'Reardon J, Amsterdam J. Treatment resistant depression: progress and limitations. Psychiatr Ann. 1998;28:634.
5. Sackeim H. The definition and meaning of treatment resistant depression. J Clin Psychiatry. 2001;62 Suppl 16:10–7.
6. Nierenberg AA, DeCecco LM. Definitions of antidepressant treatment response, remission, nonresponse, partial response, and other relevant outcomes: a focus on treatment-resistant depression. J Clin Psychiatry. 2001;62 Suppl 16:5–9.
7. Mrazek DA, Hornberger JC, Altar CA, Degtiar I. A review of the clinical, economic, and societal burden of treatment-resistant depression: 1996–2013. Psychiatr Serv. 2014;65(8):977–87.
8. Rush A. Acute and longer-term outcomes in depressed outpatients requiring one or several treatment steps: a STAR*D report. Am J Psychiatry. 2006;163(11):1905.
9. Keller MB. Time to recovery, chronicity, and levels of psychopathology in major depression. Arch Gen Psychiatry. 1992;49(10):809.
10. Fava M. Diagnosis and definition of treatment-resistant depression. Biol Psychiatry. 2003;53(8):649–59.
11. Fekadu A, Wooderson SC, Markopoulo K, Donaldson C, Papadopoulos A, Cleare AJ. What happens to patients with treatment-resistant depression? A systematic review of medium to long term outcome studies. J Affect Disord. 2009;116(1–2):4–11.
12. Berlim MT, Turecki G. Definition, assessment, and staging of treatment-resistant refractory major depression: a review of current concepts and methods. Can J Psychiatry. 2007;52(1):46–54.
13. Fava M, Davidson K. Definition and epidemiology of treatment-resistant depression. Psychiatr Clin North Am. 1996;19(2):179–200.
14. Berlim MT, Turecki G. What is the meaning of treatment resistant/refractory major depression (TRD)? A systematic review of current randomized trials. Eur Neuropsychopharmacol. 2007;17(11):696–707.
15. Souery D, Amsterdam J, de Montigny C, Lecrubier Y, Montgomery S, Lipp O, Racagni G, Zohar J, Mendlewicz J. Treatment resistant depression: methodological overview and operational criteria. Eur Neuropsychopharmacol. 1999;9(1–2):83–91.
16. Atiq R. Treatment-resistant depression. Psychiatry [Internet]. 2006;10(1):1–11.
17. Lozano AM, Mayberg HS, Giacobbe P, Hamani C, Craddock RC, Kennedy SH. Subcallosal cingulate gyrus deep brain stimulation for treatment-resistant depression. Biol Psychiatry. 2008;64(6):461–7.
18. Mayberg HS, Lozano AM, Voon V, McNeely HE, Seminowicz D, Hamani C, Schwalb JM, Kennedy SH. Deep brain stimulation for treatment-resistant depression. Neuron. 2005;45(5):651–60.
19. Bewernick BH, Hurlemann R, Matusch A, Kayser S, Grubert C, Hadrysiewicz B, Axmacher N, Lemke M, Cooper-Mahkorn D, Cohen MX, Brockmann H, Lenartz D, Sturm V, Schlaepfer TE. Nucleus accumbens deep brain stimulation decreases ratings of depression and anxiety in treatment-resistant depression. Biol Psychiatry. 2010;67(2):110–6.
20. Nelsen M, Dunner D. Treatment resistance in unipolar depression and other disorders. Diagnostic concerns and treatment possibilities. Psychiatr Clin North Am. 1993;16:541–66.
21. Weitz ES, Hollon SD, Twisk J, van Straten A, Huibers MJ, David D, DeRubeis RJ, Dimidjian S, Dunlop BW, Cristea IA, Faramarzi M, Hegerl U, Jarrett RB, Kheirkhah F, Kennedy SH, Mergl R, Miranda J, Mohr DC, Rush AJ, Segal ZV, Siddique J, Simons AD, Vittengl JR, Cuijpers P. Baseline depression severity as moderator of depression outcomes between cognitive behavioral therapy vs pharmacotherapy an individual patient data meta-analysis. JAMA Psychiatry. 2015;72(11):1102–9.
22. McClain CS, Rosenfeld B, Breitbart W. Effect of spiritual well-being on end-of-life despair in terminally-ill cancer patients. Lancet. 2003;361:1603–7.

23. Sommer BR, Roybal DJ. Treatment-resistant major depression and the capacity to terminate care. J Ethics Ment Health. 2010;5(1):1–4.
24. Alexopoulos GS, Kiosses DN, Heo M, Murphy CF, Shanmugham B, Gunning-Dixon F. Executive dysfunction and the course of geriatric depression. Biol Psychiatry. 2005;58:204–10.
25. Rizvi SJ, Grima E, Tan M, Rotzinger S, Lin P, Mcintyre RS, Kennedy SH. Treatment-resistant depression in primary care across Canada. Can J Psychiatry. 2014;59(7):349–57.
26. Tuma R, DeAngelis LM. Altered mental status in patients with cancer. Arch Neurol. 2000;57(12):1727–31.
27. Breitbart W, Rosenfeld B, Pessin H, Kaim M, Funesti-esch J, Galietta M, Nelson CJ, Brescia R. Depression, hopelessness, and desire for hastened death in terminally Ill patients with cancer. JAMA. 2000;284(22):2907–11.
28. Ganzini L, Goy ER, Dobscha SK. Prevalence of depression and anxiety in patients requesting physicians' aid in dying: cross sectional survey. BMJ. 2008;337:a1682.
29. Werth JL. The relationships among clinical depression, suicide, and other actions that may hasten death. Behav Sci Law. 2004;22(5):627–49.
30. Berghmans R, Widdershoven G, Widdershoven-Heerding I. Physician-assisted suicide in psychiatry and loss of hope. Int J Law Psychiatry. 2013;36(5–6):436–43.
31. Alexopoulos GS, Murphy CF, Gunning-Dixon FM, Latoussakis V, Kanellopoulos D, Klimstra S, Lim KO, Hoptman MJ. Microstructural white matter abnormalities and remission of geriatric depression. Am J Psychiatry. 2008;165(2):238–44.
32. Thomas AJ, Brien JTO, Davis S, Ballard C, Barber R, Kalaria RN, Perry RH. Ischemic basis for deep white matter hyperintensities in major depression. Arch Gen Psychiatry. 2002;59:785–92.
33. Baldwin RC, O'Brien J. Vascular basis of late-onset depressive disorder. Br J Psychiatry. 2002;180(2):157–60.
34. Hickie I, Scott E, Wilhelm KA, Brodaty H. Subcortical hyperintensities on magnetic resonance imaging in patients with severe depression—a longitudinal evaluation. Biol Psychiatry. 1997;42(1992):367–74.
35. Krishnan KRR. Biological risk factors in late life depression. Biol Psychiatry. 2002;52:185–92.
36. Alexopoulos GS, Borson S, Cuthbert BN, Devanand DP, Mulsant BH, Olin JT, Oslin DW. Assessment of late life depression. Biol Psychiatry. 2002;52(3):164–74.
37. Sheline YI. 3D MRI studies of neuroanatomic changes in unipolar major depression: the role of stress and medical comorbidity. Biol Psychiatry. 2000;48(8):791–800.
38. Cohen HW, Madhavan S, Alderman MH. History of treatment for depression: risk factor for myocardial infarction in hypertensive patients. Psychosom Med. 2001;63(2):203–9.
39. Jonas B, Mussolino M. Symptoms of depression as a prospective risk factor for stroke. Psychosom Med. 2000;62(4):463–71.
40. Kales HC, Maixner DF, Mellow AM. Cerebrovascular disease and late-life depression. Am J Geriatr Psychiatry. 2005;13(2):88–98.
41. Carney RM, Freedland KE, Miller GE, Jaffe AS. Depression as a risk factor for cardiac mortality and morbidity: a review of potential mechanisms. J Psychosom Res. 2002;53(4):897–902.
42. Kumar A, Mintz J, Ph D, Bilker W, Ph D, Gottlieb G. Autonomous neurobiological pathways to late-life major depressive disorder: clinical and pathophysiological implications. Neuropsychopharmacology. 2002;26(2):229–36.
43. Schatzberg AF, DeBattista C, Lazzeroni LC, Etkin A, Murphy GM, Williams LM. ABCB1 genetic effects on antidepressant outcomes: a report from the iSPOT-D trial. Am J Psychiatry. 2015;172(8):751–9.
44. Shiroma PR, Drews MS, Geske JR, Mrazek DA. SLC6A4 polymorphisms and age of onset in late-life depression on treatment outcomes with citalopram: a sequenced treatment alternatives to relieve depression (STAR*D) report. Am J Geriatr Psychiatry. 2013;22(11):1140–8.
45. Schlaepfer TE, Cohen MX, Frick C, Kosel M, Brodesser D, Axmacher N, Joe AY, Kreft M, Lenartz D, Sturm V. Deep brain stimulation to reward circuitry alleviates anhedonia in refractory major depression. Neuropsychopharmacology. 2008;33(2):368–77.

46. Riva-Posse P, Choi KS, Holtzheimer PE, McIntyre CC, Gross RE, Chaturvedi A, Crowell AL, Garlow SJ, Rajendra JK, Mayberg HS. Defining critical white matter pathways mediating successful subcallosal cingulate deep brain stimulation for treatment-resistant depression. Biol Psychiatry. 2014;76(12):963–9.
47. aan het Rot M, Collins KA, Murrough JW, Perez AM, Reich DL, Charney DS, Mathew SJ. Safety and efficacy of repeated-dose intravenous ketamine for treatment-resistant depression. Biol Psychiatry. 2010;67(2):139–45.
48. Diazgranados N, Ibrahim L, Brutsche NE, Newberg A, Kronstein P, Khalife S, Kammerer WA, Quezado Z, Luckenbaugh DA, Salvadore G, Machado-Viera R, Manji HK, Zarate CA. A randomized trial add-on trial of an N-methyl-D-aspartate antagonist in treatment-resistant bipolar depression. Arch Gen Psychiatry. 2010;67(8):793–802.
49. Newport DJ, Carpenter LL, McDonald WM, Potash JB, Tohen M, Nemeroff CB. Ketamine and other NMDA antagonists: early clinical trials and possible mechanisms in depression. Am J Psychiatry. 2015;172(10):950–66.
50. Caddy C, Amit Ben H, McCloud Tayla L, Rendell Jennifer M, Furukawa Toshi A, McShane R, Hawton K, Cipriani A. Ketamine and other glutamate receptor modulators for depression in adults. Cochrane Database Syst Rev. 2015;1–319.
51. Fabre I, Galinowski A, Oppenheim C, Gallarda T, Meder JF, De Montigny C, Olie JP, Poirier MF. Antidepressant efficacy and cognitive effects of repetitive transcranial magnetic stimulation in vascular depression: an open trial. Int J Geriatr Psychiatry. 2004;19(9):833–42.
52. Dunner DL, Aaronson ST, Sackeim HA, Janicak PG, Carpenter LL, Boyadjis T, Brock DG, Bonneh-Barkay D, Cook IA, Lanocha K, Solvason HB, Demitrack MA. A multisite, naturalistic, observational study of transcranial magnetic stimulation for patients with pharmacoresistant major depressive disorder. J Clin Psychiatry. 2014;2014(December):1394–401.
53. Nahas Z, Marangell LB, Husain MM, Rush AJ, Sackeim HA, Lisanby SH, Martinez JM, George MS. Two-year outcome of vagus nerve stimulation (VNS) for treatment of major depressive episodes. J Clin Psychiatry. 2005;66(9):1097–104.
54. Rush AJ, George MS, Sackeim HA, Marangell LB, Husain MM, Giller C, Nahas Z, Haines S, Simpson RK, Goodman R. Vagus nerve stimulation (VNS) for treatment-resistant depressions: a multicenter study. Biol Psychiatry. 2000;47(4):276–86.
55. Blazer DG. Psychiatry and the oldest old. Am J Psychiatry. 2000;157(12):1915–24.
56. Wells KB, Sherbourne CD. Functioning and utility for current health of patients with depression or chronic medical conditions in managed, primary care practices. Arch Gen Psychiatry. 1999;56(10):897–904.
57. Penninx BWJH, Leveille S, Ferrucci L, Van Eijk JTM, Guralnik JM. Exploring the effect of depression on physical disability: longitudinal evidence from the established populations for epidemiologic studies of the elderly. Am J Public Health. 1999;89(9):1346–52.
58. Appelbaum PS. Assessment of patients' competence to consent to treatment. N Engl J Med. 2007;357(18):1834–40.
59. Rudnick A. Depression and competence to refuse psychiatric treatment. J Med Ethics. 2002;28(3):151–5.
60. Joshi KG. Psychiatric advance directives. J Psychiatr Pract. 2003;9(4):303–6.
61. Khazaal Y, Manghi R, Delahaye M, Machado A, Penzenstadler L, Molodynski A. Psychiatric advance directives, a possible way to overcome coercion and promote empowerment. Front Public Health. 2014;2:37.
62. Leeman CP. Depression and the right to die. Gen Hosp Psychiatry. 1999;21(2):112–5.
63. Bruce ML, Ten Have TR, Reynolds CF. Reducing suicidal ideation and depressive symptoms in depressed older primary care patients: a randomized controlled trial. JAMA. 2010;291(9):1081–91.
64. Cohen-Mansfield J, Rabinovich BA, Lipson S, Fein A, Gerber B, Weisman S, Pawlson LG. The decision to execute a durable power of attorney for health care and preferences regarding the utilization of life-sustaining treatments in nursing home residents. Arch Intern Med. 1991;151:289–94.

65. Cicirelli VG. Relationship of psychosocial and background variables to older adults' end-of-life decisions. Psychol Aging. 1997;12:72–83.
66. Ganzini L, Lee M, Heintz R, Bloom J, Fern D. The effect of depression treatment on elderly patients' preferences for life-sustaining medical therapy. Am J Psychiatry. 1994;151:1631–6.
67. Billings JA, Block S. Depression. J Palliat Care. 1995;11(1):48–54.
68. Sullivan MD, Youngner SJ. Depression, competence, and the right to refuse lifesaving medical treatment. Am J Psychiatry. 1994;151(7):971–8.
69. Appelbaum PS, Roth LH. Competency to consent to research: a psychiatric overview. Arch Gen Psychiatry. 1982;39(8):951–8.
70. (Cal App 2d Dist). Bouvia v Superior Court, Number B019134.
71. Meisel A. The right to die. New York: Wiley; 1989.
72. Groenewould JH, Van der Mass PJ, Van der Wal G, Hengeveld MW, Tholen AJ, Schudel WJ, Ven der Heide A. Physician-assisted death in psychiatric practice in the Netherlands. N Engl J Med. 1997;336(25):1795–801.
73. Deschepper R, Distelmans W, Bilsen J. Requests for euthanasia/physician-assisted suicide on the basis of mental suffering: vulnerable patients or vulnerable physicians? JAMA Psychiatry. 2014;71(6):617–8.
74. Dees MK, Vernooij-Dassen MJ, Dekkers WJ, Vissers KC, van Weel C. "Unbearable suffering": a qualitative study on the perspectives of patients who request assistance in dying. J Med Ethics. 2011;37(12):727–34.
75. Pols H, Oak S. Physician-assisted dying and psychiatry: recent developments in the Netherlands. Int J Law Psychiatry. 2013;36(5–6):506–14.
76. Chan M. Belgian woman, 24, granted right to die by euthanasia over suicidal thoughts: "life, that's not for me". New York: New York Daily News; 2015.
77. Culang ME, Sneed JR, Keilp JG, Rutherford BR, Pelton GH, Devanand D, Roose SP. Change in cognitive functioning following acute antidepressant treatment in late-life depression. Am J Geriatr Psychiatry. 2009;17(10):881–8.
78. Yalom ID. The theory and practice of group psychotherapy. New York: Basic Books; 1995. 602 p.
79. Drane JF. Competency to give an informed consent. JAMA. 1984;252(7):925–7.
80. van der Heide A, Deliens L, Faisst K, Nilstun T, Norup M, Paci E, van der Wal G, van der Maas PJ. End-of-life decision-making in six European countries: descriptive study. Lancet. 2003;362(9381):345–50.
81. Parker M. Defending the indefensible? Psychiatry, assisted suicide and human freedom. Int J Law Psychiatry. 2013;36(5–6):485–97.

A Psychological History of Ageism and Its Implications for Elder Suicide

Alan Pope

As Heraclitus told us at the dawn of Western civilization, all phenomena are imper-manent and subject to change. We grasp this existential fact easily when speaking of rivers or even mountains, but we face tremendous emotional difficulty when applied to changes in our own bodies. Consequently, we resist the living reality of aging and death in ways that deeply impact how we perceive ourselves and relate to the world around us. One could argue, as I will, that this tendency toward denial is one of the deep underlying forces behind the widespread phenomenon of ageism in contempo-rary Western culture.

Ageism existed long before Robert Butler coined the term in 1968 [1], defining it as "a process of systematic stereotyping of and discrimination against people because they are old." Although he explicitly compared ageism with racism and sexism, there is an important structural difference. Racists and sexists define others as different from themselves on the basis of attributes (race and sex) that generally will never be bridged,[1] while ageists define others on the basis of a difference (age) that not only *can* be bridged but eventually will. That is, the qualities in the other toward whom we hold prejudice in ageism are precisely the qualities that await us in our future [2, 3]. In this way, ageism has a deep connection with *gerontophobia*, the fear of growing old [4]. The implications are profound: insofar as our personal self exists as a continuum that includes the past and the future, avoiding and deny-ing our future self is inherently self-alienating. With ageism, we therefore not only cease to identify with elders as human beings—we cease to identify with *ourselves* in the fullness of our own humanity.

This analysis reveals that ageism has a personal intimacy that racism and sex-ism generally do not.[2] Sometimes it is most difficult to see that which is closest to us. Ageist attitudes, in ourselves and other people, are accepted so widely as to go

A. Pope, Ph.D. (✉)
Department of Psychology, University of West Georgia,
1601 Maple Street, Carrollton, GA 30118, USA
e-mail: apope@westga.edu

© Springer International Publishing Switzerland 2017
R.E. McCue, M. Balasubramaniam (eds.), *Rational Suicide in the Elderly*,
DOI 10.1007/978-3-319-32672-6_5

largely unnoticed and are arguably present to some degree in everyone [5, 6]. Older adults often are regarded by individuals and portrayed in the media as incompetent and unproductive people who drain on precious resources. We celebrate youth and youthful beauty, but fail to recognize the beauty that comes with age, experience, and wisdom; instead, signs of aging are seen as ugly and a source of shame. The language we use toward elders is demeaning [7], and age discrimination commonly occurs in workplaces, medical centers, schools, and various other institutions [5]. Ageist attitudes are so pervasive that they even manifest among professional geriatric caregivers [2, 6] and, most disturbingly, elders themselves [8]. It is all too easy to align one's own attitudes and actions with those of society. Rather than resist ageist attitudes, most older persons accept and even embrace their new role in life [6], uniting to form a nonthreatening special class—namely, that of "senior citizens."

Not surprisingly, this particular demographic successfully enacts suicide at higher percentages than the rest of the adult population.[3] While the overall reasons for elder suicide are surely complex, many researchers claim that ageism is an important contributing factor [4, 11, 12]. These researchers express further concern that in an ageist culture, well-intentioned efforts to legalize voluntary euthanasia on the basis of the patient's own rational decision-making could unwittingly lead to a dystopia in which geronticide is accepted and widely practiced. Critics respond that it is nevertheless paramount that we safeguard a person's right to choose whether they live or die [13].

Rather than engage this debate directly, I wish to examine the particular historical context within which we ask these questions that we might benefit from a larger perspective and deeper understanding. And rather than focus only on social and cultural events as the causal agents in the development of attitudes toward aging and elder suicide, I wish instead to examine what such events reveal about humanity's psychological life and particularly how the hidden assumptions of our cultural worldview have given shape to the development of ageist attitudes.

For example, I have argued elsewhere that the negative image of older persons reflected by ageism has been reified into the cultural figure of "the Elderly" [14]. In earlier times, we referred to older persons as "Elders," a comparative designation that signaled a relationship and connoted respect. Now we generally refer to elders as "the elderly," a definitive form and neat abstraction into which we can easily pour our negative judgments. It also serves as a construct that separates us from living human beings—and them from us—thereby constituting the underlying source of the social class we call "senior citizens." This image of older persons maintains an archetypal function in the cultural psyche, exerting its negative influence in unconscious ways gross and subtle.

In what follows, I examine the traditional historical narrative of the development of contemporary ageism espoused within the field of social gerontology, and its limitations, before presenting a psychological interpretation aimed at understanding the psychic shift wherein "Elders" became "the Elderly." Then following a brief overview of the history of attitudes toward suicide, I consider what this analysis reveals regarding the contemporary question of elder suicide.

5.1   Traditional History of Ageism: The Lens of Social Gerontology

The standard historical narrative gracing most social gerontology textbooks places ageism as a modernist development, at which time Western culture underwent a "great transformation" in attitudes toward elders [14, 15]. According to this view, most premodern societies revered elders as the bearers of wisdom and knowledge and regarded them as authorities over their extended families [15]. But two key historical developments would lead eventually to their loss of esteem, power, and dignity. First, the invention of the printing press by Gutenberg in 1440 enabled the wide dissemination of accurately recorded information, obviating the key elder role of preserving and transmitting knowledge of culture, tradition, and history [2]. The eventual institution of formal education would essentially sound the death knell for the elders' traditional function in society [15, 16].

The second major development compromising attitudes toward elders was the Age of Revolution (1774–1848), which included the American and French revolutions and arguably the Industrial Revolution. The Industrial Revolution and its concomitant urbanization introduced new job markets which required of workers a physical strength and adaptability to new technologies that privileged youth over experience; in addition, the increasingly frequent need to relocate was difficult for older workers and put strains on the extended families over which they traditionally maintained authority [2]. In factories and offices, normal hierarchies were often reversed, as younger colleagues began to enjoy authority over their elders [15]. The political revolutions in America and Europe deepened this trend, creating an attitude of age equality that obviated the idea of venerating others on the basis of age and experience [17]. Meanwhile, medical advances extended life expectancy, which helped to generate negative attitudes toward a growing population of dependent elders for whom late life was regarded a "second childhood" [2, 18]. These attitudes would deepen in twentieth-century America with the enactment of social security legislation and the institutionalization of a retirement age [19, 20]. The once authoritative and venerated elders had become powerless, useless, and irrelevant to modern society.

Although anti-modernist in content, this narrative of the history of ageism is ironically modernist in form. Its overarching "grand narrative" oversimplifies the more complex portrait of attitudes toward aging that careful historical scholarship beginning in the 1970s would later reveal [15]. While it is clear that ageism and gerontophobia are quite pronounced in our contemporary world, historical evidence demonstrates that they have existed in various forms for various peoples through the span of Western civilization. For example, although the ancient Greeks honored elders' wisdom, they also demonstrated ageist language. In ancient Rome, elders exerted power in social and political institutions, but old age was depicted as a time of physical and mental deterioration [21]. The historical portrait we paint is always complicated by the sources we consult and the perspectives we adopt. As such, it is important to bear in mind that there are many different histories of aging [22]. I am about to tell a different one.

5.2   Psychological History of Ageism

The gerontological narrative views the unfolding of human activity as shaped almost exclusively by technological, social, and political forces. While these socio-logical elements are important, excluding the role that first-person perspective and human agency play surely provides a *limited* portrait. This is especially true when the subject is *attitudes toward older persons*, for attitudes are inherently psycho-logical and older persons evoke complex feelings and ideas regarding our own human possibilities and limitations. Therefore, it is essential to consider the role that psychological life plays in these historical developments.

Specifically, I propose that attitudes toward elders and toward aging are rooted in fundamental, collective *ways of seeing* which change over time. Our perception of self, others, and environment is shaped at a deep level by the philosophical assump-tions that we hold, certainly, as individuals, but even more powerfully as societies. These assumptions create the lenses through which we see all phenomena, includ-ing older persons. Therefore, my approach is to focus on changes in collective per-ception so as to understand the development of ageism as a psychological phenomenon that expresses and reinforces itself through sociocultural develop-ments. In doing so, I will make two arguments. First, I argue that these ways of seeing provide a deeper influence on our attitudes toward elders than the sociocul-tural events to which we ordinarily attribute them. Second, these collective ways of seeing transform long before they manifest in the sociocultural world as new phi-losophies, technologies, and sociopolitical developments.

This approach resonates with contemporary historians who believe that the sociocultural forces of modernism actually had little impact on the perceptions of old age, even as they agree that by the twentieth century, previously held respect for elders had turned into unrelenting ageism. In the words of Haber and Gratton [15]: "the key to understanding status lay in changing cultural beliefs—ones that well preceded the processes of urban and industrial change" (p. 355). Although the lan-guage and focus is different here, the basic idea applies: changes in psychological beliefs (worldview) underlie changes in attitudes toward elders and always in advance of manifest social change.

In what follows, I selectively examine changing ways of seeing throughout his-tory that explain how we have come to see "Elders" as "the Elderly." My own lens is that of *existential phenomenological psychology*, a tradition that grounds human psychology in the broad themes of human existence (existentialism) and whose method gives priority to the immediacy of lived experience, as opposed to the abstractions of naturalistic science (phenomenology).

5.2.1   Ageism as Rooted in the Fear of Death

I previously proposed that ageism is largely rooted in the *fear of death*, the latter being an important theme in existential philosophy. Some researchers tested this notion empirically using a theoretical model (*terror management theory*, or TMT), which posits that throughout history, humankind has used its worldviews, cultural productions, and even sense of self-esteem as strategies for ameliorating the terror of death awareness [23, 24]. These researchers conducted a variety of empirical studies (e.g., testing accessibility of death-related thoughts after viewing pictures of elderly people) to support their contention that ageism is largely rooted in the existential threat that older people present by reminding us of the inescapable nature of death, fallibility of the body, and impermanence of the self [24]. Terror management theory is based primarily on anthropologist Ernest Becker's 1973 landmark book *The Denial of Death* [25], which explored the notion that repression of the fear of death is even more fundamental than that of sexual conflict (à la Freud) in shaping our personality and motivating our activities. In this view, the fear of death constitutes a deeper influence on our attitudes toward elders than the sociocultural events to which we ordinarily attribute them.

But has death been feared in the same ways throughout history? The evidence clearly indicates not. For example, the ancient Greeks simply saw death as the final goal in life, accounting for their comfort in discussing topics (such as euthanasia) considered taboo by today's standards [26]. Through an extensive two-decades-long study of changing attitudes toward death in Western culture, French historian Philippe Ariès [27, 28] uncovered similar attitudes in the early Middle Ages, observing: "The old attitude in which death was both familiar and near, evoking no great fear or awe, offers too marked a contrast to ours, where death is so frightful we dare not utter its name" [27].

For Ariès, the long-standing view of death as the natural, collective destiny of humankind began to shift by the twelfth century. Over the next few centuries, death gradually came to be understood as belonging to one's own individual life and therefore something to be feared. The culmination of this incubation period was made manifest in the late sixteenth century (and continuing in the seventeenth and eighteenth centuries) when cemeteries moved from the churchyards at the center of town to marginalized areas outside of town. By the mid-nineteenth century, death, once familiar and accepted, had become shameful and forbidden; in the following century (between 1930 and 1950), dying was displaced from the home to the hospital. As if not content to eliminate death and dying from view, we likewise eliminated its precursor by moving the very old from the family home to the nursing home; eventually the institutionalization of retirement age would similarly segregate and marginalize the "young old" from everyone else [14].

This alternative narrative aligns with the gerontological account insofar as both see the same period in history as evoking transformational change. But the existential view demonstrates that the undercurrent for social and political changes began forming centuries earlier with the emergence of a stronger sense of individuality and its consequent fear of death. This understanding not only connects us with earlier periods in history; it provides a way of seeing more deeply into our own situation now.

5.2.2 Ageism as Rooted in Perception

Whereas the fear of death is rooted in how we see ourselves, this view is inseparable from how we gaze upon the world. In the fifteen century, a key psychological transformation occurred when Italian artists learned to see with *linear perspective vision*.

It seems obvious to us now that close objects appear larger than those in the distance, but it wasn't always the case. Phenomenological psychologist Robert Romanyshyn [29] argues that this new way of seeing reflected a cultural habit of mind that "[trans-formed] the landscape of the world, the geography of the soul" (p. 30). Prior to this development, we saw the world in terms of personal connection and meaning, as evidenced by pre-Renaissance art in which the relative size of objects correlated not with geographic distance but emotional closeness. That is, the world presented itself to us in terms of felt meaning rather than mathematical distance.

Brunelleschi invented linear perspective in 1425 C.E., and one decade later Alberti codified it as a technique in which the artist looks through a mathematical grid superimposed upon the landscape in order to render precisely on his page the geometrical dimensions of a vanishing point extending out to infinity. This new way of seeing gave birth to the notion of the *Archimedean point*, that place from which the world can be seen in its entirety by removing the viewer from it [30]. This is also the precursor to the grand narratives of modernism. But there is a problem. The world actually *includes* the one who views it (both bodily *and* as a constituting sub-jectivity), and thus linear perspective in actuality does not create a purely objective stance. In thinking that it does, and learning to see *only* through this lens, we iden-tify with a hegemonic eye (read "I") that is disembodied and assumes a completely passive stance toward a separate, abstract, externalized world. This seems a con-summately safe spot from which to evade concerns about aging and death. But it also necessitates seeing others in terms of size rather than meaning, separateness rather than connectedness, with the head rather than the heart. With this develop-ment, the ritual body became a technical body, the dead body a corpse. Growing old became a technical function rather than a natural one. Our loss of veneration for elders was an inevitable outcome of a more sweeping loss of veneration for our world and our embodied, relational participation in it [14, 29].

Our gaze upon the world was equally impacted by the advent of printed media [30]. The gerontological narrative explains how Gutenberg's invention of the printing press in 1440 Germany (essentially co-temporal to Italy's development of linear per-spective) eventually dislodged elders from their role as the repositories of cultural knowledge. While this is true, the deeper change occurred in the way that our oral linguistic tradition became a visual one, anchoring us, like linear perspective, to a fixed point of view [30]. Communication transformed from being a relational, embod-ied activity that partakes of the full array of senses and other living bodies to a solitary, disembodied encounter with symbolic representations [31]. The displacement of elders as bearers of knowledge reflects this deeper commitment to viewing others and the world as separate and distant, wrapping ourselves in a self-sufficient cocoon of abstractions and symbolic forms, immunized from the concerns of mortality.

5.2.3 Ageism as Rooted in How We Think

The way of seeing developed (or expressed) by the invention of linear perspective vision and the printed word in the fifteenth century would require another 200 years before reaching thematic articulation in the philosophy of Rene Descartes in the seventeenth century [29]. This historical sequencing demonstrates that collective perceptual shifts precede cognitive ones. Whereas Galileo had developed the scientific method, Descartes developed its conceptual framework [32]. Descartes' epistemological method proceeded by casting doubt on all ways of knowing so as to discern that which can be known indisputably, which he concluded to be the act of doubting itself ("I think, therefore I am"). This conclusion implied complete identification of the person with the intellect, which he characterized as immaterial and completely different in quality from all physical bodies. It is on this account that Descartes is often credited with creating the "mind-body split," completely severing the subjective life of mind from the objective physical world [33]. The hegemonic eye that two centuries earlier gazed upon the world through a geometric grid had now been made thematic as the disembodied intellect. Meanwhile, the body became a machine to be studied according to mathematical principles. This homogenizing vision undergirded the spirit of egalitarianism that arose in the eighteenth century, bringing with it the age equality that would erase any privilege that experience had previously been afforded.

Eventually the thorny problem of Descartes' dualism—namely, how immaterial mind can interact with material reality—led to adoption of *material monism*, the complete reduction of mental phenomena to physical matter [34]. Difficulties came when scientists later applied the materialistic methodologies appropriate for physics to the study of organic systems, establishing a view that first eliminated the concept of *vitalism* from biology (equivalent to the life force central to Eastern medicine) and later any nonreductive concept of *consciousness* from psychology [35]. By the twentieth century, the reductive *scientific materialist* worldview had been firmly established: the physical world is the only reality; human life has no meaning, value, or significance; and the universe is completely impersonal and indifferent to human suffering. This cultural worldview seems so natural to us that we fail to recognize that in actuality it is a *metaphysical assumption* rather than an empirical fact [36]. Unfortunately, seeing in this impoverished way has serious consequences for us and for elders. When we are nothing more than mechanical bodies, we begin to lose personal and social value the moment we pass peak physical maturity, eventually to be seen in terms of deterioration and dysfunction. This view promotes the increasingly popular medical model of aging whose basis is the stereotyping of older adults as uniquely needy [15]. When we value appearance, speed, and aggression, becoming impatient with whatever and whoever might stand in our way, elders become hindrances, which creates the conditions for gross or subtle forms of geronticide. When we value focused, linear, rational thinking in place of holistic modes of creative reflection, we privilege narrowly framed factual information over the wisdom that comes with the broadening effect of life experience.

5.3   Implications for Elder Suicide

I have demonstrated that viewing cultural-historical events as the field of human psychological life casts new light on the development of contemporary ageism. The changing nature of how we see ourselves, our bodies, and other people—whether through embodied relationship or disembodied distance—has a huge impact on how we regard and treat elders in society. What are the implications of these changing perspectives on the question of elder suicide? I will first sketch the history of changing attitudes toward suicide generally before commenting on elder suicide in our contemporary world.

5.3.1 A Brief History of Attitudes Toward Suicide

Attitudes toward suicide changed significantly through antiquity, the medieval, and modern periods. Given that the ancient Greeks and Romans regarded death as a natural event, they considered suicide a topic suitable for rational discourse. Some accepted it as potentially humane and even sensible—the Stoics in particular advocated that suicide could be rational—while others, such as Plato and Aristotle, dismissed it as against the best interests of the state [11]. The advent of Christianity eventually suppressed this environment of free inquiry when St. Augustine (354–430 C.E.) condemned suicide as a sin before God and an abomination to the state, a position that became official church doctrine and eventually law throughout the Middle Ages and one that still finds advocates today [37]. Eventually, when a new sense of individuality began to emerge in the twelfth century (as we have seen), the later Renaissance softened the condemnation on suicide and reawakened a spirit of rational discourse, first in early sixteenth-century literature (e.g., More's *Utopia*, Donne's poetry) and later eighteenth-century philosophy (e.g., Hume, Voltaire, Rousseau) [11]. But the privileged position granted to rationality waned in the nineteenth century when advances in the biological sciences envisioned mind as completely reducible to matter.

The new lens through which nineteenth-century reductive materialism would see suicide is neatly characterized by Werth [11]: "In essence, the change appears to have been from viewing suicide in theological, moral, philosophical, and legal terms to seeing suicide as a social, medical, psychological, and statistical problem" (p. 18). The newly emerging scientific psychology medicalized suicide by associating it with mental illness, thereby eliminating the possibility of rational decision-making. Meanwhile, the newly emerging discipline of sociology reduced the act of suicide to purely sociocultural factors, thereby also eliminating the possibility of free will [11]. Whether suicide's roots were conceived as organic or social, there was no genuine agency by which it could be conceived rational. In the following century, the lens of scientific materialism would further establish that life has no intrinsic meaning or moral values and that we live in fundamental isolation in a vast, indifferent universe [36].

5.3.2 Elder Suicide in Our Contemporary World

At the same time that this contemporary worldview undergirds our pronounced ageism, pragmatic factors are forcing us to revision suicide yet again. Longer life spans, exploding medical costs, and a graying population are creating pressures on individuals, families, and society to consider whether in some circumstances it is morally and rationally justified to end a life that no longer seems worth living. The specific term *rational suicide* first appeared in a leading journal in 1986 when David Mayo [38] argued that the indiscriminate use of modern, life-sustaining technologies had made it reasonable in some instances to decide to end one's life. In becoming a technical function rather than a natural one, the moment of death has been increasingly decided by doctors and hospital teams who determine when it is appropriate to discontinue life-sustaining care [27]. Consequently, a felt need has arisen for patients to make these decisions for themselves, without coercion and on the basis of rational assessment, promoting a call for physician-assisted suicide (PAS), permitted in Oregon in 1994 with the passing of the Death with Dignity Act.

At one level, this initiative seems a sensible way of counteracting the problems arising within a culture of technologically mediated dying. But a central dilemma has arisen. while condoning elder suicide (assisted or otherwise) may represent a compassionate stance aimed at eliminating unnecessary suffering, does it unwittingly open the door to systemic abuse and, potentially, geronticide [4, 12]? The latter option, often termed the *slippery slope argument*, becomes especially troubling in an ageist society, as Osgood [4] warns:

> Older people, living in a suicide-permissive society characterized by ageism, may come to see themselves as a burden on their families or on society and feel it is incumbent upon them to take their own lives or receive assisted suicide. As C. Everett Koop (1985) suggests, uncaring or greedy family members may pressure others into assisted suicide. Those who need expensive medical technology to live may be denied help and die. The right to die then becomes not a right at all, but rather an obligation which robs some members of our society of their legal right to live. (p. 168)

These are legitimate concerns, particularly given the manner in which unconscious attitudes are all too easily institutionalized. In fact, a politician in the late 1980s disturbingly suggested that terminally ill people might have not the "right to die," but the "*duty* to die" [39]. Geronticide is a genuine possibility in our culture, and in fact, Brogden [12] argues it is already present in the ways our nursing homes and medical centers engage a process of *death hastening* through indifferent care and abusive treatment.

But let us momentarily set aside these systemic concerns and return to the perspective of the individual elder contemplating suicide. In many cases, the issue is not one of deciding when to "pull the plug," but rather wanting to die long before there is a plug to pull. In the 2011 documentary, *How to Die in Oregon* [40], a woman with terminal liver cancer decides to enact physician-assisted suicide before her body has to endure the disfiguration and pain that will come with her disease. She states that she wants to die with dignity and to retain control. Although she reasons that this action will be easier for her family, her son secretly confides to the camera that it actually will be very hard to witness his mother taking the prescribed lethal "medicine" to end her life (though he defers to her wishes). As she discusses her decision for the camera, the tears streaming down her face belie that it may not have been wholly rational. As the preceding analysis would suggest, the notion of rational suicide is problematic because the reasoning we employ is likely grounded in the implicit assumptions of a culture that fails to see death properly and therefore has misguided ideas of control and dignity. But such considerations extend beyond the purview of this chapter.

5.4   Conclusion

Philosopher Martin Heidegger [42] claimed of human understanding that whenever something is revealed, something else is concealed. The modernist developments that revealed the world as a separate, homogenous field of lifeless matter (albeit enabling impressive scientific discoveries and technologies) simultaneously concealed the field of vital, interdependent connections uniting us one to the other and to the world. Conquering the natural rhythms of life by projecting a grid upon space (linear perspective) and time (mechanical clock) revealed mathematical uniformity and rational predictability, only to conceal more ambiguous, mysterious elements of life. By committing to one view over another—the material over the spiritual—our contemporary society has lost appreciation for the felt, poetic dimensions of life and the qualities of depth, patience, love, compassion, and wisdom that age and experience hold the potential to cultivate. Consequently, our narrow, linear ways of seeing have made invisible the elders we have relegated to the periphery.

The deep source of these difficulties is a profound fear of aging and dying rooted in seeing ourselves as individual selves, separate from the collective. While from one perspective (head) we are separate individuals, from another (heart) we are not. Human development requires that we concentrate on developing an individual identity early in life, only later to broaden our vision to take in the vast web of interconnected relationships within which our sense of personhood is situated. It is as if our society has not taken this next developmental step for itself, being stuck in literal ways of seeing. Opening society's vision more widely entails developing a new narrative for what it means to grow old and to die. If grounded in our natural experience of life, this narrative would recognize (as the ancient Greeks did) that death is a natural part of life and that grief and mourning hold tremendous transformative potential. With death being less feared, we might naturally see older persons once again as worthy of our respect and loving concern.

5.5   Notes

1. One exception is found in instances of sex reassignment surgery.
2. One possible exception is prejudice against persons on the basis of sexual or gender orientation, which could involve fears regarding one's own sexual nature.
3. According to the 2014 elderly suicide fact sheet of the American Association of Suicidology, persons 65 years of age and older accounted for 16.37 % of all suicides in the USA while only comprising 13.75 % of the overall population. These

figures are actually down—for example, in 1998 older adults comprised 13 % of the population while accounting for 18 % of suicide deaths (9)—but still reflect a consistent trend in which elder suicide exceeds that of other adults in the general population. Suicides among white men over the age of 85 exceed those of all age-gender-race groups and are 2.5 times higher than for men of all ages (4, 10).

References

1. Butler RN. Why survive? Being old in America. New York: Harper & Row; 1975.
2. Nelson TD. Ageism: prejudice against our feared future self. J Soc Issues. 2005;61(2):207–21.
3. Nelson TD. Ageism: the strange case of prejudice against the older you. In: Wiener RL, Willborn SL, editors. Disability and aging discrimination: perspectives in law and psychology. New York: Springer; 2010. p. 37–47.
4. Osgood N. Ageism and elderly suicide: the intimate connection. In: Tomer A, editor. Death attitudes and the older adult: Theories, concepts, and applications. Philadelphia: Brunner-Routledge; 2000. p. 157–73.
5. Levy BR, Banaji MR. Implicit ageism. In: Nelson TD, editor. Ageism: sterotyping and ageism against older persons. Cambridge, MA: MIT Press; 2002.
6. Secouler L. Physicians' attitudes toward elder suicide. New York: Garland; 1998.
7. Schaie KW. Ageist language in psychological research. Am Psychol. 1993;48(1):49–51.
8. Kimmel DC. Ageism, psychology, and public Policy. Am Psychol. 1988;43(3):175–8.
9. Mitty E, Flores S. Suicide in late life. Geriatr Nur (Lond). 2008;29(3):160–5.
10. McIntosh JL. Elder suicide: research, theory, and treatment. Washington, DC: American Psychological Association; 1994.
11. Werth JL. Rational suicide? Implications for mental health professionals. Washington, DC: Taylor & Francis; 1996.
12. Brogden M. Geronticide: killing the elderly. Philadelphia: Jessica Kingsley; 2001.
13. Szasz T. Fatal freedom: the ethics and politics of suicide. Westport: Praeger; 1999.
14. Pope A. The elderly in modern society: a cultural psychological reading. Janus Head. 1999;1(3):223–32.
15. Haber C, Gratton B. Aging in America: the perspective of history. In: Cole TR, Van Tassel DD, Kastenbaum R, editors. Handbook of the humanities and aging. New York: Springer; 1992.
16. Macnicol J. Ageism and age discrimination: some analytical issues. London: International Longevity Centre; 2010.
17. Fischer DH. Growing old in America. New York: Oxford University Press; 1977.
18. Macnicol J. Age discrimination: an historical and contemporary analysis. Cambridge: Cambridge University; 2006.
19. Conrad C. Old age in the modern and postmodern western world. In: Cole TR, Van Tassel DD, Kastenbaum R, editors. Handbook of the humanities and aging. New York: Springer; 1992.
20. Cowgill DO. The aging of populations and societies. In: Quadago JS, editor. Aging, individual and society. New York: St. Martin; 1980.
21. Falkner TR, de Luce J. A view from antiquity: Greece, Rome, and Elders. In: Cole TR, Van Tassel DD, Kastenbaum R, editors. Handbook of the humanities and aging. New York: Springer; 1992.
22. Troyansky DG. The older person in the Western world: from the middle ages to the industrial revolution. In: Cole TR, Van Tassel DD, Kastenbaum R, editors. Handbook of the humanities and aging. New York: Springer; 1992.
23. Greenberg J, Pyszczynski TA, Solomon S. The causes and consequences of a need for self-esteem: a terror management theory. In: Baumeister RF, editor. Public self and private self. New York: Springer; 1986.

24. Martens A, Goldenberg JL, Greenberg J. A terror management perspective on aging. J Soc Issues. 2005;61(2):223–39.
25. Becker E. The denial of death. New York: The Free Press; 1973.
26. Mystakidou K, Parpa E, Tsilika E, Katsouda E, Vlahos L. The evolution of euthanasia and its perceptions in Greek culture and civilization. Perspect Biol Med. 2005;48(1):95–104.
27. Ariès P. Western attitudes toward death. Baltimore: The Johns Hopkins University Press; 1974.
28. Ariès P. The hour of our death. New York: Knopf; 1981.
29. Romanyshyn R. Technology as symptom and dream. London: Routledge; 1989.
30. Romanyshyn R. The despotic eye. In: Kruger D, editor. The changing reality of modern man: essays in honour of J H van den Berg. Pittsburgh: Duquesne University Press; 1985. p. 87–109.
31. Abram D. The spell of the sensuous. New York: Vintage; 1996.
32. Wallace BA. Mind in the balance. New York: Columbia; 2009.
33. Pope KS, Singer JL. The stream of consciousness: scientific investigations into the flow of experience. New York: Plenum Press; 1978.
34. Robinson DN. An intellectual history of psychology. Madison: University of Wisconsin Press; 1995.
35. Wallace BA. Hidden dimensions: the unification of physics and consciousness. New York: Columbia University Press; 2007.
36. Wallace BA. Contemplative science: where Buddhism and neuroscience converge. New York: Columbia University Press; 2007.
37. Humble MB. Do-not-resuscitate orders and suicide attempts. Natl Cathol Bioeth Q. 2014;14(4):661–71.
38. Mayo DJ. The concept of rational suicide. J Med Philos. 1986;11(2):143–55.
39. Glascock A. Is killing necessarily murder: moral questions surrounding assisted suicide and death. In: Sokolovsky J, editor. The cultural context of aging: worldwide perspectives. 3rd ed. Westport: Praeger; 2009. p. 77–92.
40. Richardson P. How to die in Oregon. 2011.
41. Fromm E. The sane society. New York: Holt Reinhart Winston; 1965.
42. Heidegger M. Being and time. San Francisco: HarperCollins; 1927.

Rational Suicide in the Elderly: Anthropological Perspectives

6

Simon Dein

6.1   Introduction

In this chapter I examine how culture influences rational suicide in the elderly. Following a discussion of suicide and culture, generally I present a number of case studies of elderly suicide. I underscore the fact that rationality and autonomy are never free from cultural constraints. I begin with a newspaper report from the Australia: "Beverley Broadbent was not dying of a terminal illness, nor was she depressed or unhappy. But at the age of 83, she wanted to die. Over several interviews with Fairfax Media, Ms Broadbent stated she planned to take her own life so she could have a peaceful, dignified death. She said she did not want her health to deteriorate to the point where she developed dementia or found herself in a nursing home with no way out. When she explained her choice, Ms Broadbent said her fear of deteriorating to the point where she would be unable to end her life made her want to "go sooner rather than later." She said if physician-assisted suicide was legal, she might have pushed on knowing she could end her life at any time. She died at home in her bed on February 11." (http://www.theage.com.au/victoria/rational-suicide-why-beverley-broadbent-chose-to-die-20130401-2h348.html#ixzz3hgL5y5oC).

The Society for Old Age Rational Suicide (SOARS) was established, in the UK, by Michael Irwin (a former Medical Director of the United Nations and a former Chairman of the Voluntary Euthanasia Society) in 2009, on December 10th, which is observed internationally as Human Rights Day (as the UN Declaration of Human Rights was adopted on December 10, 1948). The main long-term objective of SOARS is to change the law in the UK so that very elderly, mentally competent individuals, who are suffering unbearably from various health problems (although

S. Dein, F.R.C.Psych., Ph.D. (✉)
Departments of Anthropology and Medicine, University College, London, UK

Department of Theology and Religion, Durham University, Queen's Campus, Stockon on Toon, UK
e-mail: s.dein@ucl.ac.uk

© Springer International Publishing Switzerland 2017   75
R.E. McCue, M. Balasubramaniam (eds.), *Rational Suicide in the Elderly*,
DOI 10.1007/978-3-319-32672-6_6

none of them is "terminal"), are permitted to receive a doctor's assistance to die, if this is their persistent choice. They assert that surely the decision to decide, at an advanced age, that "enough is enough" and, avoiding further suffering, to have a dignified death is the ultimate human right for a very elderly person.

In four other European countries (Belgium, Luxembourg, the Netherlands, and Switzerland), doctor-assisted dying is legal for mentally competent individuals who are terminally ill, severely disabled, or very elderly with medical problems. Data from these countries shows that the medical procedures, which are in place, work very well—with no one, who is disabled or elderly, being abused and forced to die against their will. Furthermore, in five American states (California, Montana, Oregon, Vermont, and Washington State), doctor-assisted suicide is legally possible for the terminally ill.

There are many very elderly, competent individuals who, experiencing increasing physical and psychological suffering, reach the last years of their natural lives and have to seriously consider whether dying will be much more attractive than struggling on. After eight or nine decades, many people decide that their lives have been fully lived, and now they have a life which, for them, has finally become too prolonged.

Do mental health practitioners understand rational suicide? There is little evidence that they do so. At the American Association for Geriatric Psychiatry (AAGP) 2015 Annual Meeting, a session dedicated to the issue aimed to provide guidance to clinicians who may be faced with elderly patients expressing a desire to die by suicide while they are still relatively healthy and cognitively intact. From the meeting, it was clear that the concept of suicide based on reasoned decision has been gaining acceptance, particularly in terminally ill patients. However, there has been little discussion about older people who are concerned about their failing bodies and feel that their life is already complete. The possibility of rational suicide is not discussed much in the psychiatric profession. Patients may have information about it and may have opinions, but psychiatric practitioners generally have no training about this at all.

6.2 Suicide and Culture

Suicide is a difficult phenomenon to comprehend. Not only is its demarcation somewhat problematic but it also eludes simple explanation. The societies in which suicide mortality is prevalent do not necessarily resemble each other in many ways, and neither is a single mental illness such as depression a sufficient cause to lead to suicide. Despite its statistical regularity, suicide is unpredictable at an individual level. As such, individuals make decisions in a cultural, ethical, and socioeconomic context, but this context never completely determines the decision.

I write this chapter from the viewpoint of an anthropologist who sees suicide as a form of human action. Durkheim's seminal work *La Suicide* suggests that culture—essentially, the norms and values shared by a group of people [1]—is significant in impacting rates of suicide. The act itself is determined by the sociocultural context which gives it meaning. Suicide cannot be understood merely to result from internal psychological processes and psychopathology. Few studies however have simultaneously taken account of the individual, social, anthropological, and epidemiological aspects of suicide. The micro and macro dimensions are generally divorced and prioritize either the individual or society. Suicide is not only a sign that there was something wrong with a person, but also that something might possibly be wrong with the society as a whole. Thus suicide prevention does not only or necessarily mean preventing people from committing suicide but also developing a society where there are no reasons to take one's life.

Recognizing epidemiological differences in rates of suicide across countries, scholars have examined factors predisposing to an increased risk of suicide. Few of these studies have incorporated culture or ethnicity as an important dimension impacting upon an individual's decision to take his/her own life. Kral [2] affirmed that "… suicide, like everything else that is complexly human, takes place in a powerful social context." Tseng [3] stated that "suicide, even though it is a personal act, is very much socio-culturally shaped and susceptible to socio-cultural factors." This missing area in the study of suicide has been pointed out by many scholars [4, 5].

Examining suicide through the lens of cultural and moral relativism reveals some important issues. First, not everyone contemplating suicide is irrational or mentally unwell. In some cultures suicide is viewed as the best means of fulfilling an integral life and thus as rational. Second, there are strong differences in opinion over the morality of suicide across cultures. These are prevalent and unavoidable. Finally, and perhaps most importantly, moral judgments about suicide are amenable to change.

It is essential to recognize that in seeking a rational suicide, the components that inform this decision are culturally determined, thereby introducing considerable subjectivity and possible external disagreement. Ideas of what constitute autonomy and rationality differ between cultures, and to this extent, discussions of rational suicide can never be culture-free. Furthermore the decision to end one's life is often informed by persistent suffering and is thus unlikely to be made on entirely non-emotional grounds and likely to be influenced by cognitive distortions [6]. Contends that this shift in popular thinking about suicide is just a special case of what he refers to as "the medicalization of morals," many behaviors once seen as freely chosen, but condemned as sinful (and subsequently as illegal), gradually came to be seen instead as medical issues and therefore condemned as manifestations of mental illness.

6.3   Historical Perspectives

Libanius, and his contemporaries, wrote that in Athens and the Greek colonies of Marseilles and Ceos, a supply of poison was kept by the authorities for those who would come before the Senate and plead their case for wanting to abandon life. In these cultures there was nothing particularly controversial about the fact that a "person's life might become so grim as not to be worth living, and that in these circumstance's it would be rational to end it" [7].

Seneca in AD 65 was accused of involvement in a conspiracy to overthrow Nero. After being sentenced to death, he, together with his wife and in the company of friends, cut his veins, then subsequently discussed philosophy, and gave dictation to his secretaries, before finally drinking poison in a rather dramatic reenactment of the death of Socrates. This became the model for others. The Stoics are presented as an example of rational, autonomous suicide—suicide which is reasonably considered with little emotion and without fear. What seems important in this Roman example is their desire to be in control of their death and to face up to it nobly. This can be understood in the context of their previous privileged status and their frustrated feelings of entitlement and power.

The first major opposition to suicide in our culture was religious. During the earliest centuries of Christianity, the Donatists and other Christian zealots often sought suicidal martyrdoms, maintaining that any death in the cause of the Faith guaranteed salvation. Responding to these wholesale martyrdoms, St. Augustine (during the sixth century) asserted that self-willed death was against the will of God in that it violated the Sixth Commandment. On the basis of these arguments, the Council of Braga made it a matter of Canon Law in 562 AD that funeral were rites to be refused to all suicides, and in 693 AD the Council of Toledo ruled that anyone who even attempted suicide should be excommunicated.

6.4 Anthropology and Rational Suicide

I now present an ethnographic overview of suicide in different cultural groups examining issues of rationality. More than a century after Durkheim's sociological classic placed the subject of suicide as a central concern in social science, ethnographic, cross-cultural analyses of what underlies people's attempts to take their own lives remain limited. But by highlighting how the ethnographic method privileges a certain view of suicidal behavior, we can go beyond the limited sociological and psychological approaches that define the field of suicidology in terms of social and psychological "pathology" to engage with suicide from our informants' own points of view—and in doing so redefine the problem in a new light and new terms. In particular, suicide can be understood as a kind of sociality, as a special kind of social relationship, through which people find meaning in their own lives. Anthropological studies of the native perspective indicate that in some societies, all suicides are seen as rational.

We may speculate that attitudes toward elderly suicide in any culture are associated in part with the values attributed to the elderly in that culture. In terms of value, different cultures have different attitudes and practices around aging and death, and these cultural perspectives can have a huge effect on the experience of growing older. Psychologists Erickson and Erickson [8] assert that the Western fear of aging keeps us from living full lives: "Lacking a culturally viable ideal of old age, our civilization does not really harbor a concept of the whole of life." Social factors deeply impact the ways in which the elderly view themselves. In the USA, ageism is rife. Youth is valued, whereas old age is seen as a problem. Prado [9] argues that if current attitudes toward the elderly prevail, they will come to feel that they have had their fair share in life, and suicide will become not just a possibility but even an obligation. His book *The Last Choice* argues that preemptive suicide in advanced age can be rational: that it can make good sense to evade age-related personal diminishment even at the cost of good time left.

Though attitudes toward death in contemporary American culture are largely characterized by fear, Native American cultures traditionally accept death as a fact of life. There exist over 500 Native American nations each having its own traditions and attitudes toward aging and elderly care. Significantly in many tribal communities, elders are respected for their wisdom and life experiences. As in many parts of the non-Western world, within Native American families, it's common for the elders to be expected to pass down their learnings to younger members of the family.

Similarly the Korean regard for aging derives from the Confucian principle of filial piety, a fundamental value dictating that one must respect one's parents (although Confucius was Chinese, Confucianism has a long history in Korea). Younger members of the family have an obligation to care for the aging members of the family. And even outside the family unit, Koreans are thus socialized to respect and show deference to older individuals as well as authority figures. Not only do Koreans respect the elderly, they also celebrate them. For Koreans, the 60th and 70th birthdays are significant life events, which are commemorated with large-scale family parties and feasts. As in Chinese culture, the universal expectation in Korea is that roles reverse after parents age and that it is an adult child's duty—and an honorable one at that—to look after his or her parents.

In the African-American community, death is seen as an opportunity to celebrate life. In African-American culture, death is viewed as part of the "natural rhythm of life," which diminishes the cultural fear around aging. For this reason, Karen H. Meyers writes in *The Truth About Death and Dying* [10], "African-American funerals tend to be life-affirming and to have a celebratory air intermingled with the sorrow."

At the other extreme, the elderly, imbued with little value, are killed in some cultures. Traditional nomadic tribes often abandon their elderly during their unrelenting travels. The choice for the healthy and young is to do this or carry the old and infirm on their backs—along with children, weapons, and necessities—through perilous territory. Also prone to sacrificing their elderly are societies that suffer periodic famines. One dramatic example is that Paraguay's Aché Indians assign certain young men the task of killing old people with an ax or spear or burying them alive.

There are few anthropological studies specifically focused upon suicide in the elderly. Early cross-cultural studies in anthropology attempted to explain suicide on the basis of cultural features, such as the depressiveness or aggressiveness of a culture or an ethnic personality pattern [11]. Some anthropologists have emphasized cultural emotions such as shame, anger, or loyalty as explanatory factors [12]. Other studies point to life crises, ambiguity in social roles, or institutional exclusion or abandonment. Not only does culture impact the epidemiology of suicide, but it profoundly influences its meaning. As argued by Leenaars and collaborators [13] in the preface of *Suicide: Individual, Cultural, International Perspectives:* "Individuals live in a meaningful world. Culture may give us meaning in the world. It may well give the world its theories/perspectives. This is true about suicidology. Western theories of suicide, as one quickly learns from a cultural perspective, may not be shared. Suicide has different meanings for different cultures." Douglas [14] discussed the lack of knowledge of what different cultures, and also different groups of officials who categorize deaths, mean by the term "suicide": "It is not merely the cognitive meanings of suicide that very likely vary from one society to another and from one sub-society to another. The moral meanings and the affective meanings of both the term 'suicide' and any actions either actually or potentially categorized as suicide almost certainly vary greatly as well." Colucci and Lester [4] point out that suicide is classified in many different ways in different cultures: as "(1) an unforgivable sin, (2) a psychotic act, (3) a human right, (4) a ritual obligation, and (5) an unthinkable act" (p. 33). They underscore the fact that behavior has many determinants and also highlight some universal drivers of risky behavior, such as social disorganization, cultural conflict, and the breakdown of the family.

It is worth noting that many actual suicides, which we would regard as tragic and irrational, probably contain an expressive element. Research has shown that suicide may have a different meaning in the Chinese context, especially for women with an inferior status within the family. Suicide is taken as an act of revenge in a moral and spiritual sense. The act of suicide is very powerful; it grants the woman so much power that she may achieve what she could not during her lifetime. Meng [15] saw suicide as a symbolic act of rebellion and revenge for some Chinese women.

The act of taking one's life to the benefit of others is known as altruistic suicide. One example of this is an elder ending his or her life to leave greater amounts of food for the younger people in the community. Suicide in some Eskimo cultures has been seen as an act of respect, courage, or wisdom. Williams [16] discusses American Apache Indian suicide and notes that Apaches define suicide as a voluntary intentional killing of one's body. The person killing himself/herself is considered rational and "does not care for his life."

Culture-bound suicide methods include the Japanese custom of *seppuku* (or hara-kiri), voluntary disembowelment which was performed in circumstances of disgrace and as a means of expressing loyalty to a deceased leader. Now largely of historical importance, it was performed by Yukio Mishima, three times nominated for the Nobel Prize for literature, in 1970. One form of suicide in Japan—*kakugo no jisatsu* (suicide of resolve)—is understood as an act of free will. Kitanaka [17] argues that psychiatrists in Japan are still very ambivalent about the medicalization of this phenomenon and actively distinguish between individuals who have no pathology and present rational narrative accounts as to why the attempted suicide was "worthy" and those suffering from mental illnesses.

Self-immolation is largely restricted to Iranian and Indian communities. In Iran, where the national suicide rate is around 6.2/100,000 [18], the proportion of female suicides in which self immolation is chosen varies according to region, from 25 % in Tehran to 71 % in Ilam province [19]. Moving to India, self-immolation occurred in the Hindu practice of *suttee* (or sati), the suicide of the widow on the pyre of her husband. This was a sign of respect and justified by scripture. Roop Kanwar died in this way in Rajasthan in 1987. While the practice has been outlawed, sporadic cases still occur. A recent report [20] gives the suicide rate in India as 10.3/100,000, and the proportion of suicides due to self-immolation as 8.5 % (predominantly female). There are regional variations, and in a study from Kolkata [21], the proportion of suicides due to self-immolation was 19.7 % (predominantly female). Female Indian migrants living in the UK [22] and female ethnic Indians living in Fiji (SP, personal observation) frequently deploy this method.

Thus, self-immolation is predominantly a female practice, influenced by culture and associated with a host of disadvantages including lack of education, lack of employment, and the absence of basic human rights. However, political protest suicide also usually employs self-immolation (perhaps because of its horrendous image), and these protesters are predominantly male [23]. These forms of suicide may be seen as rational in that their aim is to change the political situation (i.e., they are utilitarian).

In a similar way, a suicide attack is a political action where an attacker carries out violence against others knowing that it will result in their own death. Some suicide bombers are motivated by a desire for martyrdoms. Kamikaze missions were carried out as a duty to a higher cause or moral obligation. Murder-suicide is an act of homicide followed within a week by the suicide of the person who carried out the act. Mass suicides are often carried out under social pressure where members give up autonomy to a leader. Mass suicides can occur with as few as two people, often referred to as a suicide pact. In extenuating situations, where continuing to live would be intolerable, some people use suicide as a means of escaping. Some inmates in Nazi concentration camps are known to have killed themselves by deliberately touching the electrified fences. These suicide types discussed above can be seen as rational to the extent that they are autonomous and based upon a notion of greater utility and purpose.

6.5 Conclusion

Above I have examined how culture impacts suicide. Specifically in relation to the elderly, there is little research examining "rational suicide" cross-culturally. We need more data concerning the value attributed to the elderly in diverse cultural groups and how they define a good life. These factors are often influenced by wider religious, moral, and social contexts. It is within these contexts that elderly members of society make the decision to end their lives. One recent study [24] asked 584 students from Canada and Mainland China what constitutes a good life. The results suggested that South Asian Canadians were more oriented toward moral, spiritual, and beneficent concerns in envisioning a good life than were the Mainland Chinese and Western European Canadians. The Chinese emphasized practical, prudential, and socially defined goods. In contrast the Western European Canadians showed more preference for personally defined, internal goods. East Asian Canadians fell between Chinese and Western European Canadians in overall orientation, reflecting their biculturality. All groups placed heavy emphasis on close and enduring relationships. While there are no cross-cultural studies reported in the elderly, the above study is a good model for conducting this research in this group.

Future studies need to analyze conceptions of rationality cross-culturally and their antecedents: autonomy and utility. Ethnographic methods, with their in-depth understandings of individual and cultural motivations and values, will be central to this process.

References

1. Boyd K, Chung H. Opinions toward suicide: cross-national evaluation of cultural and religious effects on individuals. Soc Sci Res. 2013;41:1565–80.
2. Kral MJ. Suicide and the internalization of culture: three questions. Transcult Psychiatry. 1998;35:221–33.
3. Tseng W-S. Handbook of cultural psychiatry. San Diego: Academic; 2001.
4. Colucci E, Lester D, editors. Suicide and culture: understanding the context. Cambridge: Hogrefe; 2013.
5. Tortolero SR, Roberts RE. Differences in non-fatal suicide behaviors among Mexican and European American middle school children. Suicide Life Threat Behav. 2001;31:214–23.
6. Szasz T. Sex by prescription. Garden City: Doubleday Anchor; 1980.
7. Alvarez A. The savage god. New York: Random House; 1972.
8. Erickson E, Erickson J. The life cycle completed. New York: WW Norton & Company; 1998.
9. Prado CG. The last chance, pre-emptive suicide in old age. West Point: Prager; 1998.
10. Meyers K. The truth about death and dying. New York: Facts on File; 2009. p. 101.
11. Devereux G. Mohave ethnopsychiatry and suicides: the psychiatric knowledge and the psychic disturbances of an Indian tribe, Bureau of American ethnology bulletin, vol. 175. Washington, DC: GPO; 1961.
12. Firth R. Suicide and risk taking in Tikopia society. Psychiatry. 1961;2:1–17.
13. Leenaars A, Maris R, Takahashi Y, editors. Suicide: individual, cultural, international perspectives. New York: Guilford; 1997.
14. Douglas JD. The social meaning of suicide. Princeton: Princeton University Press; 1967.
15. Meng L. Rebellion and revenge: the meaning of suicide of women in rural China. Int J Soc Welf. 2002;11:300–9.
16. Williams T. Psychological anthropology. The Hague: De Gruyter Mouton; 1975.
17. Kitanaka J. Diagnosing suicides of resolve: psychiatric practice in contemporary Japan. [Case Reports, Comparative Study, Journal Article, Research Support, Non-U.S. Gov't]. Cult Med Psychiatry. 2008;32(2):152–76.
18. Akbari M, Naghavi M, Soori H. Epidemiology of deaths from injuries in the Islamic Republic of Iran. East Mediterr Health J. 2006;2:382.
19. Suhrabi A, Delpisheh A, Taghinejad H. Tragedy of women's self-immolation in Iran and developing communities: a review. Int J Burns Trauma. 2012;2(2):93–104.
20. Vijaykumar L. Indian research on suicide. Indian J Psychiatry. 2010;52 Suppl 1:S291–6.
21. Shrivastava P, Som D, Nandy S, et al. Profile of postmortem cases conducted at a morgue of a tertiary care hospital in Kolkata. J Indian Med Assoc. 2010;108:730–3.
22. Raleigh VS, Bulusu L, Balarajan R. Suicides among immigrants from the Indian Subcontinent. Brit J of Psychiatry. 1990;156:46–50.
23. Pridmore S, Walter G. Protest suicide. Australas Psychiatry. 2012;20:533–4.
24. Bonn G, Tafarodi RW. Chinese and South Asian conceptions of the good life and personal narratives. J Happiness Stud. 2014;15:741–55.

Life's Meaning and Late Life Rational Suicide

7

Jukka Varelius

7.1 Introduction

Fred used to be an active, determined, and independent person. He always took pride in his ability to take charge of things, to make reasoned decisions quickly, and to get things done. The success his aptitude brought to him in the business world was no small matter to him either. In his free time, Fred was an outdoor man, enthusiastic about hiking and fishing in demanding, even dangerous environments. Now, with age, things have changed for him. As his mental and physical abilities are deteriorating, Fred is increasingly unable to lead the kind of life he sees as worth living. Though he is not demented and the occasional fishing trip is still within his abilities, the kinds of feats that would truly excite him must now be left for others. Knowing that the decline of his abilities will continue, Fred considers his prospects discouraging and frustrating. Consequently, he often finds himself thinking that it might be best for him to end it all now, before things get even worse for him. Not only is Fred unable to see much point in his existence anymore, he has also started to question the worth of the life he has lived. Yes, he was one of the most successful building constructors of his hometown. But would it still not, he wonders, have been better for him to have pursued the interest in literature that he in his 20s rejected, with some hesitation, as financially too insecure and not quite manly enough. Perhaps, then, he could now say to himself that he has led a truly meaningful life? Then again, as he, like anybody else in light of current knowledge, will eventually die in any case, would his life not, in the end, have been futile however he had chosen?

There may be persons who are never troubled by problems of the kind that now bother Fred. Yet many people would appear to sometimes raise such questions, especially at the

J. Varelius, Ph.D. (✉)
Departments of Philosophy, Contemporary History, and Political Science,
University of Turku, Assistentinkatu 7, Turku 20014, Finland
e-mail: jukvar@utu.fi

© Springer International Publishing Switzerland 2017
R.E. McCue, M. Balasubramaniam (eds.), *Rational Suicide in the Elderly*,
DOI 10.1007/978-3-319-32672-6_7

later stages of their lives.[1] Accordingly, given the ageing of the human population, the number of such people seems likely to increase in the future. Of course, not all of these persons have led the same kind of life and had similar options as Fred. Hence, the questions they ponder are not exactly the same either. But, ultimately, the questions about the significance of life would appear to be rather similar even when the lives the people asking them have lived have been different. Are there any good answers to the questions, answers that could be helpful to persons asking the questions? Given the popular view that philosophy is about thinking about the meaning of life, it could be taken that this is a connection in which philosophers can provide definite answers. However, though related questions have been addressed in philosophy for over two thousand years, with few exceptions the history of the philosophical discussion focusing directly on the questions that now trouble Fred—henceforth questions about the meaning of life—is much shorter.[2] The questions have been systematically studied in philosophy only during the last about 40 years. And, as is common in the cases of even the more long-standing philosophical debates, no clear consensus as to how they are best answered has emerged.

Yet the philosophical debate on the problems conducted so far need not be practically useless. Despite the remaining controversies, the discussion might still help to at least formulate the most important questions and the most plausible answers to them more clearly. This promise motivates the present chapter. Hence, in what follows, I will consider Fred's case in light of the recent philosophical discussion on the meaning of life. I start by distinguishing between two importantly different questions about life's meaning and explaining how they differ from certain other issues sometimes treated as questions about the meaning of life. Then I address the two questions about the meaning of life in turn, connecting them to Fred's thoughts that his life is and has been meaningless. After that, I briefly consider how Fred's committing suicide would appear from the viewpoint of the philosophical debate on life's meaning. I conclude by summing up how the philosophical debate on the meaning of life I have referred to might help a person like Fred. Though the history of the philosophical discussion on life's meaning per se is relatively short, there is already a considerable literature on the topic. Unfortunately, I am not able to account for all of it here. Accordingly, I focus on those of the central views and arguments in the debate that have most relevance in cases like that of Fred. Needless to say, not all problems relating to such cases are philosophical ones and not all philosophical problems they give rise to relate to life's meaning.[3] Yet, without purporting to imply

[1] Empirical studies on the grounds that severely ill or injured people have for seeking assistance in dying suggest that often the main reason for their desire to die is, not the physical pain caused by their illness or injury, but things like perceived threat of loss of autonomy and dignity, inability to engage in activities that are deemed to make life worth living, and hopelessness (see, e.g., [25]).

[2] The kinds of problems that bother Fred have also been called existential questions. Besides the problems Fred is now faced with, existential questions have also been seen to include questions such as whether there is a God, what is the true nature of a human being, and is there life after death. For reasons of space, I here put these further kinds of questions aside.

[3] An example of an important question that is partly philosophical is that of how depression affects decision-making ability and whether Fred is depressive enough to be unable to competently make important life choices. For discussion related to the conceptual side of this question, see, for example, Meynen [26], Rich [24], and Schuklenk and van de Vathorst [27]. The empirical side of the question is addressed in, for example, Hindmarch et al. [28] and Kolva et al. [29].

that they would be unimportant, I here put questions other than philosophical problems directly related to life's meaning aside.[4]

7.2 Two Questions About the Meaning of Life

People may have quite different problems in mind when they speak about what they see as questions about the meaning of life. Yet often both laymen and philosophers who consider the kinds of questions that now trouble Fred would appear to ultimately focus on the question: what, if anything, makes a life worth living for the person whose life it is (cf., e.g., [1]). Accordingly, this is the question I will concentrate on below.[5] Yet, to be more precise, the question can be seen to involve two importantly distinct problems. First, it raises the problem whether a human life can have meaning at all. Perhaps, it is impossible for our lives to have any point and the view that they could, at least sometimes, be worthwhile is merely a convenient illusion? Second, it implies the problem what things or activities make a person's life meaningful, if it is possible for human lives to have meaning? As addressing the second problem would be practically rather futile if a human life could have no meaning, below I will start with the first question. But before going into it, I briefly consider how a meaningful life relates to a happy life and to a moral life.

Some people think that a life that is not a happy one can have no point.[6] According to a widespread position, a person is the happier the more pleasure and less pain she experiences. On another popular view, a person is the happier the more she gets the things she wants.[7] It would not appear to be impossible that the only thing that brings a person

---

[4] The philosophical pursuit for plausible answers to concrete evaluative problems, such as those related to life's meaning, is sometimes still seen as an endeavor primarily seeking to determine which of the traditional moral theories—utilitarianism, Kantian deontology, or Aristotelian virtue ethics—is the correct one. Yet, instead of relying on any traditional moral theory, most current philosophers working on practical moral problems rather aim to determine which answers to the problems cohere best with factual knowledge, principles of logic, and moral intuitions accepted by competent moral agents (cf., e.g., [30] and [31]). For instance, if a proposed solution to a moral problem logically implies that—to use an example presented by Ronald Dworkin [32]—torturing babies for fun is morally acceptable, that is a good reason to reject it. Some philosophers believe that plausible answers to concrete evaluative problems can be found, if at all, only after first finding out which philosophical theory about the nature of values and value judgments—which meta-ethical theory—is the correct one. Yet how the relationship between meta-ethical theories and practical evaluative problems should be conceived remains controversial. And if a meta-ethical theory logically entails, to continue with the same example, that torturing babies for fun is morally acceptable, that is a good reason to reject it. Hence, meta-ethical theories and their possible implications to concrete evaluative problems are also (to be) assessed in terms of the methodology commonly employed in addressing concrete evaluative questions in philosophy.

[5] Since the focus here is on the meaning a person's life has from her own viewpoint, what I speak of as "meaning of life" has sometimes also been referred to as "meaning in life" and as "the meaning a person's life has to her."

[6] What I say below applies also if instead of happiness the focus is on well-being.

[7] Some advocates of the first kind of theory of happiness maintain that certain pleasures and pains are more significant from the viewpoint of happiness than others (see, e.g., [33], Chap. 2; cf., e.g., [34]). And proponents of the second kind of theory of happiness mentioned above may require that the wants that count in determining happiness are the ones a person would have after being what is deemed as adequately informed about their objects and/or consequences of their satisfaction (see, e.g., [35]).

pleasure is her having a meaningful existence. A meaningful life may also be the only thing that a person wants. Yet, a happy life and a meaningful life are conceptually distinct from each other. On the one hand, consider Jack, a happy-go-lucky fellow who spends his time hanging out at the local beach with his friends, drinking beer and smoking pot. At least when other things are being equal, however happy Jack would manage to be, it is intuitively implausible that he leads a meaningful life. On the other hand, consider Mary, a teenager with two ailing parents who are unable to take care of themselves. In order to support them, Mary is forced to get a tedious job with a minimum wage. After working long hours, she goes home to attend to her parents, day in day out. Mary does not lead a happy life, but she loves her parents and takes pride in her being able to support and to take care of them. Accordingly, her life is not meaningless.

In terms of the relationship between a meaningful life and a moral life, consider that Mary however ultimately tires of her existence. Instead of continuing to take care of her parents, she decides to pursue her dream of becoming an artist, a dream her high school art teachers deemed well-grounded. At the beginning, her life is not much less of a struggle than it was previously. Yet slowly, her work starts to receive attention, beginning from small exhibitions in the local library, ultimately ending to be displayed in prestigious galleries worldwide. Intuitively plausibly, Mary's life as an artist can be a meaningful one. But it would seem to be clear that her decision to leave her parents was not the morally right choice. Leading a moral life may be more likely to be meaningful than leading an immoral life (cf., e.g., [2, 3]). Yet, the life of Mary as an artist suggests that a meaningful life and a moral life are conceptually distinct from each other.

Before going into the two questions about life's meaning distinguished above, a further clarification of the topic of this chapter is in order. One approach to answering the questions refers to one or more supernatural beings—such as God, gods, soul, spirits, etc. In a view falling within this approach, a person's life can be seen as meaningful insofar as it accords with the purpose God has given to her, the universal order imposed by a supreme spirit, etc. To some people, answers to the problems about life's meaning can only be found within this approach. Yet, people who are convinced about its correctness may not be likely to raise the kind of questions that now trouble Fred. In any case, the majority of the contemporary academic philosophical discussion on the meaning of life does not rely on supernatural points of departure. Accordingly, but without meaning to say that it would be unimportant, I here put the supernatural approach to the questions about life's meaning aside.[8]

7.3   Can a Human Life Have Meaning?

What kinds of reasons there are to think that a human life cannot have any meaning? Perhaps unsurprisingly, the main grounds to be found in recent philosophical literature refer to one or another aspect of the human constitution, often as compared with that of the universe in which we live. In light of current knowledge, the universe is

[8] For philosophical discussion related to it, see, for example, Affolter [36], Cottingham [37], and Metz [38].

billions of years old and can be infinite in volume. Our planet is one among several in a solar system that is a part of a galaxy that contains billions of stars, a galaxy that is one of the billions of galaxies in the universe. Seen from that perspective, even the biggest buildings Fred constructed are quite small. And, from that viewpoint, even if he had chosen to be an author and had managed to write something with lasting literary influence—something in the class of, say, Tolstoy or Shakespeare—the mark he would have made in the world would not have been that long-lived. Should it then be concluded that a human life can have no meaning? Not necessarily. To begin with, it seems implausible that spatial or temporal magnitude would determine worth or meaningfulness. That a pile of garbage is bigger than a work of art does not necessarily mean that it is more significant. That high-level nuclear waste exists longer than a house does not entail that it is more worthy (see also, e.g., [4]).

Requiring that our lives could have meaning only if they made a difference in cosmic terms also appears, to put it bluntly, rather megalomaniac. Accordingly, the kind of meaningfulness it would be reasonable for beings like us to expect from our lives—and whose lack could warrant sensible concerns of meaninglessness—is commonly seen in much more modest terms. This is reflected in the fact that, in the prime of his life, Fred did not raise the kinds of questions about the meaning of his existence on which he now ponders. As people need houses in which to reside, to engage in their professions, etc., by doing his work to the best of his ability Fred provided a valuable service to the society and the income that brought to him enabled him to pursue his other, nature-related interests. He did not change the universe (in any more significant terms),[9] but the life he then led was meaningful enough for him (cf. also, e.g., [5, 6]). Going a bit further, Simon Blackburn [7] writes as follows:

> The smile of her child means the earth to her mother, the touch means bliss for the lover, the turn of the phrase means happiness for the writer. Meaning comes with absorption and enjoyment, the flow of details that matter to us. The problem with life is then that it has too much meaning.[10]

Yet, as already suggested, it could be insisted that what actually grounds the meaninglessness of human life is, not that our lives do not significantly alter the history of the universe, but the fact that sooner or later we all die. This position may be based on the view that, for all we know, each individual human being will perish at some point or on the worry that our species as a whole will become extinct (or both). In terms of the latter option, the line of thinking could continue that, given the

---

[9] To be precise, that I, for instance, lift my hand from the keyboard of my computer does make the history of the universe different from what it had been had I not lifted my hand. In that sense, everything people do, or omit to do, has cosmic significance. Yet, when the difference is not significantly bigger, it most plausibly would not satisfy proponents of the view that human lives could have meaning only if the lives made a difference in terms of the history of the universe.

[10] The above division between a happy life and a meaningful life notwithstanding, the absorption and enjoyment Blackburn refers to can be seen as an element of a meaningful life. I return to this point in the next section of this chapter.

fact that the human species will become extinct, our lives could have meaning only if there were other beings in the universe that could appreciate the lives we have lived. However, though in a sense our lives could matter more if there were such beings—we could have a bigger audience, so to speak—it is not clear that having a meaningful life necessarily presupposes their existence. Someone might argue that our lives would in fact matter more if no such beings exist. For it could be maintained that the more there are beings who are able to appreciate the things we find meaningful, the more we are just ones among the many, less unique, less significant (cf., e.g., [8]). But in any case, the (assumed) facts that each individual person will sooner or later perish and in the end the human species will become extinct do not deprive human lives of the moderate kind of meaning Fred's life had before he succumbed to the existential crisis he now faces. For his death or the extinction of our species does not erase the meaning his life had then (cf. also, e.g., [4]).

Indeed, it has been argued that death after something like the current average human life-span is necessary for our lives to be meaningful. Without doing too much violence to it, the main idea of the line of argument—one initiating in the work of Bernard Williams [9], Chap. 6)—can be formulated as follows. Consider that you could become immortal, your life could continue forever. Let us assume that in your average day you would wake up in the morning, wash, eat, go to work, do what you do at work, buy groceries on your way back home, make dinner, eat again, perhaps relax a while, and then go to sleep. There would be some meaning in some of these activities and occasionally in some others, at least to begin with. But when something like that had gone on for, say, 7000 years, would you not be quite fed up with even the initially meaningful things? Or if the life you would lead would, for one reason or another, be very different from life as we know it, how could you know whether or not it would be worthwhile? Contemplating these questions, proponents of the line argument propose, shows that, for all we know, an endless life would ultimately become utterly tedious and meaningless.

The conclusion has given rise to a variety of responses. Some philosophers have found it convincing, others have expressed their willingness to live forever, or to at least try out how it would feel. Some philosophers have asked what exactly we should consider here—for example, how is the boredom in question to be understood, how does it relate to questions of life's meaning, would others too be immortal and, if yes, would that not lead to overpopulation and lethal shortage of food, water, air, etc.—and some still others have maintained that it is impossible for beings with our mental capacities to imagine what it would be like to live for even hundreds of years, not to speak of forever (see also, e.g., [10–13]). These discrepancies notwithstanding, the line of argument draws attention to what would appear to be an important point as regards the relationship between the typical human lifespan and life's meaning.

The fact that we, for all we know, ultimately die is not always in our minds (if we are lucky). Yet it gives structure to our lives and a kind of urgency to our doings. A person's life typically consists of birth, childhood, teenage years, early adulthood, adulthood, old age, and death. Generalizing again—and focusing on contemporary Western societies—each of the phases of life involves particular things, such as learning certain basic life skills and a vocation, mating, and starting a family, raising offspring and working, and retiring. It would seem that, to a significant extent, the activities we engage in during our lives get their meaning from being embedded in this kind of structure, the existence of which is ultimately based on the fact that we die approximately when we now do. True, all of us do not live lives with precisely those stages nor so that the phases involve the things that they typically contain. Yet, how even those who, say, do not have children perceive their existence is usually influenced by the expectation that at a certain stage of their lives people reproduce and raise offspring.[11] Accordingly, Michael Sigrist [14], for instance, writes as follows:

> We exist as the sort of agents that we are—agents capable of recognizing, valuing, and striving for meaning by way of forming identities—because we are aware, at some level, of our own mortality.… My possibilities get their meaning for me by my awareness that I am to realize these possibilities within the horizon of my own mortality.

Hence, it would seem that the kind of meaning that we can have in our lives is to a significant extent based on the expectation that our lives last for something like the current average human lifespan.

But it could still be maintained that, even if the kinds of thoughts briefly engaged with above could not undermine the meaningfulness of human lives, more mundane reasons related to the human condition entail that our lives cannot have meaning. It is a familiar fact that we desire many things and it would seem that we are seldom, if ever, truly satisfied. The origins of the best-known philosophical theory that grounds the meaninglessness of human life on our nature as desiring beings can be traced back to eighteenth century German metaphysics. Yet basic biology can provide what for many is a more clear and plausible basis for such a theory. If a human being in need of nutrition and hydration did not desire food and water, she would die rather soon (in the absence of outside assistance). The same would result if she had no desire to escape a freezing cold or a threatening enemy (and she was not protected by others). Accordingly, human evolution has favored the emergence and existence of mental states instrumental to our acquiring food, water, and shelter.[12] Yet, as already suggested above, it might appear that from the viewpoint of life's meaning our developing into desiring beings has been rather unfortunate. Evolution is not a precision tool. Accordingly, not only do we want what would suffice for us in terms of food, water, and shelter, but also we often desire much, much more. Given that few of us are ultimately able to get all that we want, the pessimistic conclusion is that, as long as we live, we will be dissatisfied and our lives meaningless.

However, it would seem to be clear that if we had no mental states like desires—but were like, say, stones in that respect,—it would be impossible for our lives to have meaning. If we did not want anything, our lives could not matter to us. And, as

---

[11] And even the (possible) meaningfulness of the lives of people with a similar lifespan as ours but totally different lifestyles would apparently be affected by the fact that they typically live for that period.

[12] Of course, these are not the only desires that have been explained in terms of evolutionary benefits. Yet, for the sake of simplicity, I here focus on these desires only.

already suggested, the fact that Fred is a desiring being did not make it impossible for him to be satisfied with his life in his heyday. Accordingly, at least sometimes, it is possible for humans to be satisfied enough to lead what count as meaningful lives. Moreover, and as was also already proposed above, having a meaningful life is not the same as getting all you want. Indeed, there would appear to be ways of life whose meaningfulness is to a significant extent based on the dissatisfaction of some of the central desires of those living them. Consider, for instance, the scientist wishing to unravel the most fundamental questions of her discipline. Although her satisfying the desire could be very meaningful for her, it would also deprive her of the goal the pursuit of which has given her life purpose (see also, e.g., [15]).

Finally, and not unrelated to the worries about life's meaninglessness considered above, there is a twofold concern related to arbitrariness (cf., e.g., [16]). First, people often have different options, sometimes even a wide variety of possibilities, with regard to which kind of life to pursue. And, at least when we dig deep enough, it would appear to be quite difficult for a person to provide an adequately reasoned justification for choosing in one way rather than another. Perhaps Fred's life had been more meaningful had he became an author instead of a constructor? As it was impossible for him to know which choice would result in a more meaningful life, it would seem that his choice was ultimately arbitrary. Does this kind of randomness not, in the end, undermine the meaningfulness of his existence? Second, as suggested, humans are able to look at their lives from an external viewpoint, one that transcends their own concerns. Seen from that kind of perspective, it would appear to be difficult to warrant the view that an individual's life could have any special meaning. For are not other persons' pursuits equally valuable for them? Indeed, adopting this impartial perspective, how could one at all be justified in focusing on one's own concerns?

When he made his important life choices, Fred did not know which options would in fact result in the most meaningful life. Yet, as already suggested, the arbitrariness related to his choices does not nullify the meaning involved in his life as it turned out: the life Fred led in his prime still was worthwhile. Moreover, as Sigrist suggests in the above quotation, it would seem that a person's making choices between different life options is in itself something that can bring meaning to her life. For by making such choices a person takes an active part in molding her identity and in her becoming a particular kind of person. In terms of the second part of the concern at hand, that a person leads a meaningful existence does not presuppose that it is more significant than those of other people from some external, or even from her own, viewpoint. Even if Fred's life was always less meaningful than that of, say, Mother Theresa that does not entail that the life he led in his heyday was not meaningful. Moral considerations can, of course, require a person to focus on the pursuits of others instead of those of his own. But, as — when other things are being equal — morality gives all people an equal standing, moral considerations do not obligate one to always put others before oneself. On the other hand, as already suggested, it may also be that a moral life is more likely to be meaningful than an immoral one.

In light of the above assessment of the main reasons against the view that a human life can have meaning, it is possible for our lives to be meaningful. Of course, the brief reflections are unlikely to persuade ardent proponents of the contrary view. They may continue to insist, say, that a person's life could be meaningful only if she made a dramatic difference to the history of the universe. But, as suggested, many reasonable people are willing to settle for a much more modest conception of when a human life is meaningful, one that allows our lives to have meaning, at least sometimes.

7.4   What Makes a Human Life Meaningful?

Assuming that it is possible for a human life to be meaningful, when does a person's life then have meaning? The considerations of the previous section already provided several hints on how philosophers have answered this question, but evidently many issues remain to be addressed. Below I go into some of the central ones of them and, as promised, relate them to Fred's case. The answers to the question when a person's life is meaningful to be found in recent philosophical literature can be divided into subjective and objective.[13] Some theories of the meaning of life combine subjective and objective elements with each other. According to purely subjective theories of the meaning of life, to put it briefly, a person leads a meaningful existence as long as she believes that her life is worthwhile (see, e.g., [17], Chap. 18). Hence, on these views, pursuing whatever lifestyle amounts to a meaningful life if, or insofar as, the person leading it thinks that her life has point. Purely objective conceptions of the meaning of life, in their turn, entail that a person's life is meaningful when he engages in objectively significant pursuits, whether or not she herself sees her existence as meaningful (cf., e.g., [18], Chap. 12). The theories that combine subjective and objective elements—the hybrid views, as they have been called—require that a person must both think that her life has point and engage in objectively worthwhile activities for her to lead a meaningful existence (see, e.g., [19–21]).

A person's life can evidently have worth for others even though she herself does not see it as meaningful. Consider, for instance, the time when Mary in the above example started to think that taking care of her parents cannot be her whole life. Even though Mary herself did not see her life as meaningful anymore, her tending for her parents was still valuable for them (as long as she still continued it). But that a person's life would have point from her own perspective, that it would be worthwhile *for her* presupposes that she herself sees her existence as meaningful. The subjective theories of life's meaning are plausible in that they can account for this feature of a meaningful life. Yet returning to the case of Jack—the beer-drinking, pot-smoking beach bum—suggests that purely subjective theories about life's meaning are implausible. For even if Jack managed to deem his existence

---

[13] Not all philosophers writing about the meaning of life draw the distinction between subjective and objective accounts of life's meaning in precisely the same way. Below I employ what would appear to be the most common and useful division between subjective and objective theories of life's meaning.

meaningful, as already proposed, it would be counterintuitive to maintain that he leads a worthwhile life. This problem with the purely subjective views about life's meaning provides the central motivation for the development of objective conceptions about the meaning of life.

Objective theories about the meaning of life presuppose a plausible conception of what things and activities are objectively worthwhile, where 'objectively worthwhile' is understood, roughly, as being significant from a viewpoint understandable to all rational people. Critics of the theories have, however, argued that providing such a conception is impossible. Moreover, objective theories separate a meaningful existence from the attitudes of the person leading it and, as suggested, this would appear to result in a rather alienated conception of a meaningful life. Let us briefly consider each of these two difficulties for objective theories of life's meaning in turn.[14] Among the main goods that proponents of objective theories consider as constituents of a meaningful life are such things as creativity, use of one's rational capacities, pursuit of truth and beauty, parenting and close personal relationships, appreciation of nature, and moral activity. Though not all of them are unique to humans, sometimes these goods are referred to as things that engage the distinctively human capacities. Now, critics of objective theories about life's meaning would appear to be right in that it is not clear that only these things could make a person's life meaningful. And, for reasons already presented, it would seem that moral activity, for instance, is not necessary for leading a meaningful life. But, contrary to what the critics maintain, it seems quite plausible that a life consisting of, say, engagement in close personal relationships and pursuit of truth and beauty is objectively more worthwhile than the existence of, for instance, Jack in the above example.

However, while the first of the two main problems of objective theories about life's meaning does not appear insurmountable, the second one seems much more serious. A theory that separates the meaningfulness of a life from the viewpoint of the person whose life it is arguably, if not evidently, cannot amount to a satisfactory analysis of a meaningful life understood as a life that is worthwhile for the person whose life it is. Even if a person was engaged in many objectively significant activities, her life would not have point *in that sense* unless she also herself saw it as meaningful for her (when she assessed it in light of adequate information). Together with the main problem of the purely subjective theories—the fact that they count whatever life as meaningful as long as the person living it sees it as worthwhile—this difficulty with the purely objective theories about the meaning of life has led many philosophers to endorse a hybrid theory about life's meaning. Accordingly, Susan Wolf, to use a central example, maintains that a meaningful life is one of "active engagement in projects of

---

[14] Sometimes, the first one of them is combined with the idea that the objective theories presuppose that there is one single meaningful way of life only. However, given that it is intuitively implausible that there could be only one meaningful type of existence—consider, for instance, the life of Mary as an artist and the life of Mother Theresa—objective theories about life's meaning are better construed as pluralist than as monist theories, to employ the commonly used terms.

worth" so that "subjective attraction meets objective attractiveness" (see, e.g., [19–21]). More precisely, Wolf [21] characterizes the kind of engagement she has in mind as follows:

> A person is actively engaged by something if she is gripped, excited, involved by it. Most obviously, we are actively engaged by the things and people about which and whom we are passionate. Opposites of active engagement are boredom and alienation. To be actively engaged in something is not always pleasant in the ordinary sense of the word. Activities in which people are actively engaged frequently involve stress, danger, exertion, or sorrow (consider, for example: writing a book, climbing a mountain, training for a marathon, caring for an ailing friend). However, there is something good about the feeling of engagement: one feels (typically without thinking about it) especially alive.

Instead of presenting a theory of precisely what activities and projects have objective worth, Wolf refers to lives that are often deemed as paradigm examples of meaningful lives—she mentions the lives of Gandhi, Mother Theresa, Einstein, and Cézanne—to support the view that some lives are objectively more meaningful than others [19–21]. In its objective aspect, Wolf's conception of a meaningful life would appear to accord rather closely with what proponents of objective theories of life's meaning see as objectively worthwhile lives and things. And like proponents of the purely objective theories of life's meaning, advocates of the kind of hybrid position of which Wolf's theory is a prime example sometimes disagree over precisely which activities or lives counts as objectively meaningful. Advocates of the hybrid theories of life's meaning may also have different views on exactly how the subjective attitudes relevant to a person's leading a meaningful life are to be conceived (cf., e.g., [22, 23]). Yet, in general terms, a position that combines subjective and objective elements with each other is, for the kinds of reasons presented above, the most popular one amongst philosophers currently writing on life's meaning. How, then, does Fred's case appear in light of such a conception of a meaningful life?

The above considerations already suggest an answer to this question. To begin with, in his heyday Fred was actively engaged in work that provided a valuable service to the society. Besides exciting him, Fred's hobbies also taught him to appreciate nature. Accordingly, the life Fred led then plausibly counts as a meaningful one in the hybrid view. His life might have been more meaningful if he had pursued a career in literature. Yet, he had been an utter failure as an author, the contrary would appear to be true. So, in terms of the life Fred has lived, the most popular of the current philosophical accounts of life's meaning supports the view, already suggested above, that Fred has had a meaningful life. What about his current predicament? As explained, Fred is increasingly unable to engage in the activities the pursuit of which has made life worth living for him. Does this entail that he is doomed to meaninglessness? Not necessarily. If the objectively valuable projects a person engages in were to change on, say, a daily basis, her life would probably be too chaotic to be meaningful. Yet that evidently does not entail that the activities that bring meaning to a person's existence cannot change during her life. And there would still seem to be objectively worthwhile things in which Fred could engage—such as having personal relationships and enjoying literature. It would thus seem that in principle at least, Fred could still lead a meaningful existence. Hence, Fred's thoughts about the meaninglessness of both the life he has lived and the life he could still have would appear to lack adequate grounding. Yet, given the subjective aspect of a meaningful life, whether he actually could live his remaining time meaningfully depends on whether he is able to find sufficient motivation to engage in objectively worthwhile things. Unfortunately, not all people—even the frustrated, dejected, and depressed—are able to appreciate the things and activities that in light of the above considerations could bring meaning to their lives. This emphasizes the importance of employing an interdisciplinary approach in dealing with such persons, one that besides the philosophical perspective also involves therapeutic viewpoints from psychology and psychiatry (cf., e.g., [24]).

7.5   Life's Meaning and Suicide

Consider the regrettable prospect that, despite all efforts, Fred is unable to find any point in his life anymore. He is simply too dejected by the nearing of his demise and continues to think that it would be best for him to end it all now. As the supernatural viewpoint is now put aside, Fred's committing suicide would mean no more, or less, than that his life ends. The morality and rationality of suicide has been questioned, especially earlier in the history. Yet nowadays, it is commonly—but not universally—accepted that suicide can sometimes be both rational and morally acceptable. The criteria of a morally permissible and rational suicide typically involve, at least, the requirements that a person's life is—for one reason or another—unbearable for her and that she makes her decision to end it freely, intentionally, and with sufficient understanding about its nature and consequences.[15] But how would Fred's possible suicide appear from the viewpoint of the philosophical discussion on life's meaning?

To begin with, as suggested above, meaning would appear to come in degrees, so that a person's life can be more or less meaningful. A meaningful life that could be even more meaningful is evidently not a life that is not worth living. Instead, it would seem that only a life that totally lacks meaning could provide grounds for suicide. Yet a person whose life lacks all meaning can still reasonably want to live, if she has reason to think that her life will become worth living sometime in the future. Or she may decide to pursue a life of selflessly serving others, or a cause, without expecting the life to involve the kind of subjective mental states that in view of the above considerations constitute a central element of a

---

[15] For what have been referred to as the classic philosophical arguments against suicide and criticism of them, see, for example, Feldman [39], Chap. 13. For discussion on the philosophical questions related to suicide more generally, see, for example, Cholbi [40].

meaningful life.[16] Therefore, maintaining that a person's life is not worth living is not, as such, to maintain that she has reason to commit suicide or that it is morally acceptable for her—or to others—to end her life. Sometimes suicide is opposed sternly even when a person's life is taken to irrevocably lack all meaning and she is not considered morally obligated to stay alive to meet her duties toward others. Those who do not accept suicide (even then) might argue that it just is our part as humans to suffer and that human life still has value despite being, even all in all, distressing. More positively, and for another example, people who are against suicide could instead maintain that even the bad things in life should be welcomed as parts of an overall good package. On such views, ending one's life could be seen as a despondent act that shows inadequate understanding of reality.[17] In line with this, someone might maintain that Fred's committing suicide would make his life meaningless or at least amount to a meaningless ending for his existence. Indeed, when a meaningful life is understood as a life worth living, it would seem that ending one's life could not be a meaningful act. For how could something that brings a life to an end make life worth living?

However, as already implied, even if Fred now were to commit suicide, the act would not erase the meaning his existence has had. Others might come to see his life differently than they would otherwise do, but that does not cancel the meaning Fred found in his existence in the prime of his life. Moreover, a person's ending her life is also sometimes seen as an ultimately meaningful act, one by which she can have the final say about her existence even in desperate circumstances. Seeing suicide as such an act would also appear to be compatible with the hybrid theory of life's meaning characterized above (see, however, also note 17). Interpreted in its terms, Fred's ending his life could be perceived as an act by which he brings to conclusion his main project, his life, before it loses all point it can have for him. Though it would end his life, his committing suicide would thus still be a way for him to actively engage in a project of worth. Hence, as either option would appear to be possible in light of the pertinent philosophical discussion, whether Fred's ending his life would in fact be a meaningful act rather than a desperate escape would seem to depend on his own view of his situation. If he sincerely sees his committing suicide in terms of the hybrid theory, it would seem that his ending his life could be a meaningful act. However, the philosophical debate on the moral acceptability of what can be called psychiatric-assisted suicide is as yet at its early stages only. As most jurisdictions accordingly prohibit psychiatrists from helping their patients in committing suicide, the procedure is also legally a closed option

---

[16] A person whose life is altogether meaningless can also want to continue it because she mistakenly believes that her life is worth living.

[17] Accordingly, a distressed person who is convinced about the wrongness of suicide might find meaning in continuing the struggle that she sees her life to be (cf. [41]).

in the majority of cases.[18] And, of course, the most fortunate outcome would be that Fred would after all still manage to find some things in his life that would make it worth living for him.

7.6   Conclusion

In this chapter, I have considered whether philosophical work on life's meaning could help an elderly person who is suicidal because he considers his life as meaningless. I focused on one case only—that of Fred described in the introduction—but assumed that it can throw light on several others. I proposed that, in view of the recent philosophical debate on life's meaning, there is an important sense of 'a meaningful life' in which it is possible for human lives to have meaning and that a meaningful existence in that sense is one of active engagement in objectively worthwhile pursuits. To the degree that the considerations are plausible, they undermine Fred's worry that his life has been meaningless. They also suggest that Fred might still be able to find meaning in his life, were he able to engage in other valuable pursuits than those on which he has mainly concentrated so far. It would also seem that his committing suicide would not necessarily be a meaningless act nor would it deprive his life of the significance it has had. These conclusions may unfortunately not provide sufficient consolation for a person like Fred. However, the philosophical discussion about the meaning of life is continuing and may produce more helpful answers in the future. From a different viewpoint, developments in medical science may also alter the human condition so that the questions about life's meaning we will be concerned with in the future are rather different from the ones that were considered above.[19] Yet that remains to be seen and the fact that things could be different in the future evidently does not lessen the urgency of continuing the work—philosophical, psychological, and psychiatric—on the problems cases such as that of Fred's pose now.[20]

---

[18]The contemporary debate on the moral and legal acceptability of physician-assisted dying has mainly focused on competent patients who suffer because they are severely physically ill or injured. For the main arguments presented in that debate, see, for example, [42], Chap. 1. For discussion on whether psychiatric conditions could sometimes provide moral grounds for physician-assisted suicide, see, for example, Appel [43], Cholbi [44], Parker [45], and Varelius [46]. Though Szasz famously argued against suicide-prevention (see, e.g., [47]), he did not accept physician-assisted suicide. In practice, *The Royal Dutch Association of Medicine* already allows that psychiatric reasons can warrant physician-assisted dying and in Belgium suffering unrelated to physical illness or injury is acknowledged in law as a valid basis for physician-assisted dying (see [48, 49]).

[19]In the most extreme scenarios, future technology—human enhancement technology, as it has been called—will enable us to live forever, as beings with physical, mental, and social abilities far beyond those we now have (see, e.g., [50]). If the kinds of radical scenarios would become reality, the questions about life's meaning—though to an extent similar with those considered above— would apparently be assessed with rather different faculties than the ones we now have. Unless we will have such faculties and they help us to solve the problems with climate change, sufficiency of natural resources, etc., our conceptions of the meaning of life may also be affected by rather different kinds of developments than the ones depicted in the extreme scenarios of proponents of human enhancement technology.

[20]I thank Juha Räikkä for valuable comments and the *Kone Foundation* for generous financial support.

References

1. Metz T. The concept of a meaningful life. Am Philos Q. 2001;38(2):137–53.
2. Landau I. Immorality and the meaning of life. J Value Inq. 2011;45(3):309–17.
3. Thomas L. Morality and a meaningful life. Philos Pap. 2005;34(3):405–27.
4. Trisel BA. Human extinction and the value of our efforts. Philos Forum. 2004;35(3):371–91.
5. Audi R. Intrinsic value and meaningful life. Philos Pap. 2005;34(3):331–55.
6. Metz T. The immortality requirement for life's meaning. Ratio. 2003;XVI(2):161–77.
7. Blackburn S. Being good: a short introduction to ethics. Oxford: Oxford University Press; 2001.
8. Kahane G. Our cosmic insignificance. Noûs. 2014;48(4):745–72.
9. Williams BAO. Problems of the self. Cambridge: Cambridge University Press; 1973.
10. Bortolotti L. Agency, life-extension, and the meaning of life. Monist. 2010;93(1):38–56.
11. Burley M. Immortality and meaning: reflections on the Makropoulos debate. Philosophy. 2009;84:529–47.
12. Jones WE. Venerating death. Philos Pap. 2015;44(1):61–81.
13. Smuts A. Immortality and significance. Philos Lit. 2011;35(1):134–49.
14. Sigrist MJ. Death and the meaning of life. Philos Pap. 2015;44(1):83–102.
15. Setiya K. The midlife crisis. Philos Imprint. 2014;14(31):1–18.
16. Nagel T. The absurd. J Philos. 1970;68(20):716–27.
17. Taylor R. Good and evil. New York: Prometheus Books; 2000.
18. Singer P. Practical ethics. 2nd ed. New York: Cambridge University Press; 1993.
19. Wolf S. Meaningfulness: a third dimension of the good life. Found Sci. 2014;21(2):253–69. doi:10.1007/s10699-014-9384-9.
20. Wolf S. Meaning in life and why it matters. Princeton: Princeton University Press; 2010.
21. Wolf S. Happiness and meaning: two aspects of the good life. Soc Philos Policy. 1997;14(1):207–25.
22. Kekes J. The meaning of life. Midwest Stud Philos. 2000;24(1):17–34.
23. Mintoff J. Transcending absurdity. Ratio. 2008;XXI(1):64–84.
24. Rich BA. Pathologizing suffering and the pursuit of a peaceful death. Camb Q Healthc Ethics. 2014;23(4):403–16.
25. Dees MK, Vernooij-Dassen MJ, Dekkers WJ, Vissers KC, Van Veel C. 'Unbearable suffering': a qualitative study on the perspectives of patients who request assistance in dying. J Med Ethics. 2011;37(12):727–34.
26. Meynen G. Depression, possibilities, and competence: a phenomenological perspective. Theor Med Bioeth. 2011;32(3):181–93.
27. Schuklenk U, van de Vathorst S. Treatment-resistant major depressive disorder and assisted dying. J Med Ethics. 2015;41(8):577–83.
28. Hindmarch T, Hotopf M, Owen GS. Depression and decision-making capacity for treatment or research. A systematic review. BMC Med Ethics. 2013;14:54.
29. Kolva E, Rosenfeld B, Brescia R, Comfort C. Assessing decision-making capacity at the end of life. Gen Hosp Psychiatry. 2014;36(4):392–7.
30. Cath Y. Reflective equilibrium. In: Cappelen H, Gendler TS, Hawthorne J, editors. The oxford handbook of philosophical methodology. Oxford: Oxford University Press; 2016.
31. Daniels N. Justice and justification: reflective equilibrium in theory and practice. New York: Cambridge University Press; 1996.
32. Dworkin R. Justice for hedgehogs. Cambridge: Harvard University Press; 2011.
33. Mill JS. Utilitarianism. Oxford: Oxford University Press; 1988.
34. Schaupp K. Books before chocolate? The insufficiency of Mill's evidence for higher pleasures. Utilitas. 2013;25(2):266–76.
35. Brandt R. A theory of the good and the right. Amherst: Prometheus Books; 1998.
36. Affolter J. Human nature as God's purpose. Relig Stud. 2007;43(4):443–55.
37. Cottingham J. On the meaning of life. London: Routledge; 2003.

38. Metz T. God's purpose as irrelevant to life's meaning: a reply to Affolter. Relig Stud. 2007;43(4):457–64.
39. Feldman F. Confrontations with the reaper: a philosophical study of the nature and value of death. New York: Oxford University Press; 1994.
40. Cholbi M. Suicide: the philosophical dimensions. Peterborough: Broadview Press; 2011.
41. Varelius J. Ending life, morality, and meaning. Ethical Theory Moral Pract. 2013;16(3): 559–74.
42. Battin MP. Ending life: ethics and the way we die. New York: Oxford University Press; 2005.
43. Appel JM. A suicide right for the mentally ill: a Swiss case opens a new debate. Hastings Cent Rep. 2007;37(3):21–3.
44. Cholbi M. The terminal, the futile, and the psychiatrically disordered. Int J Law Psychiatry. 2013;36(5–6):498–505.
45. Parker M. Defending the indefensible? Psychiatry, assisted suicide and human freedom. Int J Law Psychiatry. 2013;36(5–6):485–97.
46. Varelius J. Mental illness, lack of autonomy, and physician-assisted death. In: Cholbi M, Varelius J editors. New directions in the ethics of assisted suicide and euthanasia. New York: Springer; 2015. p. 59–77.
47. Szasz T. Suicide prohibition: the shame of medicine. Syracuse: Syracuse University Press; 2011.
48. Royal Dutch Association of Medicine. Termination of life. 2011. http://knmg.artsennet.nl/Publicaties/KNMGpublicatie-levenseinde/100696/Position-paper-The-role-of-the-physician-in-the-voluntary-termination-of-life-2011.htm. Accessed 7 Oct 2015.
49. Naudts K, et al. Euthanasia: the role of the psychiatrist. Br J Psychiatry. 2006;188(5):405–9.
50. Savulescu J, Bostrom N, editors. Human enhancement. Oxford: Oxford University Press; 2009.

Baby Boomers and Rational Suicide

8

Robert E. McCue

> *What a drag it is getting old.* –Keith Richards and Mick Jagger,
> "Mother's Little Helper"
>
> © Abkco Music, Inc.

8.1   Introduction

In 2012, Peter Levitan, a 60-year-old advertising executive and self-identified Baby Boomer, informed the world in his book, *Boomercide* [1], that he would kill himself at age 80. At the time, Mr. Levitan was in good health, financially comfortable, and happily married with two children. However, he realized the likelihood that at some point in his old age, his health would deteriorate to the extent that he would be unable to participate in the things that he found meaningful and would require care that would deplete his financial resources. For him, it was better to pick a definite time to die, plan accordingly, and enjoy things in the meantime. What is one to make of this plan to kill himself? From his writings and self-description, Mr. Levitan does not seem mentally ill. Could it have something to do with his being a Baby Boomer?

In the coming decades, clinicians treating older adults will have Baby Boomers as patients. This cohort is so large that it will profoundly affect how the elderly live and die in our society. In this chapter, we will examine the connection between aging Baby Boomers and suicide, particularly rational suicide. Like Peter Levitan, many Baby Boomers will not consider rational suicide to be an outlier act of questionable morality, but an option for having the kind of death suitable for their needs and wishes.

R.E. McCue, M.D. (✉)
Department of Psychiatry, New York University School of Medicine,
1 Park Avenue, New York, NY 10016, USA
e-mail: Robert.mccue@nyumc.org

© Springer International Publishing Switzerland 2017
R.E. McCue, M. Balasubramaniam (eds.), *Rational Suicide in the Elderly*,
DOI 10.1007/978-3-319-32672-6_8

8.2   What Is so Special About the Baby Boomers?

Beginning in the 1920s, the United States had a relatively stable fertility rate of about 19 births/1000 population. This ended in 1946 when fertility rates abruptly rose. They remained high for 18 years, until 1964. At the peak in 1947, the fertility rate was 26.5 births/1000 population. The boom ended in the mid-1960s when the fertility rate dropped to 15. The 72.5 million Americans born during this unprecedented period of increased births are called the Baby Boomers [2]. This large number of births skewed the age distribution of the American population in ways that are still being felt today. From immigration, the number of Baby Boomers has further increased, totaling 78.5 million by 1999. Today, 76 million Americans are Baby Boomers (about 65 million were born in the United States during the period) constituting 24 % of the population.

After World War II, the United States was the world's major industrial, military, and economic power. Economic growth and low unemployment produced conditions conducive to marrying and raising a family. Coupled with this was the Servicemen's Readjustment Act of 1944 (also known as the GI Bill) that subsidized housing, education, and business loans to returning soldiers. With the automobile, housing could be further away from the workplace, allowing the formation of suburbs. The new housing developments were filled with young couples capable of having and supporting larger families. The Baby Boom followed. Many other countries also had increases in births after World War II, but unless otherwise specified, this chapter will refer to the Baby Boom generation of the United States as it has been studied much more.

Baby Boomers are a heterogeneous group with remarkable variability in class and race [3]. However, Schuman and Scott [4] found that, despite heterogeneity, generational cohorts have distinct characteristics that form from major events occurring when the population is between 17 and 25 years old. Baby Boomers are no exception and have identifiable and enduring characteristics. Schewe et al. [5] divide the Baby Boomers into two groups, the Early and Late Boomers. The Early Boomers, born 1946–1954, were the subject of focused attention by advertisers from the start. The enormous success of Dr. Benjamin Spock's *Baby and Child Care*, published in 1946, showed the benefit of marketing to the needs of this group. Early Boomers came of age in 1963–1972 and experienced the assassinations of John Kennedy, Martin Luther King, Jr., and Robert Kennedy; the Vietnam War and campus unrest; the Civil Rights movement; the widespread availability of television; the threat of nuclear annihilation by the Soviets; and a healthy economy. In 1964, 37 % of the American population were Baby Boomers. They overwhelmed all other age groups and defined "The Sixties" with its emphasis on youth, idealism, self-indulgence, sexual freedom, distrust of authority, experimentation with drugs, and concern about unequal rights. The typical Early Boomer values youth, individualism, idealism, stimulation, questioning the established authority, and advocating for causes [6]. Late Boomers, born 1955–1964, were exposed to Watergate, the Arab oil embargo, and a failing economy. While sharing characteristics of Early Boomers, they are also purported to be more narcissistic, inclined to self-help, and,

since the use of credit cards had become acceptable, willing to use debt to satisfy
their consumer needs and desires.

The Sixties are long gone, and Baby Boomers are getting old. In the mid-
twentieth century, about 8–10 % of the United States population was over the age of
65. In 2010, this age group was 13.0 % of the population and is predicted to rise to
18 % by 2030 when all Baby Boomers will be over age 65 [7]. From 2000 to 2010,
the fastest growing age group in the United States was those between the ages of
85–94. As the first Baby Boomers began turning 65 in 2011, these late-age groups
of "old-old" will grow even more over the next decades. The huge number of old
Baby Boomers, many of whom will need specialized services, is expected to exceed
the institutional and financial capacity to provide them. In 1945, there were 12 older
adults being supported by 100 working-age adults; however, in 2030, there will be
35 being supported by 100 of working age. The established programs and customs
to care for the elderly will be insufficient and will meet a generation of older adults
more than willing to cast aside them aside for something better. What comes next
will be determined by people whose values and identity were established during the
1960s and 1970s. Just as they caused a social revolution when young, Baby Boomers
will have a similar impact on the "Golden Years," including the treatment of
advanced age and death.

8.3   Attitudes Toward Youth and Aging

From the generation's name, youth is clearly essential to the identity of Baby Boomers.
This was the first generation to be treated as a distinct cohort by advertisers. They
were studied by marketers; clothes, food, music, literature, and other recreational
items uniquely preferred by the young were produced and sold to them. A close relationship was established between Baby Boomer consumers who demanded items
suitable to their view of life and the producers of consumer goods who were more than
willing to supply this large, generally affluent group with what they wanted or were
told they needed. Youth was paramount. It was not a culture of idle youth, though.
Young Baby Boomers were an idealistic and politically active group whose activities
led to profound changes in society: the end of the war in Vietnam, the abolition of the
draft, environmental awareness, the sexual revolution, the expansion of rights to
women and minorities, the partial acceptance of drug use, and classic rock music.
With their legacy of defining the social desirability of youth, Baby Boomers retain a
strong identification with the youth culture. Studies [8, 9] have shown that over 60 %
of Baby Boomers report feeling younger than their age by about 7–10 years.

How are Baby Boomers dealing with aging? They are the first generation to
observe the increase in longevity since the 1960s and are aware that they will live
many more years than did their grandparents. Just as they fought against the established ways of doing things when young, they do not intend to conform to the traditional ways of being an older adult. A 2002 marketing report [10] emphasized that
in midlife, both men and women Baby Boomers are seeking ways to renew and
preserve their youth. Ever attuned to the needs of this cohort, business is willing to

oblige. The global market in antiaging products is expected to be $191.7 billion in 2019 [11], a 57 % increase over 2013. Antiaging skin products, marketed to Baby Boomers who feel "young at heart," are a $3.6 billion market in the United States, growing by 24 % over 5 years [12]. Other means used to prolong youthfulness are exercise programs, hair coloring, prescription medications (e.g., sildenafil, finasteride), nutraceuticals, growth hormone injections, hobbies identified with youth (e.g., motorcycling), and cosmetic surgery. In addition to looking young, many Baby Boomers intend to remain active and engaged during late life, even after the traditional retirement age of 65. Personal fulfillment, over institutional or establishment obligations, remains very important to Baby Boomers. The path to fulfillment will vary but will include continuing with full-time work, part-time work, travel, periodic education, or the return to hobbies and passions that were not realized in the past. This period in later life will offer opportunities for adventure and exploration. It may be called a Third Age [13], anything but the dreaded term, old age.

Despite efforts to the contrary, Baby Boomers will reluctantly enter a period clearly identifiable as old age. Jones et al. [14] studied the identity processes of mid-age Baby Boomers and found that many are becoming victims of the culture of youth that they created. In their research, Baby Boomers are prone to use identity accommodation to deal with aging. As a result, small signs of aging become exaggerated as definitive evidence of being "old." This leads to hopelessness and discouragement around the aging process. In a 2004 survey [15], British midlife Baby Boomers had very negative associations with being old. Many believed that old age started around age 80, when there are clear signs of physical or cognitive disability. Being old was seen as being decrepit and marginalized. The 2009 Pew Research Center study [16] reported that most American adults agreed that one was old when there was failing health, inability to live independently, inability to drive, and difficulty with stairs. Baby Boomers who were interviewed believed that old age did not start until at least 72. Negative attitudes toward being old are also found among French middle-aged adults [17]. These negative attitudes toward old age were formed by the relatively new phenomenon of having a parent live long enough to enter decrepitude, the result of increased longevity. Caring for aging parents in deteriorating health has been a focus of many mid-age Baby Boomers [18]. In 1800, a 60-year-old woman would have had a 3 % chance of having a living parent; in 1980, this probability was 80 % [19]. The prolonged exposure to an aging parent in poor health and increased dependency has presented a picture of old age that is terrifying to many Baby Boomers. Above all is the fear of dementia or Alzheimer's disease. A 2007 study by Suhr and Kinkela [20] found that personal experience with Alzheimer's disease, particularly with someone with whom you are genetically related, is strongly associated with a fear of developing the disease. Fear of the disease was also associated with depression and negative views of aging. Despite having themselves cared for an aging parent, Baby Boomers are fearful of being a burden to their own family or friends [15]. It remains to be seen if the Baby Boomers' negative view of old age will change as they approach 72 or 80. However, it would not be surprising that some believe suicide is a rational alternative to such an undesirable state.

8.4   Baby Boomers and Death

Baby Boomers cannot ignore the inevitability of death. Just as this group desired to live on its own terms, it will also be important to die on its own terms. They will examine conventions surrounding death and retain or discard them depending on what is personally meaningful. Baby Boomers do accept death, but a prolonged dying process is feared and to be avoided. A "good death" is desirable. What is a "good death"? Charles Garfield [21], an expert on providing emotional support to people with life-threatening illnesses, characterizes a good death in the following manner:

- Experience as little pain as possible.
- Recognize and resolve interpersonal conflicts.
- Satisfy any remaining wishes that are consistent with their present condition.
- Review life to find meaning.
- Hand over control to a trusted person, someone committed to helping them have the kind of death they desire.
- Be protected from needless procedures that serve to only dehumanize and demean without much or any benefit.
- Decide how social and how alert they want to be.

For many Baby Boomers, this was not how their elderly parents or other loved ones died. The ideal death should be quick, peaceful, at home, and dignified. Baby Boomers will take control of the dying process, insist on death with dignity, and not leave this to chance [22]. For some, suicide will be an acceptable and dignified way to avoid a significant decline in the quality of life and realize a "good death" [23].

Baby Boomers are leading the way in bringing death and dying into the open and under their control. Since 2011, the Death Cafe movement has been gaining ground, and over 2500 Death Cafes have taken place worldwide [24]. These are non-clinical groups where people gather to "eat cake, drink tea, and discuss death" with the goal "to increase awareness of death with a view to helping people make the most of their (finite) lives." As a generation courted and catered to by marketers, Baby Boomers believe that the death and mourning processes can and should be personalized to suit the needs of the individual. This may involve a nontraditional funeral ceremony [25] or being allowed to legally make a decision to end their life. A May 2015 poll by Gallup [26] found that 68 % of Americans support legalization of physician-assisted suicide for terminally ill patients, a nearly 20-point increase since 2013. This increasing support is being driven by Baby Boomers who insist on the right to exercise control over their bodies [27]. The issue of control is crucial to Baby Boomers. Peter Levitan mentioned it as an important factor in his decision to kill himself. Skaff [28] hypothesized that the Baby Boomers' enhanced sense of control developed from having grown up in a time of affluence and opportunity and having seen the impact that they had on society when young. In any case, there will be more than a few Baby Boomers intent on *not* dying as their parents did, but taking control of their life's end, even if it means killing themselves.

8.5 Baby Boomers and Suicide Risk in Late Life

Baby Boomers have had a long-standing relationship with suicide. Their suicide rate during adolescence, particularly among young white males, was much higher than previous generations [29]. This increase was attributed to drug use, depression, and competition among a large cohort for finite resources [30]. The high rate of suicide among Baby Boomers continues. From 1999 to 2010, the suicide rates of adults between ages 50–59 increased 50 % to over 19 per 100,000 population [31]. Middle-age is typically a time of lower suicide rates, but apparently not for aging Baby Boomers. Hempstead and Phillips [32] attributed this increase partly to the financial and employment problems stemming from the Great Recession and partly to being a member of a cohort that has a lower threshold than older generations for resorting to suicide when times get tough. As Baby Boomers enter old age, they will encounter circumstances that increase the risk of suicide. While some may be unavoidable factors of aging, others will be specific to the Baby Boom generation.

8.5.1 Social Isolation

Social isolation [33, 34] and unmarried status, particularly for men [30, 35], are well-known risk factors for suicide. In the past, people entered late life being married. This is not true for Baby Boomers. A 2009 survey found that one-third were unmarried in midlife [36]. Most were divorced or had never married. Unlike previous generations when marriage was the norm, Baby Boomers chose other options such as foregone marriage, divorce, cohabitation outside of marriage, and non-marital childbearing [37]. Many Baby Boomers will end up living alone in late life [19], but in need of assistance as cognitive and physical problems develop. Traditionally, a spouse or family member provided this care. For Baby Boomers who are unmarried, this responsibility will fall on their children or, lacking available children, most likely strangers who are paid to provide care. Baby Boomers had fewer children than their parents, and, with the increased rate of divorce, their children may have with a weakened sense of filial obligation [38]. Therefore, children will not be a reliable source of support. Paid care providers may suffice for some, but will be financially or personally unacceptable for others. Van Orden et al. [39] proposed an interpersonal theory of suicide with the major factors leading to suicide being thwarted belongingness (lack of social connectedness) and perceived burdensomeness. These two speak to the many Baby Boomers in old age who will be living alone and in need of care that may not be easily provided. For them, thoughts of suicide will not be rare.

8.5.2 Substance Use

Baby Boomers were the "turned on" generation. Substance abuse rates are highest for those born between 1953 and 1964 [40]. The use of drugs was an acceptable means of recreation and enlightenment. Baby Boomers have had less substance abuse since leaving young adulthood, but it is still comparatively high. There has been a dramatic increase in the rate of accidental drug overdoses in mid-age Baby Boomers [41, 42]. A group comfortable with using psychoactive drugs now has access to widely abused opioid analgesics. Colliver et al. [43] project that from 2000 to 2020, there will be over 50 % increase in the rate of illicit drug use in people over age 50. Duncan et al. [44] examined admissions for alcohol and substance abuse in people 55 years of age and older from 1998 to 2006. Admissions for alcohol abuse remained stable, while those for other substances increased substantially. Aging Baby Boomers are using mood-altering drugs at much higher rates than previous cohorts of similar age. Substance use is highly associated with suicide [45], and the unprecedented degree of drug use among aging Baby Boomers will be another factor increasing this generation's risk for suicide.

8.5.3 Chronic Illnesses

Having a chronic debilitating physical illness in old age is associated with increased suicide risk [46, 47]. In general, Baby Boomers are wealthier and better educated than previous generations, but their old age is likely to be one plagued by poor health. Our longer life expectancy has led to a prolonged period at the end of life with severe health problems. In addition, while some baby Boomers are embarking on a program of exercise and healthy living to prolong their youthfulness and vitality, as a whole, this cohort at midlife is in poorer health than previous generations. Martin et al. [48] looked at the health and functioning in mid-age of Baby Boomers compared to previous cohorts. Although Baby Boomers initially had less mortality and poor health from 1982 to 2006, since 1997 there have been increases in the rates of cardiovascular disease, obesity, lung problems, and diabetes mellitus. These increases may be partially accounted for by increased awareness and reporting, but the authors conclude that given their educational opportunities and the advancement in medical science, the Baby Boomers should be doing better health-wise. In 2013, King et al. [49] reported that after controlling for age, sex, race, and socioeconomic factors, 46–64-year-olds had significantly more obesity, diabetes mellitus, hypertension, and hypercholesterolemia than the prior generation. One-half of Baby Boomers surveyed had no regular physical exercise. Other studies have borne out that late-life Baby Boomers will have higher rates of chronic disease and disability than their parents. Wang et al. [50] predict that by 2030, 86.3 % of adults will be overweight or obese. The United States is not unique; Wild et al. [51] looked at the worldwide prevalence of diabetes mellitus and estimate that in 2030 nearly 50 % of adults over age 65 in developed countries will have diabetes, even if current rates of obesity are unchanged. Nemetz et al. [52] examined the autopsy findings of 3237 younger residents (ages 16–64) of Olmsted County, Minnesota, from 1981 to 2004 who died from external causes. From 1981 to 1995, the grade of coronary artery disease declined in the autopsy specimens; however, after 2000, it increased. The authors attributed this unexpected finding to the increased prevalence of obesity and diabetes mellitus. If these findings are confirmed, aging Baby Boomers may be faced with increasing morbidity secondary to cardiovascular disease, reversing a trend that started in the 1960s.

A major concern among the aging Baby Boomer population is cognitive impairment and dementia. The Aging, Demographics, and Memory Study [53, 54] estimated that for people over the age of 71, the prevalence of dementia is 13.9 %, of Alzheimer's disease is 9.7 %, and of cognitive impairment but not dementia is 22.2 %. At these rates, in 2030, 9.7 million elderly Baby Boomers will have with dementia and another 15.5 million will have mild cognitive impairment. To the Alzheimer's Association, Baby Boomers are "Generation Alzheimer's" and will be defined by the disease. For Baby Boomers who have watched their parents or elderly relatives decline with a dementing illness, this is a frightening prospect. The media has reported on some notable cases [55, 56] where suicide was a way of avoiding ending up in the regressed and helpless state of late-stage dementia. Studies [57–59] have shown an increase in suicide attempts after the diagnosis of Alzheimer's disease, often unrelated to the coexistence of a mood disorder. A failing of the body and mind with advanced age will not be a rare occurrence to Baby Boomers. For a group that prizes youth and fulfillment, suicide may seem like a reasonable choice over what is perceived as helpless decrepitude.

8.5.4   Financial Difficulties

For some Baby Boomers, late life will be a time to work at will, travel, explore interests, invest in a hobby, or relax in comfort [13, 60]. While wealthier than previous generations, a 2005 [61] report from the Pew Research Center found significant financial disparity among Baby Boomers. Of the over 3000 interviewed, 24 % expected to have just enough money to meet basic expenses when old, and another 17 % did not expect to have even that much. Among 954 Baby Boomers interviewed in a 2011 AARP survey [9], 44 % were dissatisfied with what they saved for retirement. By the life path models of the Employee Benefit Research Institute [62], over 40 % of Baby Boomers will not have sufficient resources to pay for basic retirement expenses and uninsured health costs. Longevity risk, nursing home expenses, and home health-care costs can compromise the financial resources of even those Baby Boomers who have diligently saved for retirement [63]. While some may choose to work longer, currently 50 % of retirements are not planned or expected [64]; many people leave work because of physical disability, family care responsibilities, and employer changes. Willis and Schaie [65] studied the cognitive functioning of mid-age Baby Boomers and question whether the large number who wants to continue working into their 70s will be cognitively competent to do so.

Late Boomers (1955–1964) appear to be saving less for retirement than Early Boomers [66]. Rhee and Boivie [67] found that 40.7 % of heads of household between the ages of 55–64 do not even have a retirement account. Baby Boomers have had the financial advantages of a prosperous economy during the 1950s and 1960s, good educational opportunities, and, for some, a defined benefit pension plan. These financial advantages have been countered by being the first generation to be isolated by advertisers and encouraged to buy and also being the first group of adults to have easy access to credit cards. While the median income of Baby Boomers is higher than other adult age groups, the number of bankruptcy filings has been rising faster in this group (even before the Great Recession) [68]. Among Baby Boomers, those who are minorities, less educated, and less employed will have higher poverty rates in old age [69]. Eggebeen and Sturgeon [70] found a substantial portion of midlife Baby Boomers with low or modest income (60 % of whites, 80 % of blacks, 80–85 % of Hispanics).

On a higher level are the persistent reports of fiscal catastrophe as the large number of Baby Boomers claim Social Security and Medicare. In 2030, these two expenditures are estimated to cost an unaffordable 15 % of the United States' economic output [68]. Possibly as a result, Baby Boomers [9] are more pessimistic about the future economy. A large group of Baby Boomers will have insufficient financial assets in old age and will have to take drastic measures to reduce their standard of living. That this will lead to suicide for some is already evidenced by the increased rate of suicide in Baby Boomers since 1999 that has been partly attributable to the Great Recession [32]. The projected depletion of his financial assets by age 83 was one reason that Peter Levitan chose age 80 to kill himself.

8.6 Conclusions

Suicide rates were relatively high for the Baby Boom generation during their youth and mid-age and are expected to remain so when they are elderly. In many cases, suicide will be secondary to substance abuse or depression. These are treatable. Efforts to identify and appropriately intervene should be able to prevent some of these suicides where judgment is likely impaired.

However, Baby Boomers are likely to face other circumstances related to increased suicide risk such as social isolation, deteriorated physical and cognitive health, and exhausted financial resources. It is debatable whether these are amenable to mental health interventions. Faced with these circumstances and little realistic hope of improvement, some Baby Boomers will question whether continuing to live is worthwhile and decide to kill themselves. This will be rational suicide. Baby Boomers will decide that their parents' manner of dying, prolonged and at the mercy of institutions and medical technology, is no longer acceptable. Life is about youth, freedom, activity, and self-fulfillment. If one can no longer live like this, death becomes an option, and dying at the time and manner of one's choosing is an even more reasonable option.

The Baby Boom generation is so large and diverse that although most Baby Boomers did not become hippies, take LSD, go to Woodstock, march in Civil Rights protests, or confront police on campus, the minority who did had a large impact on society. Similarly, the conclusion of this chapter is not that most Baby Boomers will consider rational suicide. Rather, because of external circumstances or personal belief, a significant minority will consider suicide to be an intelligent and rational act in the face of an irreversible worsening in the quality of life. We will soon be encountering older patients or clients who present suicide in a manner that is outside the realm of our typical clinical experience. While we may agree or disagree with the rationality of these beliefs, it is our responsibility to address them in a compassionate and therapeutic manner. How to do so can be found in the other chapters of this book. The aging of the Baby Boom generation will cause us to modify our clinical approach to "geriatric" patients. We, like the rest of society, will also be forced to evaluate our preconceptions about old age and how we deal with dying and death in the face of increased longevity.

References

1. Levitan P. Boomercide: from Woodstock to suicide. Portland: Portlandia Press; 2012.
2. Colby SL, Ortman JM. The Baby Boom cohort in the United States: 2012 to 2060. In: Current Population Reports. U.S. Census Bureau, Washington, DC. 2014. http://www.census.gov/content/dam/Census/library/publications/2014/demo/p25-1141.pdf. Accessed 7 Nov 2015.
3. Morgan DL. Facts and figures about the baby boom. Generations. 1998;22(1):10–5.
4. Schuman H, Scott J. Generations and collective memories. Am Soc Rev. 1989;54(3):359–81.
5. Schewe CD, Noble SM. Market segmentation by cohorts: the value and validity of cohorts in America and abroad. J Mark Manage. 2000;16:129–42. doi:10.1362/026725700785100479.
6. Stewart AJ, Torges CM. Social, historical, and developmental influences on the psychology of the baby boom at midlife. In: Whitbourne SK, Willis SL, editors. The Baby Boomers grow up: contemporary perspectives on midlife. Mahwah: Lawrence Erlbaum Associates; 2006. p. 23–44.
7. Werner CA. The older population: 2010. U.S. Census Bureau, Washington, DC. 2011. http://www.census.gov/prod/cen2010/briefs/c2010br-09.pdf. Accessed 9 Nov 2015.
8. Cohn D, Taylor P. Baby Boomers approach 65—Glumly. In: Social & Demographic Trends Report. Pew Research Center, Washington, DC. 2010. http://www.pewsocialtrends.org/2010/12/20/baby-boomers-approach-65-glumly/. Accessed 9 Nov 2015.
9. AARP and GFK Custom Research North America: Baby Boomers envision what's next? AARP, Washington, DC. 2011. http://assets.aarp.org/rgcenter/general/boomers-envision-retirement-2011.pdf. Accessed 9 Nov 2015.
10. Weiss MJ. Chasing youth. Am Demogr. 2002;24(9):34–41.
11. Anti-aging Market—Global Industry Analysis, Size, Share, Growth, Trends and Forecast, 2013–2019. Transparency Market Research, Albany, New York. 2014. http://www.transparencymarketresearch.com/anti-aging-market.html. Accessed November 9, 2015.
12. Alexander A. Anti-aging rides wave of sales from Baby Boomers. 2013. http://www.drugstorenews.com/article/anti-aging-rides-wave-sales-baby-boomers. Accessed 2 Nov 2015.
13. Sadler W. The third age: six principles of growth and renewal after forty. Boston: Da Capo Press; 2001.
14. Jones KM, Whitbourne SK, Skultety KM. Identity processes and the transition to midlife among baby boomers. In: Whitbourne SK, Willis SL, editors. The Baby Boomers grow up: contemporary perspectives on midlife. Mahwah: Lawrence Erlbaum Associates; 2006. p. 149–63.
15. Harkin J, Huber J. Eternal youths: how the Baby Boomers are having their time again. London: Demos; 2004.
16. Taylor P, Morin R, Parker K, Cohn D, Wang WW. Growing old in America: expectations vs. reality. Pew Research Center, Washington, DC. 2009. http://www.pewsocialtrends.org/2009/06/29/growing-old-in-america-expectations-vs-reality/. Accessed 10 Nov 2015.
17. Nicholson H. French Revolution. The Times (London). 2002.
18. Fingerman KL, Dolbin-MacNab M. The Baby Boomers and their parents: cohort influences and intergenerational ties. In: Whitbourne SK, Willis SL, editors. The Baby Boomers grow up: contemporary perspectives on midlife. Mahwah: Lawrence Erlbaum Associates; 2006. p. 237–59.

19. Pillemer K, Suitor JJ. Baby boom families: relations with aging parents. Generations. 1998;22(1):65–9.
20. Suhr JA, Kinkela JH. Perceived threat of Alzheimer disease (AD): the role of personal experience with AD. Alzheimer Dis Assoc Disord. 2007;21(3):225–31. doi:10.1097/WAD.0b013e31813e6683.
21. Garfield C. Seven keys to a good death. In: Family & Couples. The Greater Good Science Center, University of California at Berkeley, Berkeley. 2014. http://greatergood.berkeley.edu/article/item/seven_keys_to_good_death. Accessed 14 Nov 2015.
22. Kadlec D. A good death: how Boomers will change the world a final time. In: TIME. Time Inc.,NewYork.2013.http://business.time.com/2013/08/14/a-good-death-how-boomers-will-change-the-world-a-final-time/. Accessed 2 Nov 2015.
23. Carlson WL, Ong TD. Suicide in later life: failed treatment or rational choice. Clin Geriatr Med. 2014;30(3):553–76. doi:10.1016/j.cger.2014.04.009.
24. Death Cafe. http://deathcafe.com/what/. Accessed 5 Dec 2015.
25. Queenan J. I don't do grief. Am Spect. 2001;34(5):53–8.
26. Dugan A. In U.S., support up for doctor-assisted suicide. Gallup Inc., Washington, DC. 2015. http://www.gallup.com/poll/183425/support-doctor-assisted-suicide.aspx. Accessed 14 Nov 2015.
27. Pettypiece S. Boomers push doctor-assisted dying in end-of-life revolt. 2013. http://www.bloomberg.com/news/articles/2013-04-11/boomers-push-doctor-assisted-dying-in-end-of-life-revolt. Accessed 14 Nov 2015.
28. Skaff MM. The view from the driver's seat: sense of control in the Baby Boomers at midlife. In: Whitbourne SK, Willis SL, editors. The Baby Boomers grow up: contemporary perspectives on midlife. Mahwah: Lawrence Erlbaum Associates; 2006. p. 185–204.
29. Suicide—United States, 1970–1980. Morbidity and Mortality Weekly Report. Centers for Disease Control, Atlanta. 1985;34(24):353–357.
30. Phillips JA, Robin AV, Nugent CN, Idler EL. Understanding recent changes in suicide rates among the middle-aged: period or cohort effects? Public Health Rep. 2010;125(5):680–8.
31. Sullivan EM, Annest JL, Luo F, Simon TR, Dahlberg LL. Suicide among adults aged 35–64 years—United States, 1999–2010. Morb Mortal Wkly Rep. 2013;62(17):321–325.
32. Hempstead KA, Phillips JA. Rising suicide among adults aged 40–64 years: the role of job and financial circumstances. Am J Prev Med. 2015;48(5):491–500. doi:10.1016/j.amepre.2014.11.006.
33. Durkheim E. Suicide: a study in sociology. Glencoe: Free Press; 1951 (Original work published 1897).
34. Breault KD. Suicide in America: a test of Durkheim's theory of religious and family integration, 1933–1980. Am J Sociol. 1986;92(3):628–56. doi:10.1086/228544.
35. Denney JT, Rogers RG, Krueger PM, Wadsworth T. Adult suicide mortality in the United States: marital status, family size, socioeconomic status, and differences by sex. Soc Sci Q. 2009;90(5):1167–85. doi:10.1111/j.1540-6237.2009.00652.x.
36. Lin I-F, Brown SL. Unmarried boomers confront old age: a national portrait. Gerontologist. 2012;52(2):153–65. doi:10.1093/geront/gnr141.
37. Cherlin AJ. Demographic trends in the United States: a review of research in the 2000s. J Marriage Fam. 2010;72(3):403–19. doi:10.1111/j.1741-3737.2010.00710.x.
38. Fingerman KL, Pillemer KA, Silverstein M, Suitor JJ. The Baby Boomers' intergenerational relationships. Gerontologist. 2012;52(2):199–209. doi:10.1093/geront/gnr139.
39. Van Orden KA, Witte TK, Cukrowicz KC, Braithwaite SR, Selby EA, Joiner Jr TE. The interpersonal theory of suicide. Psychol Rev. 2010;117(2):575–600. doi:10.1037/a0018697.
40. Piazza JR, Charles ST. Mental health among the Baby Boomers. In: Whitbourne SK, Willis SL, editors. The Baby Boomers grow up: contemporary perspectives on midlife. Mahwah: Lawrence Erlbaum Associates; 2006. p. 111–48.
41. Warner M, Chen LH, Makuc DM, Anderson RN, Miniño AM. Drug poisoning deaths in the United States, 1980–2008. NCHS Data Brief. 2011;81:1–8.
42. Elinson Z. Aging Baby Boomers hold on to drug habits. Wall Street J. 2015.

43. Colliver JD, Compton WM, Gfroerer JC, Condon T. Projecting drug use among aging Baby Boomers in 2020. Ann Epidemiol. 2006;16(4):257–65. doi:10.1016/j.annepidem.2005.08.003.
44. Duncan DF, Nicholson T, White JB, Bradley DB, Bonaguro J. The Baby Boomer effect: changing patterns of substance abuse among adults ages 55 and older. J Aging Soc Policy. 2010;22(3):237–48. doi:10.1080/08959420.2010.485511.
45. Borges G, Walters EE, Kessler RC. Associations of substance use, abuse, and dependence with subsequent suicidal behavior. Am J Epidemiol. 2000;151(8):781–9. doi:10.1093/oxfordjourn-als.aje.a010278.
46. Fässberg MM, Cheung G, Canetto SS, et al. A systematic review of physical illness, functional disability, and suicidal behaviour among older adults. Aging Ment Health. 2015;20(2):166–94. doi:10.1080/13607863.2015.1083945.
47. Wiktorsson S, Berg AI, Wilhelmson K, Van Orden K, Duberstein P, Waern M. Assessing the role of physical illness in young old and older old suicide attempters. Int J Geriatr Psychiatry. 2016;31(7):771–4. doi:10.1002/gps.4390.
48. Martin LG, Freedman VA, Schoeni RF, Andreski PM. Health and functioning among Baby Boomers approaching 60. J Gerontol B Psychol Sci Soc Sci. 2009;64(3):369–77. doi:10.1093/geronb/gbn040.
49. King DE, Matheson E, Chirina S, Shankar A, Broman-Fulks J. The status of Baby Boomers' health in the United States: the healthiest generation? [letter]. JAMA Intern Med. 2013;173(5): 385–6.
50. Wang Y, Beydoun MA, Liang L, Caballero B, Kumanyika SK. Will all Americans become overweight or obese? Estimating the progression and cost of the US obesity epidemic. Obesity. 2008;16(10):2323–30. doi:10.1038/oby.2008.351.
51. Wild S, Roglic G, Green A, Sicree R, King H. Global prevalence of diabetes estimates for the year 2000 and projections for 2030. Diabetes Care. 2004;27(5):1047–53. doi:10.2337/diacare.27.5.1047.
52. Nemetz PN, Roger VL, Ransom JE, Bailey KR, Edwards WD, Leibson CL. Recent trends in the prevalence of coronary disease: a population-based autopsy study of nonnatural deaths. Arch Intern Med. 2008;168(3):264–70. doi:10.1001/archinternmed.2007.79.
53. Plassman BL, Langa KM, Fisher GG, et al. Prevalence of dementia in the United States: the aging, demographics, and memory study. Neuroepidemiology. 2007;29(1–2):125–32. doi:10.1159/000109998.
54. Plassman BL, Langa KM, Fisher GG, et al. Prevalence of cognitive impairment without dementia in the United States. Ann Intern Med. 2008;148(6):427–34. doi:10.7326/0003-4819-148-6-200803180-00005.
55. Henig RM. The last day of her life. The New York Times. 2015.
56. Fallon C. Terry Pratchett, Popular Fantasy Author, Dead at 66. 2015. http://www.huffington-post.com/2015/03/12/terry-pratchet-dead_n_6489502.html. Accessed 5 Dec 2015.
57. Barak Y, Aizenberg D. Suicide amongst Alzheimer's disease patients: a 10-year survey. Dement Geriatr Cogn Disord. 2002;14(2):101–3. doi:10.1159/000064931.
58. Erlangsen A, Zarit SH, Conwell Y. Hospital-diagnosed dementia and suicide: a longitudinal study using prospective, nationwide register data. Am J Geriatr Psychiatr. 2008;16(3):220–8. doi:10.1097/01.JGP.0000302930.75387.7e.
59. Seyfried LS, Kales HC, Ignacio RV, Conwell Y, Valenstein M. Predictors of suicide in patients with dementia. Alzheimers Dement. 2011;7(6):567–73. doi:10.1016/j.jalz.2011.01.006.
60. Bass SA. Emergence of the third age: toward a productive aging society. J Aging Soc Policy. 2000;11(2–3):7–17. doi:10.1300/J031v11n02_02.
61. Taylor P, Funk C, Kennedy C. Baby Boomers approach age 60: from the Age of Aquarius to the age of responsibility. Pew Research Center, Washington, DC. 2005. http://www.pewsocial-trends.org/2005/12/08/baby-boomers-from-the-age-of-aquarius-to-the-age-of-responsibility/. Accessed 10 Nov 2015.
62. VanDerhei J. Retirement income adequacy for Boomers and Gen Xers: evidence from the 2012 EBRI Retirement Security Projection Model®. EBRI Notes. 2012;33(5):2–14.

63. VanDerhei J. Retirement savings shortfalls: evidence from EBRI's Retirement Security Projection Model®. Employee Benefit Research Institute, Washington, DC. 2015. http://www.ebri.org/pdf/briefspdf/EBRI_IB_410_Feb15_RSShrtfls.pdf. Accessed 28 Nov 2015.
64. Helman R, Copeland C, VanDerhei J. The 2015 Retirement Confidence Survey: having a retirement savings plan a key factor in Americans' retirement confidence. In: EBRI Issue Brief. Employee Benefit Research Institute, Washington, D.C. April 2015. http://www.ebri.org/pdf/briefspdf/EBRI_IB_413_Apr15_RCS-2015.pdf. Accessed 28 Nov 2015.
65. Willis SL, Schaie KW. Cognitive functioning in the Baby Boomers: longitudinal and cohort effects. In: Whitbourne SK, Willis SL, editors. The Baby Boomers grow up: contemporary perspectives on midlife. Mahwah: Lawrence Erlbaum Associates; 2006. p. 205–34.
66. DeVaney SA, Chiremba ST. Comparing the retirement savings of the Baby Boomers and other cohorts. U.S. Bureau of Labor Statistics, Washington, DC. 2005. http://stats.bls.gov/opub/mlr/cwc/comparing-the-retirement-savings-of-the-baby-boomers-and-other-cohorts.pdf. Accessed 7 Nov 2015.
67. Rhee N, Boivie I. The continuing retirement savings crisis. National Institute on Retirement Security, Washington, DC. 2015. http://laborcenter.berkeley.edu/pdf/2015/RetirementSavingsCrisis.pdf. Accessed 7 Nov 2015.
68. Greenblatt A. Aging Baby Boomers. CQ Researcher. 2007;17(37):865–88.
69. Butrica BA, Toder EJ, Toohey DJ. Boomers at the bottom: how will low income Boomers cope with retirement? AARP Public Policy Institute, Washington, DC. 2008. http://www.urban.org/sites/default/files/alfresco/publication-pdfs/1001217_low-income_boomers.pdf. Accessed 17 Nov 2015.
70. Eggebeen DJ, Sturgeon S. Demography of the Baby Boomers. In: Whitbourne SK, Willis SL, editors. The Baby Boomers grow up: contemporary perspectives on midlife. Mahwah: Lawrence Erlbaum Associates; 2006. p. 3–22.

Who Are the Elderly Who Want to End Their Lives?

9

Gary Cheung and Frederick Sundram

> *"There is but one truly serious philosophical problem, and that is suicide"*
>
> Albert Camus

Steve was 66 years old when he was given a diagnosis of terminal prostate cancer and had 18 months to live. His wife of 20 years suffered from Parkinson's disease. Following the cancer diagnosis, Steve and his wife decided to form a suicide pact. They followed the plastic bag method described in Derek Humphrey's book "Final Exit" (Chapter 22) because neither euthanasia nor physician-assisted suicide was legal in their country. They left a suicide note clearly documenting they had decided to die because of their suffering. Steve's wife died but he survived; and he was later charged by the police for aiding his wife with ending her life. He appeared in court a year later. By now he had another 6 months to live. He was physically weak and suffered from a lot of pain. The media coverage of the court case started to bother him. He decided to hang himself in the garage.

John was 80 years old and lived a happy life with his wife in a retirement village until he was diagnosed with terminal bladder cancer. He had multiple visits to the hospital in the 6 months leading up to his death. John had always been a strong supporter of euthanasia but neither euthanasia nor physician-assisted suicide was legal in his country. In the month prior to his death, his quality of life was poor. He was suffering from a number of physical symptoms including shortness of breath, difficulty swallowing, and pain. He requested the local hospice service to stop his

G. Cheung, F.R.A.N.Z.C.P. (✉) • F. Sundram, Ph.D., F.R.C.Psych.
Department of Psychological Medicine, The University of Auckland, Level 12,
Auckland Hospital Support Building, Grafton, Auckland 1142, New Zealand
e-mail: g.cheung@auckland.ac.nz; f.sundram@auckland.ac.nz

© Springer International Publishing Switzerland 2017
R.E. McCue, M. Balasubramaniam (eds.), *Rational Suicide in the Elderly*,
DOI 10.1007/978-3-319-32672-6_9

treatment so it would "hurry things up a bit". It was particularly stressful the day before John decided to end his life. He vomited in bed and his wife had to clean up the "mess". The next morning, he was found dead in his car in the garage. He died of carbon monoxide poisoning.

These cases are examples of what may be considered a *rational decision* to proceed with suicide; and there are many more but these cases serve as illustrative examples. The coroners who investigated these cases gave a suicide verdict. These were in a country where euthanasia and/or physician-assisted suicide (PAS) was not available for people suffering from a terminal medical condition.

9.1   Definition of Rational Suicide

Siegel listed three criteria for rational suicide (1) a realistic assessment of the situation; (2) mental processes unimpaired by psychological illness or severe emotional distress; and (3) a motivational basis that would be understandable to uninvolved observers [1]. Werth and Cobia also provided a similar definition for rational suicide which is (1) an unremittingly hopeless condition; (2) a suicidal decision made as a free choice; (3) an informed decision-making process [2]. Although one cannot speculate on whether these two men had unimpaired mental processes, their decision to end their lives is understandable given their ongoing suffering, expected future deterioration and the terminal nature of their conditions. These two men would likely have fulfilled the criteria for euthanasia/PAS if they lived in a country where these practices were legal. For example, the Dutch's "Termination of Life on Request and Assisted Suicide (Review Procedures) Act" (2002) states that euthanasia and PAS are not punishable if the attending physician acts in accordance with criteria of due care:

1. The patient's request should be voluntary and well considered.
2. The patient's suffering should be unbearable and without prospect of improvement.
3. The patient should be informed about his situation and prospects.
4. There are no reasonable alternatives.
5. Another independent physician should be consulted.
6. The termination of life should be performed with due medical care and attention.

Mak and Elwyn suggested that suffering is multi-dimensional and related to the patient's illness experience; and an euthanasia request is an expression of suffering [3]. Rational suicide is by no means a Sisyphean task and in order to gain insight and address the question "Who are the elderly who want to end their lives?", we reviewed the rational suicide and euthanasia/PAS literature in older people, particularly from countries where these practices are legal.

The euthanasia/PAS literature in older people was derived from four sources (1) euthanasia/PAS cases and statistics in countries/states where these practices are legal; (2) requests for euthanasia/PAS in people with terminal illness; (3) attitudes towards euthanasia/PAS in patients without terminal illness; and (4) attitudes towards euthanasia/PAS in the general public. Hypothetical scenarios are often used in research exploring attitudes towards euthanasia/PAS; however, it is important to note that hypothetical scenarios may not correspond to actual reactions of those who are terminally ill or wanting death [4].

9.2   Epidemiology

The incidence of rational suicide is unknown but a recent systematic literature review found the rates of PAS among all deaths ranged from 0.1 to 0.2 % in the US states (Oregon, Washington, and Montana) and Luxembourg to 1.8–2.9 % in the Netherlands [5]. The total number of reported cases and the percentage of reported assisted deaths of all deaths increased over time in countries and states where euthanasia/PAS has been legal for longer periods (Belgium, the Netherlands, Switzerland, and Oregon). However, this observation is likely to be a result of more complete reporting to the authorities.

9.3   Age and Ageing

The literature on euthanasia and PAS from the Netherlands, Belgium, and Oregon suggests the oldest old (age ≥85) do not die as a result of cuthanasia and/or PAS [6–12]. Moreover, it has been suggested that some older people may believe they are more vulnerable to possible abuses if euthanasia became an acceptable practice [13].

Most of the 1684 cases of euthanasia/PAS in the Netherlands from 1984 to 1993 were performed in the 70–79 age group (27 %) and 60–69 age group (25 %), followed by the 50–59 age group (16 %) and 80+ age group (14 %) [6]. Similarly, the findings of five Dutch studies from 1991 to 1997 concluded that euthanasia and PAS occurred most frequently in the age group of 65–79 years, followed by the age group of 50–64 years [8]. In the first 5 years after euthanasia was legalised in 2002 in the Netherlands and Belgium, the majority of the cases were in the 60–79 age group (the Netherlands: 53 % and Belgium: 53 %), whereas 12 % of the cases in the Netherlands and 18 % in Belgium were in the oldest old group (age ≥80) [9]. Smets et al. reported people older than the age of 80 were under-represented among euthanasia cases in Belgium between 2002 and 2007 [10]. In the US, participants of the Death with Dignity Act who died in Oregon and Washington from 2009 to 2012 were highest in the 65–74 age group, followed by the 75–84 and 55–64 age groups [12].

In regard to attitude towards euthanasia/PAS, participants in the Longitudinal Ageing Study Amsterdam (aged ≥64; $n=3615$, longitudinal sampling over three time-points from 2001 to 2009) were asked whether they could imagine requesting their physician to end their life ("euthanasia"), or imagine asking for a pill to end their life if they became tired of living in the absence of a severe disease ("end-of-life pill") [14]. They found the 64–74 age group was more likely to have a positive attitude towards euthanasia (OR = 1.71, 95 % CI = 1.25–2.34) compared to the ≥85 age group; however, there was no significant difference between the 75–84 age group and ≥85 age group.

The age factor is different in Switzerland. The Swiss "Right-to-Die" society EXIT was founded in 1982 to assist suicide by providing terminally ill members with a lethal dosage of barbiturates on request. Frei et al. reported that EXIT assisted suicides from 1992 to 1997 (n = 35) had a significantly higher mean age (men: 75 vs. 50 and women: 74 vs. 52) compared with non-EXIT suicides (n = 425) [15]. A more recent Swiss study with a larger sample of assisted suicide from 2003 to 2008 (age 25–64: n = 439 and age 65–94: n = 862) found that the rates of assisted suicide increased with increasing age in every 10-year age-band between the ages of 25–34 years (0.3 per 100,000 95 % CI = 0.2–0.5) and 85–94 years (38.9 per 100,000 95 % CI = 32.8–46.2) [16]. Fischer et al. also found the proportions of older people who had assisted suicide and suffering from non-fatal diseases showed a steady increase over a 15-year period (from 1990 to 2004) in Switzerland [17]. They suggested that "weariness of life" may be a more common reason for assisted suicide. In the Netherlands, request for euthanasia and PAS in the absence of a severe disease was investigated in a sample of nursing home physicians, general practitioners, and clinical specialists [18]. Twenty-nine such requests (age ≥60) were identified and they were most common in the 80–89 age group (38 %), followed by the 70–79 age group (31 %), 90–97 age group (21 %), and 60–69 age group (10 %). Their reasons for the requests were being through with life (55 %), physical decline (55 %), tired of living (48 %), and no purpose in life (41 %). In another Dutch study, general practitioners reported that "being tired of living" also played a major role in 28 % of the people who requested euthanasia but they had no severe physical or psychiatric disease [19].

It has been argued that age in itself may not be the most important predictor of attitude towards euthanasia/PAS, but it is mediated by religious beliefs. A US study (n = 1311; age 18–29: 40 %; age 30–49: 33 %; age 50–64: 15 %; and age 65–96: 11 %) found older peoples' greater focus on religious beliefs was significant in explaining their lower levels of acceptance of PAS, as compared to younger people [20]. Another US study (n = 5534) with data collected in a general survey of participants over a 15-year period from 1977 to 1991 found the youngest age group (age 45–49) had the lowest percentage (39 %), whereas the oldest group (age 80–85) had the highest percentage (48 %) against euthanasia [13]. However, the most significant predictors of euthanasia found in this study were attendance at religious services. Similarly, a study in Texas, US (age ≥60; Mini Mental State Examination ≥18; Mexican American: n = 100; and non-Hispanic White: n = 108) found age was not a significant factor for supporting PAS; whereas religiosity plays a role in non-Hispanic White but not Mexican American [21]. Religious factors and euthanasia/PAS are discussed in more detail in a later section.

9.4   Gender

Specific information on gender and euthanasia/PAS in older people is not routinely reported in the literature, but the majority of reported euthanasia/PAS cases (of all ages) in the Netherlands, Belgium, Oregon (except in 2011), and Washington were men (range 50.6–57%) [5, 12]. Battin et al. found the rate ratio of PAS (of all ages) was 1.0 in women and 1.1 in men in Oregon from 1998 to 2006 and 1.0 in women and 1.3 in men in the Netherlands in 2005 [11]. In the nursing home setting, a Dutch survey of physicians found euthanasia and PAS ($n=69$; mean age$=71$) was performed on more men (65%) than women (35%) [22].

The situation in Switzerland is different where more women than men died by assisted suicide. For example, a Swiss study of EXIT deaths from 1990 to 2000 found women were overrepresented (in comparison with all other deaths and all other suicides) in the 65–84 year group [23]. In the ≥85 year group, men were overrepresented in comparison with all other deaths, whereas women were overrepresented in comparison with all other suicides. The 2003–2008 Swiss study also found for the 65–94 age group that assisted suicide was more likely in women than in men (OR$=1.66$, 95% CI$=1.40$–1.96) [16].

In regard to attitude towards euthanasia, participants in the Longitudinal Ageing Study Amsterdam found no difference between males and females [14]. However, the Texas study found men were more likely to support PAS among the older Mexican Americans, but not non-Hispanic White [21].

9.5   Marital Status

There are less consistent findings on marital status and euthanasia/PAS. Most people (of all ages) who died of euthanasia/PAS were married, followed by the widowed and divorced; however, it is difficult to interpret these data without knowing the distribution of marital status among all deaths [5]. The Dutch nursing home survey of euthanasia and PAS cases found more women than men were "previously married", whereas more men than women were married or "living with a partner" [22].

The 2003–2008 Swiss study of assisted suicide found for the 65–94 age group marital status (married vs. single vs. widowed vs. divorced) or children status were not significant factors. However, assisted suicide was more likely in 1-person households (OR$=1.44$, 95% CI$=1.11$–1.87) than ≥2 persons households [16].

The Longitudinal Ageing Study Amsterdam found that participants who were divorced were more likely to have a positive attitude towards euthanasia, but no statistical differences were found between the widowed vs. married and never married vs. married [14]. Similarly, the Texas study found marital status was not a significant factor in people's agreement with PAS [21].

9.6   Ethnicity

The relationship between euthanasia/PAS and ethnicity is not well researched in older people. Participants (of all ages) of the Death with Dignity Act who died in Oregon and Washington from 2009 to 2012 were predominantly White [12]. The 2003–2008 Swiss study found for the 65–94 age group assisted suicide was more likely in people who lived in the French-speaking region (OR = 1.27, 95 % CI = 1.06–1.51) than people who lived in the German-speaking region; but there was no difference between Italian-speaking and German-speaking regions [16].

A Hawaiian study (older people: $n = 125$, mean age = 73; adult children: $n = 120$, mean age = 42) compared the response to "Are there conditions under which physician-assisted death should be permitted?" in five ethnic groups (Caucasian, Chinese, Filipino, Hawaiian, and Japanese) found no significant differences in the responses between the two generations [24]. However, the responses varied significantly by ethnicity. The Fillipnos (54 %) and Hawaiians (44 %) were more likely to say "NO"; compared to Caucasian (21 %), Chinese (18 %), and Japanese (8 %). The authors did not measure the interaction between ethnicity and religion, but 88 % of Filipinos were Catholic, 59 % of Japanese were Buddhists, and the majority of others were Protestants. It is interesting to note that Chinese and Japanese in Hawaii have the longest life expectancy, whereas Hawaiians have the shortest. In contrast, the Texas study found more Mexican American (52.7 %) supported PAS, compared to 33.7 % of non-Hispanic White [21].

9.7   Religion

Older people with religious beliefs are less likely to support euthanasia/PAS. For example, the Texas study found religiosity was significantly higher in people who disagreed with PAS [21]. Similarly, a Dutch study of 76 older people living independently and 56 older people living in nursing homes found those who were affiliated with a church more frequently rejected euthanasia [25]. A US study of general medical hospital patients (age $\geq$ 60; $n = 158$) also found religious coping was significantly correlated with less interest in PAS when they were presented with two hypothetical scenarios [26]. Lastly, the 1977–1991 US general survey concluded that the lower acceptance of euthanasia among older people stemmed from their greater religiosity [13].

A New Zealand qualitative study of 11 older people (age $\geq$ 65) found "religious reasoning and beliefs" was one of the four main themes in the older people who opposed physician-assisted dying [27]. Similarly, three of the 26 participants with Alzheimer's disease (Mini Mental State Examination $\geq$ 17; mean age = 78) in a US study gave religious reasons for opposing PAS [28]:

"The Lord will take you when he wants to."
"My body would burn in hell if I killed myself."

In terms of religious affiliation, Catholics are less likely, whereas Buddhists are more likely to support euthanasia/PAS. The findings in Protestants are mixed. For example, a Swiss study of assisted suicide from 2000 to 2005 found that in both older men and women (age 65–94) religion was protective but most significantly in Catholics [29]. The 2003–2008 Swiss study found assisted suicide was more likely in older people (age 65–94) with no affiliation (OR = 6.63, 95 % CI = 5.29–8.32) and Protestants (OR = 2.05, 95 % CI = 1.68–2.50) than in Catholics [16]. The Hawaiian study found Buddhists and Protestants were significantly more likely to support physician-assisted death than Catholics [24]; whereas the Longitudinal Ageing Study Amsterdam found older people who were Dutch reformed/protestant, Catholic or with other religions were less likely to have a positive attitude towards euthanasia [14].

A Belgian qualitative study explored the attitudes towards voluntary euthanasia, assisted suicide and non-voluntary euthanasia in a sample of older (age 60–75, mean = 65; n = 23) Hasidic,[1] non-Hasidic Orthodox, and secularised Orthodox Jewish women [30]. They found almost all of the secularised Orthodox Jewish respondents were in favour of voluntary euthanasia, but all Hasidic respondents were found to be absolute opponents. For all of the non-Hasidic Orthodox respondents, euthanasia was found to be irreconcilable with being an Orthodox Jew, as this treatment decision is forbidden by Jewish law. The participants emphasised that although Jews are free to make choices, in the end their actions will be judged by God.

9.8   Spirituality

Spirituality is a multi-dimensional construct that includes components of meaning, purpose, and hope, and can exist separately from religiousness. Unlike religion, its relationship with euthanasia/PAS is not well studied. An Oregon study found a significantly lower level of spirituality in a group of terminally ill patients who were seriously pursuing and/or requesting lethal medication under Oregon's Death with Dignity Act (n = 55; mean age = 65.3) when compared to patients with advanced disease but no interest in pursuing physician-assisted dying (n = 39; mean age = 60.9) [31]. In spirituality terms, it was suggested that people who pursued physician-assisted dying may lack an expectation of meaning in the dying process, and they may not see any opportunities remaining and pursue physician-assisted dying as a manner to circumvent suffering that has no value.

---

[1] For Orthodox (Hasidic and non-Hasidic) Jews being Jewish means following the stipulations of Jewish law, secularised Orthodox Jews interpret their Jewish identity in ethnic and cultural terms. For them, being Jewish essentially means that they belong to the Jewish community and strive for its continuation by passing on the Jewish tradition and culture. They characterise themselves as "traditionalist" or "non-practising" Jews, referring to a reduced Jewish praxis which is maintained out of habit or tradition.

9.9   Education

Older people with a higher education are more likely to support euthanasia/PAS [14, 16, 24, 32]. For example, the 2003–2008 Swiss study found assisted suicide was more likely in older people who had tertiary or higher education (OR=2.74, 95% CI=2.15–3.43) and secondary education (OR=1.74, 95% CI=1.45–2.10) than those with less education [17]. The Longitudinal Ageing Study Amsterdam also found participants who had secondary or tertiary education were more likely to have a positive attitude for euthanasia than those who had primary education or less [14].

The only exception to this association was reported in the Texas study where older people with an education of less than Grade 10 were more likely to agree with PAS than people with an education of high school or higher (OR=2.08, 95% CI=1.05–4.12) [21].

9.10   Social Support

An Australian study based on the palliative care service of a tertiary referral hospital reported six requests (age=44, 58, 70, 71, 71, and 78) for euthanasia out of their 490 new referrals in 2000 [33]. Social isolation was reported in four of these six patients. A Dutch study found isolation was a factor in 59% of the 29 older people (in the absence of a severe disease) when they made a request to their general practitioner for euthanasia and PAS [18]. In an US study, caregivers (age <65: n=79 and age ≥65: n=136) of terminally ill patients who had moderate or many supports were less likely to support euthanasia and PAS than caregivers who had few or no support (OR=0.63, 95% CI=0.44–0.90) [34].

Social support, however, does not appear to have a role in euthanasia/PAS in studies with large sample sizes. For example, the US study of general medical hospital patients found perceived social support (including the availability of instrumental, emotional, and financial support) was not associated with an interest in PAS [26]. A study of patients with advanced cancer in Oregon (n=161; mean age=61.6, SD=11.7; Mini Mental State Examination >23) following the enactment of the Oregon Death with Dignity Act (1997) found social support (measured by the Duke-University of North Carolina Functional Support Scale) was not associated with an interest in requesting a lethal prescription in the previous 2 weeks [35]. Another Oregon study of a group of terminally ill patients, who were seriously pursuing and/or requesting lethal medication, also reported a similar finding [31]. Lastly, a Swiss study found social isolation (defined as limited or no friends, no loved-ones) was not associated with assisted suicide in their older people (age ≥65) [36].

9.11   Physical Problems and Ill Health

9.11.1 Cancer/Malignancy

Cancer/malignancy is the most common reason for older people to request euthanasia and/or PAS. The Dutch nursing home survey found 53% of the euthanasia and

PAS cases had a malignant neoplasm (digestive tract, respiratory tract, bones/connective tissue/skin/breast, and urogenital tract), followed by diseases of the nervous system and sense organs (multiple sclerosis, motor neurone disease, and Parkinson's disease; 21 %), diseases of the circulatory system (12 %) and diseases of the respiratory system (9 %) [22]. The Oregon study of patients with advanced cancer found 57 % supported or strongly supported the legalisation and 9 % had a serious interest in physician-assisted dying in the previous 2 weeks [35]. An Australian study of 228 outpatients attending an oncology clinic found no differences in general and personal support for euthanasia and PAS in the <55 and ≥55 age groups: 68 % vs. 69 %, respectively [37]. However, this study used ambulant outpatients with low levels of disability attending clinic and so would not be representative of inpatients or terminally ill cancer patients.

9.11.2 Pain

Participants in the Hawaiian study felt that physician-assisted dying was acceptable for an individual with untreated pain, especially if they were also terminally ill [24]. Similarly, a study involving six sites in the US found pain was associated with being more likely for terminally ill patients (mean age = 66.5) to consider euthanasia or PAS in a hypothetical situation [34]. Pain was also frequently given as a reason for euthanasia in the Dutch study of older people living independently and in nursing homes [25]. A US study examined the characteristics of women (age ≥55) who committed suicide and women whose death were assisted by Dr Jack Kevorkian[2] from 1995 to 1997. They found assisted suicide cases were more likely to have a decline in health, pain, and neurological diseases (including multiple sclerosis and amyotrophic lateral sclerosis) [38].

9.11.3 Alzheimer's Disease/Cognitive Impairment

The US study of patients with Alzheimer's disease found more than 50 % of the participants answered "YES" when asked if they would want to have PAS as a personal option [28].

"I want the choice because my mother [a patient with Alzheimer's disease] had a long death—dying inch by inch. I don't want that to happen to me."

"My grandfather and my mother both had Alzheimer's disease, and I saw what they went through, the agony it is, and I don't want to put my family through that. I want to be remembered some other way."

"We should have the ability to choose. I don't want the burden on my family. There should be an understanding between the doctor and myself."

---

[2] Jacob "Jack" Kevorkian was an American pathologist and euthanasia activist. He is best known for publicly championing a terminal patient's right to die via physician-assisted suicide; he claimed to have assisted at least 130 patients to that end. He was often portrayed in the media as "Dr. Death". In 1999, Kevorkian was arrested and tried for his direct role in a case of voluntary euthanasia.

9.11.4 Sensory Impairment

The 2001–2004 Swiss study found the older age group (age ≥65) was significantly more likely to list visual and hearing impairment by the decedents (OR = 3.45, 95 % CI = 1.06–11.2) and physicians (OR = 3.88, 95 % CI = 1.21–12.50) as one of the reasons to justify assisted suicide [36].

9.12 Depression and Euthanasia/PAS

The relationship between depression, the wish to die, and attitude towards euthanasia in older people is complex. For example, depressed participants in the Longitudinal Ageing Study Amsterdam were statistically more likely to have a positive attitude towards euthanasia [14].

9.12.1 Depression/Depressive Symptoms in the Context of Medical Problems

The US study of general medical hospital patients found that older people who were depressed were 13 times more likely to accept PAS when compared to those who were not depressed [26]. A Dutch study found 41 % of heart failure patients (n = 61; mean age = 80) reported feeling of worthlessness, whereas 36 % reported feeling depressed at the time of request for euthanasia or PAS [39].

9.12.2 Depression in the Context of Terminal Illness

Depression can play a role in terminally ill people requesting euthanasia/PAS. Ganzini et al. found 26 % of the 58 Oregonians (mean age = 66, SD = 12) who had requested physician-assisted dying (mostly terminally ill with cancer or amyotrophic lateral sclerosis) met the diagnostic criteria for depression [40]. In another Oregon report, terminally ill patients who seriously pursued and/or requested lethal medication under the Death with Dignity Act had significantly higher subjective levels of depression (as measured by the Hospital Anxiety and Depression Scale: depression subscale) and hopelessness (as measured by the Beck Hopelessness Scale) than patients with advanced disease but no interest in pursuing PAD [31]. However, in a Dutch study, depressive feelings did not seem to be an important discriminating factor of terminally ill cancer patients who died after euthanasia (n = 106; <45 years: 17 %; 45–60 years: 25 %; 61–75 years: 43 %; and >75 years 16 %) and terminally ill cancer patients who did not request euthanasia (n = 64; <45 years: 6 %; 45–60 years: 25 %; 61–75 years: 50 %; and >75 years: 19 %) [41].

    Brown et al. asserted that it was depression (rather than having a terminal illness) that caused patients to desire death [42]. His study of 44 terminally ill Canadian patients (mean age = 63, range 29–82) reported the majority (77 %) never wished death to come early,whereas three were suicidal and seven desired death. All ten patients desiring death were reported to be suffering from DSM-III major depression. Chochinov et al. studied 200 terminally ill patients (mean age = 70.9, SD = 10.6, range = 31–94) and found that desire for death was correlated most significantly with measures of depression [43]. Among those patients who desired death, 58.8 % were diagnosed with depressive syndromes. In comparison, 7.7 % of those not wanting to die were depressed.

However, there is one US study that did not find a strong relationship between PAS, depression, and terminal illness. This relatively small sample of 35 people (prospective cohort: $n = 12$, mean age = 72; retrospective cohort: $n = 23$, mean age = 66) with incurable disease who were pursuing PAS, seriously seeking out or were reported to have had a hastened death found none of the subjects met the DSM-IV criteria for probable major depressive episode [44]. Three patients were described as having possible major depressive episode. A history of major depressive episode was documented in one patient who had been in psychiatric treatment for several years prior to and up to his death.

9.12.3 Depression and Stability of Attitudes Towards Euthanasia/PAS

A US study explored the stability of attitudes towards euthanasia/PAS in older cognitively intact medically hospitalised patients (age $\geq$60; Mini Mental State Examination $\geq$24) who had a life expectancy of greater than 6 months [45]. They were interviewed about their interest in euthanasia/PAS in the event of an unexpected life-threatening event followed by treatment which "would likely restore you to your current condition". Interest in euthanasia or PAS was also determined in five other hypothetical outcomes (terminal condition, limited mobility, Alzheimer's disease, nursing home care, and coma). This study used the Center for Epidemiologic Studies Depression Scale to measure depressive symptomatology and found patients who had been depressed at baseline were significantly more likely to change their minds and reject euthanasia and PAS for the current condition 6 months later.

An Australian study followed up 22 older people (mean age = 76.9) diagnosed with major depression and their preferences regarding voluntary euthanasia [46]. They found before treatment for their depression, 44 % indicated an initial desire for voluntary euthanasia, but after treatment only 11 % desired voluntary euthanasia. They suggested the possibility that depressed older patients may utilise voluntary euthanasia as an alternative to suicide.

9.13   Personality Factors

Research on personality factors and attitudes towards euthanasia/PAS is limited, particularly in older people. One study found 44 % of the patients who completed PAS described themselves or were reported to have an unusually high need for control [44]. Similar results were found in an Oregon study exploring physicians' perceptions of patients who requested assisted suicide [47]. 35 physicians were interviewed, but the age of their patients in this study was not reported. These physicians reported that patients who requested assisted suicide often had a pervasive coping style of a strong desire to remain independent and in control.

If we assume personality is a stable construct across one's lifespan, studies with younger people may provide some understanding of the significance of personality and attitudes towards euthanasia/PAS in older people. For example, an Iranian study investigated personality factors and attitudes towards euthanasia in 165 university students (mean age = 23.3) [48]. This study used the HEXACO Personality Inventory which has the following dimensions [49]:

1. Honesty-humility: sincerity, fairness, greed avoidance, and modesty
2. Emotionality: fearfulness, anxiety, dependence, and sentimentality
3. Extraversion: social self-esteem, social boldness, sociability, and liveliness
4. Agreeableness: forgiveness, gentleness, flexibility, and patience
5. Conscientiousness: organisation, diligence, perfectionism, and prudence
6. Openness to experience: aesthetic appreciation, inquisitiveness, creativity, and unconventionality

After controlling for religiosity and spirituality, unconventionality (part of the openness factor) was the only positive correlate of acceptance of euthanasia. The authors suggested that having non-conformist opinions is definitive of unconventionality that reflects a readiness to re-examine social, political, and religious values. Similarly, an Australian study ($n = 168$; mean age = 29, range 16–61) found, regardless of the participants' level of religiosity, low levels of conservatism was associated with positive attitudes towards euthanasia [50].

9.14 Psychological Factors: Life Satisfaction and Burden on Others

The 1977–1991 US general survey found acceptance of euthanasia was greater among older people who were less satisfied with their own lives (due to poor health, low income, etc.) and more anomic [32]. A Hong Kong qualitative study (age ≥60; $n = 18$) found the following major themes behind the support for euthanasia: fear of burden to family members, fear of pain and suffering, and feeling of uselessness in old age [51]. The "familistic" orientation of Chinese people may explain the older participants' worry about being a burden to the family. Another Hong Kong qualitative study of six participants (age 54–83) in a palliative care unit found the desire for euthanasia incorporates hidden existential yearnings for connectedness, care, and respect, understood within the context of the patients' lived experience [3]. The Australian study of six euthanasia requests in a palliative care service also found fear of being a burden/dependent and autonomy/control were the most common underlying factor [33].

Attachment style was investigated in two groups of patients: (1) a group of terminally ill patients who seriously pursued and/or requested lethal medication under Oregon's Death with Dignity Act ($n = 55$; mean age = 65.3, SD = 11.6), and (2) patients with advanced disease but no interest in pursuing PAS ($n = 39$; mean age = 60.9, SD = 13.2) [31]. They found the first group of patients had significantly higher levels of dismissive attachment. The authors suggested that those with dismissive styles of attachment may identify with features of self-reliance, autonomy, and independence, often at the expense of intimacy. When confronted with threats to security, they may recoil at the idea of relying on others for care, and an option that allows avoidance of dependency, such as PAS, might be attractive. Thus, PAS may be a way for individuals to maintain an ultimate sense of control and autonomy within a process that allows very little opportunity for either. Emile Durkheim's concept of anomie in sociology may also be a contributor to an individual's sense of futility, despair, emptiness, and a lack of purpose when taken in the context of not fulfilling social standards or values.

The Interpersonal Theory of Suicide proposes two proximal causes of the desire for suicide (thwarted belongingness and perceived burdensomeness, collectively referred as social disconnectedness) and this suicidal desire must be accompanied by an acquired capability for suicide [52]. Thwarted belongingness is *a painful mental state that results from an unmet need to belong—a need to feel connected to others in a positive and caring way* [53]. Perceived burdensomeness involves *"the mental calculation"*, *"My death is worth more than my life to others"*, and involves *the presence of interpersonal connections that are negatively valenced and this do not meet the need to belong* [53]. An acquired capacity for suicide is *acquired through habituation to the pain and fear involved in suicidal behaviour if lethal (or near-lethal) suicidal behaviours are to result* [53]. It involves the degree to which a person is able to initiate a suicide attempt.

9.15   Conclusions

The decision to proceed with rational suicide, euthanasia or PAS in older people is complex and there are often several interacting factors why this might arise. The statistics on the occurrence of this is presently unclear but likely to increase with ageing populations across most countries. There are variations in legislation which might affect how this area is studied and described. "Weariness of life" is becoming a common reason for older people requesting euthanasia/PAS and when this is coupled with declining health, impaired functioning, and dependency, an older person may perceive being a burden on others. When depression is present, it results in cognitive distortions and heightens this perception of burdensomeness. Studies of marital status and gender are inconsistent, but support for euthanasia/PAS is generally more common in men who often have a smaller social network than women. An older person with a dismissive attachment style tends to avoid relationships and this can further increase the risk of social disconnectedness; whereas religiosity is a protective factor of euthanasia/PAS and also in promoting social connectedness.

Lastly, an educated older person with an unconventional view of the world is more likely to consider the choice of euthanasia/PAS when he/she is experiencing thwarted belongingness and perceived burdensomeness. Additionally, threats to one's independence and sense of self-control are reasons why an individual may consider an earlier demise.

References

1. Siegel K. Psychosocial aspects of rational suicide. Am J Psychother. 1986;40(3):405–18.
2. Werth JL, Cobia DC. Empirically based criteria for rational suicide: a survey of psychotherapists. Suicide Life Threat Behav. 1995;25(2):231–40.
3. Mak YYW, Elwyn G. Voices of the terminally ill: uncovering the meaning of desire for euthanasia. Palliat Med. 2005;19(4):343–50.
4. Mishara BL. Synthesis of research and evidence on factors affecting the desire of terminally ill or seriously chronically ill persons to hasten death. Omega (Westport). 1999;39(1):1–70.
5. Steck N, Egger M, Maessen M, Reisch T, Zwahlen M. Euthanasia and assisted suicide in selected european countries and US states: systematic literature review. Med Care. 2013;51(10):938–44.
6. Onwuteaka-Philipsen BD, Muller MT, Van der Wal G. Euthanasia and old age. Age Ageing. 1997;26(6):487–92.
7. Onwuteaka-Philipsen BD, Rurup ML, Pasman HRW, Van Der Heide A. The last phase of life: who requests and who receives euthanasia or physician-assisted suicide? Med Care. 2010;48(7):596–603.
8. Muller MT, Kimsma GK, Van Der Wal G. Euthanasia and assisted suicide: facts, figures and fancies with special regard to old age. Drugs Aging. 1998;13(3):185–91.
9. Rurup ML, Smets T, Cohen J, Bilsen J, Onwuteaka-Philipsen BD, Deliens L. The first five years of euthanasia legislation in Belgium and the Netherlands: description and comparison of cases. Palliat Med. 2012;26(1):43–9.
10. Smets T, Bilsen J, Cohen J, Rurup ML, Deliens L. Legal euthanasia in Belgium: characteristics of all reported euthanasia cases. Med Care. 2010;48(2):187–92.
11. Battin MP, van der Heide A, Ganzini L, van der Wal G, Onwuteaka-Philipsen BD. Legal physician-assisted dying in Oregon and the Netherlands: evidence concerning the impact on patients in "vulnerable" groups. J Med Ethics. 2007;33(10):591–7.
12. Carlson WL, Ong TD. Suicide in later life. Failed treatment or rational choice? Clin Geriatr Med. 2014;30(3):553–76.
13. Leinbach RM. Euthanasia attitudes of older persons: a cohort analysis. Res Aging. 1993;15(4):433–48.
14. Buiting HM, Deeg DJH, Knol DL, Ziegelmann JP, Pasman HRW, Widdershoven GAM, et al. Older peoples' attitudes towards euthanasia and an end-of-life pill in the Netherlands: 2001–2009. J Med Ethics. 2012;38(5):267–73.
15. Frei A, Schenker T-A, Finzen A, Kräuchi K, Dittmann V, Hoffmann-Richter U. Assisted suicide as conducted by a "right-to-die"-society in Switzerland: a descriptive analysis of 43 consecutive cases. Swiss Med Wkly. 2001;131(25–26):375–80.
16. Steck N, Junker C, Maessen M, Reisch T, Zwahlen M, Egger M. Suicide assisted by right-to-die associations: a population based cohort study. Int J Epidemiol. 2014;43(2):614–22.
17. Fischer S, Huber CA, Imhof L, Mahrer Imhof R, Furter M, Ziegler SJ, et al. Suicide assisted by two Swiss right-to-die organisations. J Med Ethics. 2008;34(11):810–4.
18. Rurup ML, Muller MT, Onwuteaka-Philipsen BD, Van Der Heide A, Van Der Wal G, Van Der Maas PJ. Requests for euthanasia or physician-assisted suicide from older persons who do not have a severe disease: an interview study. Psychol Med. 2005;35(5):665–71.

19. Rurup ML, Onwuteaka-Philipsen BD, Jansen-Van Der Weide MC, Van Der Wal G. When being 'tired of living' plays an important role in a request for euthanasia or physician-assisted suicide: patient characteristics and the physician's decision. Health Policy. 2005;74(2):157–66.
20. Hare J, Skinner D, Riley D. Why older age predicts lower acceptance of physician-assisted suicide. WMJ. 2000;99(7):20.
21. Espino DV, MacIas RL, Wood RC, Becho J, Talamantes M, Finley MR, et al. Physician-assisted suicide attitudes of older Mexican-American and non-hispanic white adults: does ethnicity make a difference? J Am Geriatr Soc. 2010;58(7):1370–5.
22. Muller MT, Van der Wal G, Van Eijk JTM, Ribbe MW. Active euthanasia and physician-assisted suicide in Dutch nursing homes: patients' characteristics. Age Ageing. 1995;24(5):429–33.
23. Bosshard G, Uhlrich E, Bär W. 748 cases of suicide assisted by a swiss right-to-die organisation. Swiss Med Wkly. 2003;133(21–22):310–7.
24. Braun KL. Do Hawaii residents support physician-assisted death? A comparison of five ethnic groups. Hawaii Med J. 1998;57(6):529–34.
25. Segers JH. Euthanasia in The Netherlands. Elderly persons on the subject of euthanasia. Issues Law Med. 1988;3(4):407–24.
26. Blank K, Robison J, Doherty E, Prigerson H, Duffy J, Schwartz HI. Life-sustaining treatment and assisted death choices in depressed older patients. J Am Geriatr Soc. 2001;49(2):153–61.
27. Malpas PJ, Wilson MK, Rae N, Johnson M. Why do older people oppose physician-assisted dying? A qualitative study. Palliat Med. 2014;28(4):353–9.
28. Daskal FC, Hougham GW, Sachs GA. Physician-assisted suicide: Interviews with patients with dementia and their families. Ann Long-Term Care. 1999;7(8):293–8.
29. Spoerri A, Zwahlen M, Bopp M, Gutzwiller F, Egger M. Religion and assisted and non-assisted suicide in Switzerland: National Cohort Study. Int J Epidemiol. 2010;39(6):1486–94.
30. Baeke G, Wils J-P, Broeckaert B. 'We are (not) the master of our body': elderly Jewish women's attitudes towards euthanasia and assisted suicide. Ethn Health. 2011;16(3):259–78.
31. Smith KA, Harvath TA, Goy ER, Ganzini L. Predictors of pursuit of physician-assisted death. J Pain Symptom Manage. 2015;49(3):555–61.
32. Ward RA. Age and acceptance of euthanasia. J Gerontol. 1980;35(3):421–31.
33. Virik K, Glare P. Requests for euthanasia made to a tertiary referral teaching hospital in Sydney, Australia in the year 2000. Support Care Cancer. 2002;10(4):309–13.
34. Emanuel EJ, Fairclough DL, Emanuel LL. Attitudes and desires related to euthanasia and physician-assisted suicide among terminally ill patients and their caregivers. J Am Med Assoc. 2000;284(19):2460–8.
35. Ganzini L, Beer TM, Brouns M, Mori M, Hsieh Y-C. Interest in physician-assisted suicide among Oregon cancer patients. J Clin Ethics. 2006;17(1):27–38.
36. Fischer S, Huber CA, Furter M, Imhof L, Imhof RM, Schwarzenegger C, et al. Reasons why people in Switzerland seek assisted suicide: the view of patients and physicians. Swiss Med Wkly. 2009;139(23–24):333–8.
37. Carter GL, Clover KA, Parkinson L, Rainbird K, Kerridge I, Ravenscroft P, et al. Mental health and other clinical correlates of euthanasia attitudes in an Australian outpatient cancer population. Psychooncology. 2007;16(4):295–303.
38. Roscoe LA, Malphurs JE, Dragovic LJ, Cohen D. Antecedents of euthanasia and suicide among older women. J Am Med Womens Assoc. 2003;58(1):44–8.
39. Maessen M, Veldink JH, Van Den Berg LH, Schouten HJ, Van Der Wal G, Onwuteaka-Philipsen BD. Requests for euthanasia: origin of suffering in ALS, heart failure, and cancer patients. J Neurol. 2010;257(7):1192–8.
40. Ganzini L, Goy ER, Dobscha SK. Prevalence of depression and anxiety in patients requesting physicians' aid in dying: cross sectional survey. Br Med J. 2008;337(7676):973–5.
41. Georges J, Onwuteaka-Philipsen BD, van der Wal G, van der Heide A, van der Maas PJ. Differences between terminally ill cancer patients who died after euthanasia had been

performed and terminally ill cancer patients who did not request euthanasia. Palliat Med. 2005;19(8):578–86.

42. Brown MB, Henteleff P, Barakat S, Rowe CJ. Is it normal for terminally ill patients to desire death? Am J Psychiatr. 1986;143(2):208–11.

43. Chochinov HM, Wilson KG, Enns M, Mowchun N. Desire for death in the terminally ill. Am J Psychiatr. 1995;152(8):1185–91.

44. Bharucha AJ, Pearlman RA, Back AL, Gordon JR, Starks H, Hsu C. The pursuit of physician-assisted suicide: role of psychiatric factors. J Palliat Med. 2003;6(6):873–83.

45. Blank K, Robison J, Prigerson H, Schwartz HI. Instability of attitudes about euthanasia and physician assisted suicide in depressed older hospitalized patients. Gen Hosp Psychiatry. 2001;23(6):326–32.

46. Hooper SC, Vaughan KJ, Tennant CC, Perz JM. Preferences for voluntary euthanasia during major depression and following improvement in an elderly population. Australas J Ageing. 1997;16(1):3–7.

47. Ganzini L, Dobscha SK, Heintz RT, Press N. Oregon physicians' perceptions of patients who request assisted suicide and their families. J Palliat Med. 2003;6(3):381–90.

48. Aghababaei N. Attitudes towards euthanasia in Iran: the role of altruism. J Med Ethics. 2014;40(3):173–6.

49. Lee K, Ashton MC. Psychometric properties of the HEXACO personality inventory. Multivar Behav Res. 2004;39(329):358.

50. Ho R, Penney RK. Euthanasia and abortion: personality correlates for the decision to terminate life. J Soc Psychol. 1992;132(1):77–86.

51. Fok S, Chong AM. Euthanasia and old age: the case of Hong Kong. Hallym Int J Aging. 2003;5(1):41–53.

52. Van Orden KA, Witte TK, Cukrowicz KC, Braithwaite SR, Selby EA, Joiner Jr TE. The interpersonal theory of suicide. Psychol Rev. 2010;117(2):575–600.

53. Van Orden K, Conwell Y. Suicides in late life. Curr Psychiatry Rep. 2011;13(3):234–41.

Psychological Issues in Late-Life Suicide 10

Elissa Kolva and Darryl Etter

10.1 Introduction

The debate surrounding rational suicide stems from the question "what is a good death?" and the idea that some people believe that individuals should be able to control the circumstances surrounding their own deaths. Siegel [1] defined rational suicide as a desire for suicide (1) resulting from a realistic assessment of life circumstances, (2) where the individual is free from psychological and severe emotional distress, and (3) where the motivation for suicide is understandable by others. Werth [2] elaborated that rational suicide must involve the presence of an unremittingly hopeless condition, the decision for suicide must be made as a free choice, and it must be the result of an informed decision-making process. It also may include the involvement of others and occur over a considerable deliberation period. The debate surrounding rational suicide has primarily focused on suicide in the context of a terminal illness. These discussions need to be extended to include rational suicide in the absence of a terminal diagnosis.

When healthy older adults express a desire to end their lives, there is a role for mental health professionals to play. However, working with an older adult who has expressed a desire for death by suicide, particularly in the absence of a terminal illness or significant mental illness, can be very stressful for mental health providers. This clinical situation can trigger conflicts related to the clinician's ethical and

E. Kolva, Ph.D. (✉)
Division of Medical Oncology, Department of Medicine, University of Colorado School of Medicine, 12801 E. 17th Avenue, Mail Stop 8117, Research 1, South Aurora, CO 80045, USA
e-mail: elissa.kolva@ucdenver.edu

D. Etter, Psy.D.
Department of Primary Care—Mental Health Integration, VA Eastern Colorado Health Care System, 1055 Clermont Street, Denver, CO 80220, USA
e-mail: Darryl.etter@va.gov

© Springer International Publishing Switzerland 2017
R.E. McCue, M. Balasubramaniam (eds.), *Rational Suicide in the Elderly*,
DOI 10.1007/978-3-319-32672-6_10

religious beliefs. Discussion of rational suicide in both the literature and in popular media has engendered impassioned responses from mental health professionals. While no mental health provider should be forced to provide care in opposition to his/her values [3], the provider is responsible for conducting an assessment or risk and identifying appropriate interventions for patients at risk [4]. "Staying out of it," or avoiding discussions of suicidality can ultimately lead to increased suffering for patients.

While rational suicide is understandably a controversial issue, as healthcare providers it is crucial not to reduce the patient to merely a "side" in an ongoing national debate. As outlined by the relevant ethics codes and licensing bodies, mental health professionals have a responsibility to care for their patients to the best of their abilities. The aim of this chapter is to provide an overview of psychological issues that may play a role in expressions of rational suicide. This includes guidelines for conducting suicide risk assessments, hybrid psychological/legal issues like decision-making capacity, and lessons learned from health psychology—specifically the field of psycho-oncology. Obtaining a better understanding of these constructs and the role they play in suicide in medically ill patients will aid case conceptualization, suicide risk assessment, and intervention planning.

As stated by Siegel [1] and Ho [5], rational suicide does not always occur in the context of mental illness, irrationality, or diminished capacity. Research consistently demonstrates that mental illness is a major factor in 90 % of all deaths from suicide [6]. We are focused on the factors that contribute to the other 10 %. As a result, this chapter does not have a strong focus on the role of mental illness, but focuses on other psychosocial issues that can increase risk for suicide. The reasons behind expressions of rational suicide are often logical (e.g., fear of inevitable decline in functioning) and are more closely connected to, and may be better conceptualized as, desire for hastened death (DHD). The goal of the assessment provided in this chapter is not to prevent all expression of rational suicide, but to better understand issues experienced by patients and to aid in the development of a strategy for intervention that can maximize quality and, if possible, length of life.

10.2   Psychological Theories of Suicide

Within the field of mental health, suicide, or the expression of a wish for death, is viewed as a symptom or feature of a disorder [7]. There are many different theories for why people die by suicide, often based on larger therapeutic orientations. These causes, whether it is hopelessness, from a cognitive-behavioral approach [8], or unconscious drives, from a psychodynamic approach [9], often dictate the course of assessment and treatment. However, until recently, there was no overarching theory to help mental health professionals understand and conceptualize suicidality.

Joiner's [10] interpersonal theory of suicidal behavior attempted to fill that gap and is now widely accepted and well known. The theory proposes that desire for suicide is caused by two interpersonal constructs: thwarted belongingness and perceived burdensomeness. Thwarted belongingness involves feelings of disconnection from others and social isolation. Perceived burdensomeness is driven by the belief that one is a burden on family, friends, and society [11]. Joiner's theory separates itself from other theories of suicidality in that, in addition to attending to cognitive and affective factors that cause suicidal ideation, it focuses on an individual's ability to enact a lethal self-injury [12]. The model proposes that the desire for suicide is separate from the capability to engage in suicidal behavior. Individuals build their capacity to engage in self-harm through repeated exposures to painful or frightening experiences. This results in habituation, high pain tolerance, and low fear of death. Over time, through practicing behaviors, individuals can increase their capacity for suicide. According to the interpersonal theory, individuals who possess both the desire and the capability are at highest risk for death by suicide [13], so assessment of suicide risk seeks to address both of these factors.

10.3 Rational Suicide Risk Assessment

The assessment and management of patients who express suicidal ideation is one of the most stressful tasks for clinicians [14]. However, it is becoming a more prevalent part of a clinician's job with the dramatic rise in suicide rates over the past 45 years [15]. Conducting a comprehensive and accurate assessment of suicide risk can be a daunting challenge as it has the potential for significant medical, legal, and ethical consequences. When discussing suicide risk assessment, Britton and colleagues [4] stated "clinicians are in the precarious position of being legally responsible for failing at an extremely demanding task (p. 53)." Mental health professionals are vulnerable to lawsuits should a patient die by suicide, and as a result they may be more likely to err on the side of more aggressive, restrictive interventions like hospitalization, or in contrast, shy away from assessing suicide risk all together.

Conducting a suicide risk assessment with an older adult who is not mentally or terminally ill can be particularly challenging for clinicians. Traditional methods of suicide assessment may fall short as they tend to focus on the role of psychiatric symptoms in suicide risk. Therefore, in this section, in addition to reviewing traditional suicide risk assessment, we review additional assessment strategies that focus on the individual experience of the patient rather than on symptoms of mental illness. These empirically supported, collaborative approaches may result in a more accurate and comprehensive assessment. These strategies can aid in case conceptualization and identify initial areas for intervention for older adults expressing a desire for rational suicide.

10.3.1 Traditional Suicide Risk Assessment

Traditional suicide risk assessment involves obtaining information about risk factors, protective factors, and warning signs of suicide. This information is integrated and used in a clinical formulation of suicide risk [16]. The American Psychiatric Association [17, 18] provided general guidelines for the psychiatric assessments of patients with suicidal behavior, both to inform practice and as a means to protect clinicians from litigation. First, the clinician should conduct a comprehensive psychiatric evaluation including assessing for signs and symptoms of mental illness, assessing history of suicidal behavior (i.e., intent, ideation, and past attempts), review the patient's psychiatric history (including family mental health history), consider psychosocial risk factors such as financial and relationship difficulty, and assess psychological strengths and vulnerabilities. Following the psychiatric evaluation, clinicians should focus on assessing the patient's *current* suicidal ideation, plans, and behaviors. This includes assessing level of intent and lethality of proposed plan. These assessments can be used to determine a level of suicide risk. It is also critical that the suicide risk assessment always be documented in the medical record.

The American Psychological Association [19] proposed specific practice guidelines for clinicians working with older adults, including attention to risk factors for suicide. These guidelines focus primarily on recognizing and treating depression as a major risk factor for suicide, so thus may not be perfectly relevant for older adults who do not meet diagnostic criteria for depression. They also promote the use of an interdisciplinary assessment of the patient. Clinicians should incorporate into their assessment an appreciation of the medical, social, and environmental (i.e., housing situation) factors for each patient.

10.3.2 Motivational Interviewing

When assessing a patient at risk for suicide, it is often, if not explicitly, the clinician's goal for the patient's behavior to change. Thus, a Motivational Interviewing (MI; [20]) approach, based on Prochaska and DiClementi's [21] stages of change, or transtheoretical model, is applicable. MI is collaborative and inherently respectful of patient autonomy. It is not wedded to the outcome of the intervention, as it honors a patient's responsibility for his/her own life. This spirit of promoting patient autonomy and responsibility is shared by the recent literature on rational suicide [5]. Rollnick, Miller, and Butler [22] profess that this detachment from focus on outcome actually encourages patients to make changes. Overall, the spirit of MI is characterized by a resistance to "right" or direct patients, a desire to understand patients' motivation, empathetic listening, and a commitment to encouraging hope and optimism in patients.

An MI approach to rational suicide assessment focuses on detecting and then highlighting any ambivalence surrounding the desire for death by suicide in the context of a positive therapeutic relationship while gathering relevant information about suicide risk [7]. This approach prioritizes patient autonomy, which is particularly important when working with older adults. According to Zerler [7], "because the client ultimately will survive by his or her own agency, adopting a posture that promotes self-efficacy may be more prudent and potentially more effective than a stance that assumes the client is helpless in the face of imminent harm and assumes the role of rescuer."

MI in practice focuses on adherence to four core skills [20]. The first skill is to ask *open-ended questions* that encourage reflection. This serves as an opportunity for the clinician to listen for change talk, or a patient's desire to engage in intervention. These questions are not merely aimed at gathering information, but at understanding the patient and strengthening the therapeutic relationship. The second skill is *affirming* the client as a person with the capacity to take responsibility for his/her life. It is particularly useful in suicidal patients, because this can help overcome initial judgments or strongly held beliefs about the ethics or morals inherent in the decision, resulting in a more authentic interaction. The third core skill is *reflective listening*. Reflective listening statements serve the purpose of ensuring that the clinician and patient are on the same page. Finally, *summarizing* allows the clinician to move along the process toward change. They integrate the patient's motivation and intention for change. These strategies can be integrated into a traditional suicide risk assessment and result in a more patient-centered approach to assessment.

10.3.3   Self-Determination Theory

Britton and colleagues [4] integrated MI strategies with self-determination theory (SDT) for the assessment and treatment of patients with suicidal ideation. SDT [23] posits that human beings are naturally intrinsically motivated to engage in healthy activities. In fact, providing extrinsic rewards reduced the likelihood that individuals would continue to engage in intrinsically rewarding activities [24]. This framework states that individuals have basic needs for autonomy, competence, and relatedness and that satisfaction of these needs is related to improved treatment engagement and health behaviors [25, 26].

The goal of the integration of SDT and MI principles into assessment of suicidal ideation is to resolve the inherent tension between respecting patient autonomy and protecting patients from harm [4]. Britton and colleagues recommend that when working with patients who express suicidal ideation clinicians should:

1. Acknowledge the client's perspective.
2. Convey to clients that they have choices: this highlights respect for patient autonomy.
3. Provide a meaningful rationale for engaging in intervention.
4. Support every client's individuality and autonomy.
5. Support clients' perceived competence.
6. Emphasize the relational aspects of the therapeutic relationship.

The integration of SDT and MI strategies maintain respect for patient autonomy in the context of a thorough risk assessment, thus complying with relevant legal standards. The authors proposing these interventions do acknowledge the need for the involuntary hospitalization of patients who cannot be safely treated on an outpatient basis, but only as a last resort [4].

10.3.4 Collaborative Assessment and Management of Suicidality (CAMS)

The Collaborative Assessment and Management of Suicidality (CAMS; [27]) is a conceptual framework that can be applied to suicide risk assessment. Jobes [27] stressed that CAMS is, like MI, both a philosophy of care and a series of clinical techniques designed to improve patient quality of life. The CAMS approach holds that suicidal ideation and behaviors are often sensible and serve a function for the patient, making it especially applicable to cases of rational suicide; however, these beliefs are also worrisome and thus call for intervention. Suicide is never endorsed as a recommended treatment option, and the clinician expresses commitment to the relevant legal and ethical codes.

As an approach to suicide risk assessment, CAMS is composed of five steps that rely heavily on the development of a strong therapeutic alliance between clinician and patient and uses this alliance to enhance motivation for change [7, 27]. Overall, it integrates multiple theoretical orientations (i.e., cognitive, psychodynamic, humanistic, existential, and interpersonal; [28]). *Step one* is to identify risk for suicide. This can occur through clinical interview or brief self-report measures. The CAMS approach recommends that clinicians aim to identify suicidal ideation within the first 10 min of the session. *Step two* involves collaborative assessment. The patient and clinician complete the Suicide Status Form (SSF) together, often sitting side by side. The SSF uses both Likert and open-ended questions to assess psychological pain, stress, agitation, hopelessness, self-hate, and overall suicide risk [29]. The SSF provides information specific to the individual patient's suicidality. *Step three* is collaborative treatment planning. The information learned through completion of the SSF is used to develop a plan that will reduce the potential for self-harm and ensure safety. The patient must complete a "Crisis Response Plan," which involves plans for reducing access to lethal means, and connect the patient to others [30]. *Step four* of CAMS involves maintaining the patient on Suicide Status. This involves on-going monitoring of risk for suicide using patient self-report on the SSF, and continual evaluation of the treatment plan. *Step five* involves the resolution of suicide risk. Once the patient has three consecutive sessions without reporting suicidal thoughts, feelings, or behaviors, the risk is thought to be resolved.

10.3.5 Structured Assessments

The use of self-report measures could supplement and guide clinical assessments of suicide risk. In response to the increased risk for suicide faced by older adults and the fact that the majority of older adults who died by suicide had met with their primary care providers in the 30 days prior to their death [31–33], Edelstein and colleagues [34] developed the Reasons For Living—Older Adults Scale (RFL-OA). Rather than focusing primarily on risk factors (i.e., demographics, clinical variables, and behaviors), they recommended an assessment approach that focuses on identifying reasons for living. This approach can promote resiliency and provides avenues for clinical intervention [35]. The Geriatric Suicide Ideation Scale (GSIS; [36]) is a shorter self-report measure of suicidal ideation in older adults. Even passing familiarity with these measures can enhance the accuracy of the risk assessments performed by clinicians who have only been trained in traditional suicide risk assessment.

10.3.6 Medical Decision-Making Capacity

Werth [2] stated that in order for suicide to be rational, the patient must be capable of making a competent decision. The question of capacity to decide to hasten death bears strongly on ethical, legal, and treatment decisions a clinician must make, so clinicians working with older adults at risk for suicide should be familiar with the guidelines for basic decision-making capacity assessment. Importantly, assessment of decisional capacity examines the process of decision making rather than the outcome or "rightness" of the decision. Because a patient may make a decision that does not seem "right" to the clinician, decision-making capacity assessment seeks to resolve the tension that clinicians face in trying to promote patient autonomy while simultaneously protecting patients from harm [37, 38].

Decision-making capacity assessments are guided by the prevailing legal standards. Legal scholars have distilled the standards used across jurisdictions into four major categories [37, 39, 40]. Clinicians should assess a patient's ability to express a consistent *choice*. Clinicians should assess the patient's ability to *understand* information relevant to the decision they are being asked to make. Ability to *appreciate* the implications of the treatment decision and the impact it will have on his/her life should be assessed. Finally, the clinician should evaluate the patient's ability to rationally manipulate information relevant to the treatment decision, or *reason* about the relative risks and benefits of the proposed decision.

When conducting a comprehensive suicide risk assessment, clinicians should be aware of the cognitive capacities involved in medical decision making. It is important for clinicians to be aware that older adults [41–43] and adults with medical illness (particularly when admitted to the hospital; [44, 45]) are particularly vulnerable to impaired decisional capacity due to the effects of aging, hospitalization, and/or medical illness. Use of standardized measures of decision-making capacity can improve the reliability and validity of capacity assessments. The MacArthur Competence Assessment Tool for Treatment (MacCAT-T; [46]) and The Aid to Capacity Evaluation (ACE; [47]) can both be adapted to the decision at hand and used to improve the quality of clinicians' assessment of decisional capacity.

10.4 Lessons from Psycho-Oncology

To our knowledge, there are no published studies on the psychological risk factors that increase risk for rational suicide. Thus, it is necessary to borrow from other fields. There are certainly lessons to be learned from "traditional suicide" and the role of psychological distress including symptoms of anxiety and depression. There is no doubt that these symptoms play a role in suicide and thus should be included in any suicide risk assessment. However, for our purposes, we are conceptualizing rational suicide as often occurring in the absence of mental illness, so it is necessary to expand our horizons in attempting to understand relevant psychological risk factors.

Psycho-oncology developed over the last quarter of the twentieth century. As a field, it has overcome stigma associated with talking about both cancer and mental health issues and emerged as a discipline committed to studying and treating the psychosocial and behavioral aspects of cancer [48]. The incidence of death by suicide in patients with cancer is nearly twice that of the general U.S. population [49, 50]. Patients with cancer are often faced with declining health status, physical symptoms, and uncertainty about the future. This section draws on several existing reviews of risk factors for suicide in patients with cancer [51–53].

In our work in psycho-oncology, it was not uncommon to meet with patients with advanced or incurable cancer who expressed significant suicidal ideation that was quite rational. The idea that death is a rational response to current circumstances is more approachable in this population [5], allowing both researchers and patients to more candidly explore a topic that otherwise can carry stigma. Research in this area has focused on redefining and conceptualizing psychological distress associated with coping with serious health threats.

10.4.1 Desire for Hastened Death

Desire for hastened death (DHD) is thought to be the construct underlying suicidality in medically ill patients. It is characterized by the desire for death to occur faster or sooner than it would by natural disease progression [54]. DHD ranges in acuity from a fleeting desire for death to occur quickly to a specific thought regarding ending one's life to formulating or enacting a plan for actively hastening death [55]. Death can be hastened through both passive (i.e., nonadherence to life-sustaining medications) and active measures (i.e., suicide).

DHD is fairly common in patients with terminal cancer. Prevalence estimates range from 44.5 % of terminally ill cancer patients who reported a fleeting desire for death, to 25 % with serious thoughts, to 8.5–17 % who reported a more persistent wish for hastened death [54, 56, 57]. Longitudinal analyses revealed that DHD fluctuates over time, even over the last few weeks of life [58, 59] and is unrelated to level of pain or functional impairment [60]. Significant positive correlations have been found consistently between DHD and cognitive impairment, low social support, low spiritual well-being, depression, and hopelessness [55, 56, 60–63]. A study of terminally ill patients with both high DHD and high depression found that effective treatment for depression also reduced DHD [51, 52]. When assessing DHD, clinicians recommend assessing fear of pain and anticipated emotional suffering, social or personal factors that may influence DHD, and direct thoughts about facilitating one's death [64, 65]. There are several instruments developed to measure

DHD. Most notably, Chochinov et al.'s [54] Desire for Death Rating Scale (DDRS) and Rosenfeld and colleagues' [64, 65] Schedule of Attitudes toward Hastened Death (SAHD). Both have been used in research on DHD and could also be incorporated into clinical assessments.

The construct DHD has direct relevance to better understanding rational suicide in older adults. It may be useful for clinicians to conceptualize desire for hastened death as a wish for death sooner than it would occur as the result of *any* process, including the natural aging process. In fact, there are many similarities between reasons for DHD and for rational suicide. After conducting a systematic review of the literature, Hudson and colleagues [55] concluded that patients with advanced disease often express DHD because of their perceptions of how they may feel in the future. In a qualitative study of patients receiving palliative care for a terminal illness, Pestinger et al. [66] found that patients expressed DHD because they were trying to balance time remaining and anticipated agony. They viewed DHD as a coping strategy for managing emotional and cognitive experiences. This is similar to many of the reasons older adults express desire for rational suicide.

Conceptualizing rational suicide as a form of DHD has the potential to change the way clinicians assess and treat older adults who express a seemingly rational desire to die sooner than might occur through the natural progression of time. By adopting this approach when working with patients, clinicians may be less likely to judge the patient's experience and more likely to build empathy. This provides opportunity to explore other options and identify areas for intervention.

10.4.2 Hopelessness

Definitions of the construct of hopelessness differ based on theoretical orientation. Hopelessness was originally conceptualized as a symptom of depression [67]. Beck and colleagues [8] defined hopelessness as the presence of negative expectations and a pessimistic attitude toward the future. From a psychodynamic point of view, hopelessness is defined as "an inability to retain a good object feeling and to generate self-soothing, self-affirming responses in the face of disappointment" [68]. It can also be considered a form of anticipatory grief [67]. Hopelessness can also be viewed as a consequence of helplessness. The hopeless individual is characterized by his conviction that nothing can turn out well for him [69]. This difficulty identifying solutions to unbearable psychological pain can lead hopeless individuals to consider suicide [70], and hopelessness has, indeed, been found to be a major contributor to suicidality [69].

Within the field of psycho-oncology, hopelessness has been identified as an important construct influencing desire for hastened death, suicidal ideation, and requests for assisted suicide. In fact, a study in patients with advanced cancer found that depression and hopelessness provided independent, unique contributions to the prediction of desire for hastened death [56]. In a qualitative study of hope and hopelessness at the end of life, terminally ill patients described hopelessness as a dark and dangerous state akin to death [71]. Hopelessness fits well into our conceptualization of rational suicide because, although hopelessness is a symptom of depression, it is not in itself a mental illness.

The Beck Hopelessness Scale (BHS; [8]) is considered the gold standard in the assessment of hopelessness. However, recent critiques of the measure note that it may not be specific enough to capture the experience of older adults [72] or medically ill adults [73]. Fry [74] developed the Geriatric Hopelessness Scale (GHS) specifically to assess hopelessness in older adults. The Hopelessness Assessment in Illness (HAI; [73]) was developed to address some of the perceived shortcomings of the BHS in terminally ill patients (i.e., some of the scale items are simply not true for terminally ill patients). Given our recommended conceptualization of rational suicide as a form of desire for hastened death in older adults, the HAI may be an appropriate measure to use when working with this population.

Hopelessness should always be assessed when conducting a suicide risk assessment with an older adult. It is important not to shy away from assessing hopelessness. Directly asking patients if they feel hopeless and then assessing the strength of that feeling, and associated cognitions is very useful in determining risk for suicide.

10.4.3 Burdensomeness, Helplessness, and Loss of Control

Declines in functional ability are inevitable as adults age. This can result in loss of independence and the need to rely on others for assistance. Loss of control and feelings of helplessness play a role in suicidality in the seriously ill. For example, patients with cancer who report more concern about loss of autonomy are at higher risk for DHD [55]. In a study of patients with terminal cancer who died by suicide while receiving home palliative care services, Filiberti and colleagues [75] highlighted the significance of loss of autonomy at the end of life. In their sample, all five participants who died by suicide had been concerned about loss of autonomy and were wary of needing to rely on others. In addition, the majority of participants ($n=4$) cited awareness of a terminal prognosis, hopelessness, fear of suffering, and worry about becoming a burden on others, as contributing factors. Many of these characteristics are not unique to terminal illness and are relevant for older adults facing possible declining health and functional status.

The literature has consistently demonstrated a relationship between being perceived as a burden and risk for death by suicide [76, 77]. Cukrowicz and colleagues [78] examined the impact of perceived burdensomeness on suicidal ideation in a community sample of older adults. They found that perceived burdensomeness significantly accounted for variance in suicidal ideation after controlling for depressive symptoms, hopelessness, and functional impairment. In a study of terminally ill patients who died by assisted suicide in Oregon, Sullivan, Hedberg, and Hopkins [79] found that 63 % of patients believed that they had become a burden on their families and caregivers. These, and additional findings [80, 81], echo Joiner's [12] assertion that perceived burdensomeness drastically increases risk for death by suicide.

As many of the case studies presented in the other chapters of this book detail, older adults who express rational suicidal ideation often express concern about declines in functioning and needing to rely heavily on others. Thus, as a part of the assessment of psychosocial factors in a comprehensive suicide risk assessment, it is very important to pay attention to factors related to loss of control, fear of dependency, and perception of burdensomeness. Not only are these factors that place a patient at higher risk for suicide, but they are also areas that are ripe for intervention. Connection with social services including home safety evaluations and interventions can help older adults to be and feel safer in their homes. Family and couples interventions can help to clarify caregiver needs and perceptions of burden.

10.4.4 Social Support

Social support concerns both the extent to which a person feels (and actually is) cared for and is part of a social network. There are many different sources, or types, of social support, including emotional, informational, instrumental, and social companionship [82]. Social support has been found to be protective for both emotional and physical health in patients with cancer [83, 84]. Social isolation and alienation, or thwarted belongingness, is one of the strongest, most consistent, risk factor for experiencing suicidal ideation [12]. As noted above, studies have consistently demonstrated a relationship between low levels of social support and high DHD in patients with cancer [54, 56, 62]. A number of self-report measures have been developed to assess social support [85–88].

Assessing social support is an important part of a complex suicide risk assessment. Suicidal ideation was significantly associated with lower perceived social support and lower social interaction patterns in older adults [89]. Again, low perceived social support is an easily assessed for risk factor and one that is modifiable. Referrals to group psychotherapy interventions can aid sense of connection to others and reduce social isolation. Interdisciplinary coordination with social work services may also be useful.

10.4.5 Existential Distress

Clinicians should also consider the role of existential issues (i.e., loss of meaning, purpose, dignity, regret, and unfinished business) as it may contribute to higher levels of DHD and risk of suicide [90]. Existential distress is common in patients with terminal cancer and is not necessarily consistent with a mental health diagnosis. Existential psychotherapy is purposely antireductionistic and thus cautions clinicians against assigning diagnoses, instead focusing on the patient's experience. Yalom [91] conceptualized existential distress as arising from four ultimate concerns: death, freedom, isolation, and meaninglessness. Kissane [92] expanded upon Yalom's ultimate concerns and identified death, meaning, grief, aloneness, freedom, and dignity as existential challenges faced by terminally ill patients. These concerns can result in different forms of existential distress including death anxiety, loss of control, loneliness, demoralization (combination of hopelessness, loss of meaning, and desire for hastened death), complicated grief, worthlessness, conflict and alienation, and spiritual doubt and despair.

There are several self-report measures that are primarily used for research purposes that address existential issues. The Functional Assessment of Chronic Illness Therapy-Spiritual Well-Being Scale (FACIT-Sp; [93]) contains Meaning and Peace subscales in addition to other aspects of spirituality and is used often in studies of medically ill patients. The Meaning in Life Questionnaire (MLQ; [94]) assesses presence of meaning and search for meaning in life. Clinicians who are unfamiliar with assessing existential distress may benefit from becoming familiar with these measures.

It can be argued that the existential challenges experienced by medically ill patients are also faced by adults as they age regardless of the presence of a terminal illness. Due to physical and mental degradation, retirement, empty-nesting, and death of friends and loved ones, issues of meaning, isolation, aloneness, dignity, etc. are particularly relevant to older adults. During a suicide risk assessment, when assessing other relevant constructs, such as hopelessness, clinicians may benefit from asking patients about the things that give their lives meaning and purpose. This assessment can also involve assessing spirituality and spiritual suffering. Incorporating existential issues into a suicide risk assessment will allow the clinician to better understand the source of desire for rational suicide and to identify potential areas for intervention.

10.5 Practice Guidelines

The goal of this chapter was to highlight the importance of conducting a comprehensive assessment of risk for suicide that is informed by both an understanding of assessment strategies and relevant psychological issues. It is important that the clinician should ask direct questions, and not shy away from discussing suicidal ideation, intent, and plan. Conducting a thorough assessment does not increase risk for suicide [95]. Furthermore, we have found in our work in psycho-oncology that a good assessment can often act as an intervention.

We believe that it may be helpful for clinicians to conceptualize expressions of rational suicidal ideation as a form of DHD. Hudson and colleagues [96] recommend a two-phase approach to responding to expressed desire for hastened death. This approach shares many values with the MI, self-determination theory, and CAMS approaches described earlier in the chapter. The first phase involves taking time to explore the background of the desire for hastened death. The second phase involves considering broader information and initiating interventions. These approaches concern the both the spirit and procedures of a suicide risk assessment. Valuing the patient's experience and joining, rather than judging, builds a strong therapeutic relationship and reduces the likelihood of impulsive behavior, providing patients with the time and therapeutic space to explore alternatives and receive intervention.

When thinking about rational suicide assessment, most of the general principles of suicide risk assessment apply. Traditional suicide risk assessment often focuses on distress in the form of mental illness or cognitive impairment. Clinicians should expand upon this when assessing rational suicidal ideation. Once the immediate safety of the patient has been ensured, the clinician should adopt an attitude of openness and respect. This can be done through the integration of MI, SDT, or CAMS techniques and will facilitate the development of the therapeutic relationship. We also believe integrating knowledge from psycho-oncology is beneficial to make sure that we are not missing other forms of distress. In these cases, Block and Billings [97] recommend that the clinician conduct a thorough assessment of the following six areas:

1. Physical suffering: including the assessment of uncontrolled pain as well as the somatic symptoms of anxiety and depression.
2. Psychological suffering: this combines aspects of traditional suicide assessment with assessment of hopelessness, desire for hastened death, and anticipatory grief.
3. Decision-making capacity: this assessment is guided by relevant legal standards.
4. Social suffering: including assessment of social isolation as well as feelings of burdensomeness and general social support.
5. Existential/spiritual suffering: this also draws on lessons learned from psycho-oncology and may incorporate issues of spirituality and meaning in life.
6. Dysfunction in the physician/patient relationship: Clinicians should explore patient concerns about safety and confidence in the treatment plan.

Although these guidelines were created for working with terminally ill patients who expressed a wish for euthanasia or assisted suicide, they are particularly applicable for older adults who express a desire for death in the absence of a terminal illness.

It is important for clinicians to remember that just because a patient expresses a desire for death that is rational, the patient is not untreatable. Block and Billings [97] asserted that many terminally ill patients who express a wish for death by suicide or euthanasia are actually asking for assistance in life. This is underscored by reviewing lessons learned from the Oregon Death with Dignity Act [98], the first law in the United States to permit physicians to write a prescription for lethal drugs to competent, terminally ill patients. One of the most striking pieces of information to come out of studies of the ODDA is that, only 541 prescriptions were written in the first 10 years and only 341 were used [99]. Some have argued that the numbers of patients utilizing the ODDA are low because having the option of physician-assisted death served as a catalyst for improving end-of-life care, including improved pain control practices and greater integration of palliative care services. In kind, increasing our understanding of rational suicidal ideation and our level of comfort discussing it could similarly serve as a catalyst for improving care to older patients who are suffering, even in the absence of mental or terminal illness.

10.5.1 Interdisciplinary Intervention

Following a thorough assessment of suicide risk, the clinician is tasked with formulating a plan for intervention. In addition to selecting the most appropriate psychotherapeutic intervention, clinicians must consider interdisciplinary intervention. *Social workers* can facilitate connection with community resources. This can result in improved independence and reduced sense of burdensomeness. They can facilitate connection with social programs that can reduce social isolation and increase sense of belongingness. Referring patients to *physical and occupational therapy* can result in improved physical functioning. These specialists can also conduct home safety evaluations that can foster a sense of independence and allow patients to live in a way that is more consistent with their values for longer. Clinicians should also refer patients to *spiritual support services* when appropriate. Finally, effective collaboration with the *medical team* is crucial. The majority of older adults at risk for suicide are connected with primary care providers [31–33]. Medical providers can ensure that physical symptoms are appropriately controlled.

10.6 Conclusion

Assessing older adults who express a desire for hastened death in the absence of mental illness or terminal disease is a complex process. However, a critical, and simple, guideline is that conducting a thorough assessment will offer the clinician the best opportunity to connect with the patient and institute interventions that will improve quality of life—and if used properly, the assessment itself can function as an important intervention. Suicide risk assessment should draw on the existing literature and involve an approach that is collaborative and seeks to understand patient motivation. This allows the patient to maintain responsibility for his/her own life [5]. We also believe that lessons and tools from psycho-oncology are applicable in informing assessment of rational suicide. Finally, when conducting suicide risk assessments, clinicians should actively work to identify avenues of psychological and interdisciplinary intervention.

References

1. Siegel K. Psychosocial aspects of rational suicide. Am J Psychother. 1986;40(3):405–18.
2. Werth Jr JL. Rational suicide and AIDS: considerations for the psychotherapist. Couns Psychol. 1992;20:645–59.
3. Werth JL, Holdwick DJ. A primer on rational suicide and other forms of hastened death. Couns Psychol. 2000;28(4):511–39.

4. Britton PC, Williams GC, Conner KR. Self-determination theory, motivational interviewing, and the treatment of clients with acute suicidal ideation. J Clin Psychol. 2008;64(1):52–66. doi:10.1002/jclp.20430.
5. Ho AO. Suicide: rationality and responsibility for life. Can J Psychiatry. 2014;59(3):141–7.
6. Clark DC, Fawcett J. Review of empirical risk factors for evaluation of suicidal patient. In: Bongar B, editor. Suicide: guidelines for assessment, management, and treatment. New York: Oxford University Press; 1992.
7. Zerler H. Motivational interviewing in the assessment and management of suicidality. J Clin Psychol. 2009;65(11):1207–17. doi:10.1002/jcp.20643.
8. Beck AT, Weissman A, Lester D, Trexler L. The measurement of pessimism: the hopelessness scale. J Consult Clin Psychol. 1974;42:861–5. doi:10.1037/h0037562.
9. Menninger K. Man against himself. London: Harvest Books; 1938.
10. Joiner T. Why people die by suicide. Cambridge: Harvard University Press; 2005.
11. Joiner TE, Pettit JW, Walker RL, Voelz ZR, Cruz J. Perceived burdensomeness and suicidality: two studies on the suicide notes of those attempting and those completing suicide. J Soc Clin Psychol. 2002;21(5):531–45.
12. Joiner T. The interpersonal-psychological theory of suicidal behavior: Current empirical status. Psychological Science Agenda. Americal Psychological Associaion. 2009. http://www.apa.org/science/about/psa/2009/06/sci-brief.aspx
13. Van Orden KA, Witte TK, Cukrowicz KC, Braithwaite SR, Selby EA, Joiner TE. The interpersonal theory of suicide. Psychol Rev. 2010;117(2):575–600.
14. Jobes DA. The challenge and the promise of clinical suicidology. Suicide Life Threat Behav. 1995;25:437–49.
15. Fowler JC. Suicide risk and assessment in clinical practice: pragmatic guidelines for imperfect assessments. Psychotherapy. 2012;49(1):81–90.
16. Shea SC. Suicide assessment. Psychiatric Times. 2009;26(12):1–6.
17. American Psychiatric Association. Practice guidelines for the assessment and treatment of patients with suicidal behaviors: a quick reference guide. 2003.
18. American Psychiatric Association. Practice guideline for the assessment and treatment of patients with suicidal behaviors. 2010
19. American Psychological Association. Guidelines for psychological practice with older adults. Am Psychol. 2014;69(1):34–65. doi:10.1037/a0035063.
20. Miller WR, Rollnick S. Motivational interviewing: helping people change. New York: Guilford; 2012.
21. Prochaska J, DiClemente C. Stages and processes of self-change in smoking: toward an integrative model of change. J Consult Clin Psychol. 1983;5:390–5.
22. Rollnick S, Miller WR, Butler CC. Motivational interviewing in health care: helping patients change behavior. New York: Guilford; 2008.
23. Deci L. Intrinsic motivation. New York: Plenum; 1975.
24. Deci EL. Effects of externally mediated rewards on intrinsic motivation. J Pers Soc Psychol. 1971;18:105–15.
25. Ryan RM, Deci EL. An overview of self-determination theory. In: Deci EL, Ryan RM, editors. Handbook of self-determination research. Rochester: University of Rochester Press; 2002. p. 3–33.
26. Ryan RM, Deci EL, Grolnick WS, LaGuardia JG. The significance of autonomy and autonomy support in psychological development and psychopathology. In: Cicchetti D, Cohen D, editors. Developmental psychopathology, Theory and methods, vol. 1. 2nd ed. New York: Wiley; 2006. p. 295–849.
27. Jobes DA. The CAMS approach to suicide risk: philosophy and clinical procedures. Suicidologi. 2009;14:3–7.
28. Jobes DA, Drozd JF. The CAMS approach to working with suicidal patients. J Contemp Psychother. 2004;34(1):73–85.

29. Jobes DA, Wong SA, Conrad AK, Drozd JF, Neal-Walden T. The collaborative assessment and management of suicidality versus treatment as usual: a retrospective study with suicidal outpatients. Suicide Life Threat Behav. 2005;35(5):483–97.
30. Jobes DA. Managing suicidal risk: a collaborative approach. New York: Guilford; 2006.
31. Conwell Y, Olsen K, Caine EE, Falnnery D. Suicide in late life: psychological autopsy findings. Int Psychogeriatr. 1991;3:59–66.
32. Diekstra RFW, van Egmond M. Suicide and attempted suicide in general practice, 1979–1985. Acta Psychiatr Scand. 1989;79:268–75.
33. Luoma JB, Martin CE, Pearson JL. Contact with mental health and primary care providers before suicide: a review of the evidence. Am J Psychiatr. 2002;159:909–16.
34. Edelstein BA, Heisel MJ, McKee DR, Martin RR, Koven LP, Duberstein PR, Britton PC. Development and psychometric evaluation of the reasons for living—older adults scale: a suicide risk assessment inventory. Gerontologist. 2009;49(6):736–45.
35. Linehan MM, Goodstein LJ, Nielsen SL, Chiles JA. Reasons for staying alive when you are thinking of killing yourself: the reasons for living inventory. J Consult Clin Psychol. 1983;51:276–86.
36. Heisel MJ, Flett GL. The development and initial validation of the geriatric suicide ideation scale. Am J Geriatr Psychiatr. 2006;14(9):742–51.
37. Appelbaum PS, Lidz CW, Meisel A. Informed consent: legal theory and clinical practice. New York: Oxford University Press; 1987.
38. Faden RR, Beauchamp TL, King NMP. A history and theory of informed consent. New York: Oxford University Press; 1986.
39. Appelbaum PS, Grisso T. Assessing patients' capacities to consent to treatment. N Engl J Med. 1988;319:1635–8. doi:10.1056/NEJM198812223192504.
40. Roth LH, Meisel A, Lidz CW. Tests of competency to consent to treatment. Am J Psychiatr. 1977;134:279–84.
41. Taub HA. Informed consent, memory and age. Gerontologist. 1980;20:686–90. doi:10.1093/geront/20.6.686.
42. Taub HA, Baker MT. The effect of repeated testing upon comprehension of informed consent materials by elderly volunteers. Exp Aging Res. 1983;9:135–8. doi:10.1080/03610738308258441.
43. Taub HA, Baker MT, Sturr JF. Informed consent for research. Effects of readability, patient age, and education. J Am Geriatr Soc. 1986;34:601–6.
44. Cassell EJ, Leon AC, Kaufman SG. Preliminary evidence of impaired thinking in sick patients. Ann Intern Med. 2001;134:1120–3.
45. Fitten LJ, Waite MS. Impact of medical hospitalization on treatment decision making capacity in the elderly. Arch Intern Med. 1990;150:1717–21.
46. Grisso T, Appelbaum PS, Hill-Fotouhi C. The MacCAT-T: a clinical tool to assess patients' capacities to make treatment decisions. Psychiatr Serv. 1997;48:1415–9.
47. Etchells E, Darzins P, Silberfeld M, Singer PA, McKenny J, Naglie G, Katz M, Guyatt GH, Molloy DW, Strang D. Assessment of patient capacity to consent to treatment. J Gen Intern Med. 1999;14:27–34.
48. Holland JC. History of psycho-oncology. In: Holland JC, Breitbart WS, Jacobsen PB, Ledgerberg MS, Loscalzo MJ, McCorkle R, editors. Psycho-oncology. 2nd ed. New York: Oxford University Press; 2010.
49. Anquiano L, Mayer DK, Piven ML, Rosenstein D. A literature review of suicide in cancer patients. Cancer Nurs. 2012;35(4):14–25. doi:10.1097/NCC.0b013e31822fc76c.
50. Misono S, Weiss NS, Fann JR, Redman M, Yueh B. Incidence of suicide in persons with cancer. J Clin Oncol. 2008;26(29):4731–8. http://doi.org/10.1200/JCO.2007.13.8941.
51. Breitbart W, Pessin H, Kolva E. Suicide and desire for hastened death in patients with cancer. In: Kissane D, Maj M, Sartorius N, editors. Depression in cancer. Chichester: Wiley-Blackwell; 2010.
52. Breitbart W, Rosenfeld B, Gibson C, Kramer M, Li Y, Tomarken A, Nelson C, Pessin H, Esch J, Galietta M, Garcia N, Brechtl J, Schuster M. Impact of treatment for depression on desire

for hastened death in patients with advanced AIDS. Psychosomatics. 2010;51:98–105. doi:10.1176/appi.psy.51.2.98.

53. Pessin H, Amakawa L, Breitbart WS. Suicide. In: Holland JC, Breitbart WS, Jacobsen PB, Lederberg MS, Loscalzo MJ, McCorkle R, editors. Psycho-oncology. 2nd ed. New York: Oxford University Press; 2010.

54. Chochinov HM, Wilson KG, Enns M, Mowchun N, Lander S, Levitt M, Clinch JJ. Desire for death in the terminally ill. Am J Psychiatr. 1995;152:1185–91.

55. Hudson PL, Kristjanson LJ, Ashby M, Kelly B, Schofield P, Hudson R, Street A. Desire for hastened death in patients with advanced disease and the evidence base of clinical guidelines: a systematic review. Palliat Med. 2006;20:693–701. doi:10.1177/0269216306071799.

56. Breitbart W, Rosenfeld B, Pessin H, Kaim M, Funesti-Esch J, Galietta M, Nelson CJ, Brescia R. Depression, hopelessness, and desire for hastened death in terminally ill patients with cancer. JAMA. 2000;284:2907–11. doi:10.1001/jama.284.22.2907.

57. Emanuel EJ, Fairclough DL, Daniels ER, Clarridge BR. Euthenasia and physician-assisted suicide: a comparative study of physicians, terminally-ill cancer patients, and the general population. Lancet. 1996;347:1805–10.

58. Nissim R, Gagliesse L, Rodin G. The desire for hastened death in individuals with advanced cancer: a longitudinal qualitative study. Soc Sci Med. 2009;69(2):165–71. doi:10.1016/j.socscimed.2009.04.021.

59. Rosenfeld B, Pessin H, Marziliano A, Sorger B, Abbey J, Olden M, Brescia R, Breitbart W. Does desire for hastened death change in terminally ill cancer patients? Soc Sci Med. 2014;111:35–40. doi:10.1016/j.socscimed.2014.03.027.

60. O'Mahony S, Goulet J, Kornblith A, Abbatiello G, Clarke B, Kless-Siegel S, Breitbart W, Payne R. Desire for hastened death, cancer pain and depression: report of a longitudinal observational study. J Pain Symptom Manage. 2005;29:446–57. doi:10.1016/j.jpainsymman.2004.08.010.

61. Pessin H, Rosenfeld B, Burton L, Breitbart W. The role of cognitive impairment in desire for hastened death: a study of patients with advanced AIDS. Gen Hosp Psychiatry. 2003;25:194–9. doi:10.1016/S0163-8343(03)00008-2.

62. Rodin G, Zimmermann C, Rydall A, Jones J, Shepherd FA, Moore M, Fruh M, Donner A, Gagliese L. The desire for hastened death in patients with metastatic cancer. J Pain Symptom Manage. 2007;33:661–75. doi:10.1016/j.jpainsymman.2006.09.034.

63. Tiernan E, Casey P, O'Boyle C, Birkbeck G, Mangan M, O'Siorain L, Kearney M. Relations between desire for early death, depressive symptoms and antidepressant prescribing in terminally ill patients with cancer. J R Soc Med. 2002;95:386–90.

64. Rosenfeld B, Breitbart W, Galietta M, Kaim M, Funesti-Esch J, Pessin H, Nelson CJ, Brescia R. The schedule of attitudes toward hastened death: measuring desire for death in terminally ill cancer patients. Cancer. 2000;88:2868–75. doi:10.1002/1097-0142(20000615)88:12.

65. Rosenfeld B, Breitbart W, Stein K, Funesti-Esch J, Kaim M, Krivo S, Galietta M. Measuring desire for death among patients with HIV/AIDS: the schedule of attitudes toward hastened death. Am J Psychiatr. 1999;156:94–100.

66. Pestinger M, Steil S, Elsner F, Widdershoven G, Voltz R, Nauck F, Radbruch L. The desire to hasten death: using grounded theory for a better understanding "When perception of time tends to be a slippery slope". Palliat Med. 2015;29(8):711–9. doi:10.1177/0269216315577748.

67. Sullivan MD. Hope and hopelessness at the end of life. Am J Geriatr Psychiatr. 2003;11(4):393–405.

68. Levine R. Treating idealized hope and hopelessness. Int J Group Psychother. 2007;57(3):297–317.

69. Burgy M. Phenomenological investigation of despair in depression. Psychopathology. 2008;41:147–56.

70. Pearson JL, Brown GK. Suicide prevention in late life: directions for science and practice. Clin Psychol Rev. 2000;20(6):685–705.

71. Sachs E, Kolva E, Pessin H, Rosenfeld B, Breitbart W. On sinking and swimming: the dialectic of hope, hopelessness, and acceptance in terminal cancer. Am J Hosp Palliat Care. 2013;30(2):121–7. doi:10.1177/1049909112445371.
72. Heisel MJ, Flett GL. A psychometric analysis of the geriatric hopelessness scale (GHS): towards improving assessment of the construct. J Affect Disord. 2005;87(2–3):211–20.
73. Rosenfeld B, Pessin H, Lewis C, Abbey J, Olden M, Sachs E, Amakawa L, Kolva E, Brescia R, Breitbart W. Assessing hopelessness in terminally ill cancer patients: development of the Hopelessness Assessment in Illness Questionnaire (HAI). Psychol Assess. 2011;23:325–36. doi:10.1037/a0021767.
74. Fry PS. Development of a geriatric scale of hopelessness: implications for counseling and intervention with the depressed elderly. J Couns Psychol. 1984;31:322–31.
75. Filiberti A, Ripamonti C, Totis A, Ventafridda V, DeConno F, Tamburini M. Characteristics of terminal cancer patients who committed suicide during a home palliative care program. J Pain Symptom Manage. 2001;22(1):544–53.
76. Van Orden KA, Bamonti PM, King DA, Duberstein PR. Does perceived burdensomeness erode meaning in life among older adults? Aging Ment Health. 2012;16(7):855–60. doi:10.10 80/13607863.2012.657156.
77. Wilson KG, Curran D, McPherson CJ. A burden to others: a common source of distress for the terminally Ill. Cogn Behav Ther. 2005;34(2):115–23. doi:10.1080/16506070510008461.
78. Cukrowicz KC, Cheavens JS, Van Orden KA, Ragain RM, Cook RL. Perceived burdensomeness and suicide ideation in older adults. Psychol Aging. 2011;26(2):331–8. doi:10.1037/a0021836.
79. Sullivan AD, Hedberg K, Hopkins D. Legalized physician-assisted suicide in Oregon, 1998–2000. N Engl J Med. 2001;344(8):605–7.
80. Kelly B, Burnett P, Pelusi D, Badger S, Varghese F, Robertson M. Factors associated with the wish to hasten death: a study of patients with terminal illness. Psychol Med. 2003;33(1):75–81.
81. Street A, Kissane DW. Dispensing death, desiring death: an exploration of medical roles and patient motivation during the period of legalized euthanasia in Australia. Omega (Westport). 1999–2000;40: 272–280.
82. Cohen S, Wills TA. Stress, social support, and the buffering hypothesis. Psychol Bull. 1985;98:310–57.
83. Kroenke C, Kubzansky L, Schernhammer ES, Holmes MD, Kawachi I. Social networks, social support, and survival after breast cancer diagnosis. J Clin Oncol. 2006;24:1105–11.
84. Ringdal GI, Ringdal K, Jordhøy MS, et al. Does social support from family and friends work as a buffer against reactions to stressful life events such as terminal cancer? Palliat Support Care. 2007;5:61–9.
85. Broadhead WE, Gehlbach SH, DeGruy FV, et al. The Duke–UNC functional social support questionnaire: measurement of social support in family medicine patients. Med Care. 1988;26:709–23.
86. Cyranowski JM, Zill N, Bode R, Butt Z, Kelly MAR, Pilkonis PA, Salsman JM, Cella D. Assessing social support, companionship, and distress: NIH toolbox adult social relationship scales. Health Psychol. 2013;32(3):293–301. doi:10.1037/a0028586.
87. Sarason IG, Levine HM, Basham RB, Sarason BR. Assessing social support: the social support questionnaire. J Pers Soc Psychol. 1983;44(1):127–39. doi:10.1037/0022-3514.44.1.127.
88. Zimet GD, Dahlem NW, Zimet SG, Farley GK. The multidimensional scale of perceived social support. J Pers Assess. 1988;52(1):30–41. doi:10.1207/s15327752jpa5201_2.
89. Rowe JL, Conwell Y, Schulberg HC, Bruce ML. Social support and suicidal ideation in older adults using home healthcare services. Am J Geriatr Psychiatr. 2006;14(9):758–66.
90. Breitbart W. Spirituality and meaning in supportive care: spirituality- and meaning- centered group psychotherapy interventions in advanced cancer. Support Care Cancer. 2002;10(4):272–80.
91. Yalom ID. Existential psychotherapy. New York: Basic Books; 1980.
92. Kissane DW. Psychospiritual and existential distress. Aust Fam Physician. 2000;29:1022–5.
93. Peterman AH, Fitchett G, Brady MJ, Hernandez L, Cella D. Measuring spiritual well-being in people with cancer: The Functional Assessment of Chronic Illness Therapy–Spiritual Well-Being Scale (FACIT–Sp). Ann Behav Med. 2002;24:49–58. doi:10.1207/S15324796ABM2401_06.

94. Steger MF, Frazier P, Oishi S, Kaler M. The meaning in life questionnaire: assessing the presence of and search for meaning in life. J Couns Psychol. 2006;53:80–93.
95. Dazzi T, Gribble R, Wessely S, Fear T. Does asking about suicide and related behaviours induce suicidal ideation? What is the evidence? Psychol Med. 2014;44(16):3361–3.
96. Hudson PL, Schofield P, Kelly B, O'Connor M, Kristjanson LJ, Ashby M, Aranda S. Responding to desire to die statements from patients with advanced disease: recommendations for health professionals. Palliat Med. 2006;20(7):703–10.
97. Block SD, Billings JA. Patient requests for euthanasia and assisted suicide in terminal illness: the role of the psychiatrist. Psychosomatics. 1995;36:445–57.
98. Oregon Revised Statutes. The Oregon death with dignity act. 1994. https://public.health.oregon.gov/ProviderPartnerResources/EvaluationResearch/DeathwithDignityAct/Documents/statute.pdf. Accessed 16 Dec 2015 from the Oregon state web site.
99. Campbell CS. Ten years of "Death with Dignity." The New Atlantic. Fall 2008; 33–46.

A Psychodynamic Perspective on Suicidal Desire in the Elderly

11

Meera Balasubramaniam

11.1 The Case of Ms. A

Ms. A was a 93-year-old lady, a sprightly retired middle-school teacher who presented to the Emergency Room (E.R.) of a local teaching hospital complaining of dizziness. She reported with much concern that she had fallen twice within the past month. She used a walker to ambulate. A thorough medical evaluation by the physician in the E.R and a few tests soon followed and ruled out all major medical causes for her dizziness. She was advised to reduce the dose of her antihypertensive medication and follow up with her primary care doctor. The nurse in the emergency room went over the discharge plan, when Ms. A casually told her about "the helium hood" she had purchased. She explained that she planned to execute the "final exit" someday. She denied thoughts of wanting to hurt herself at the present time but added that she "will do it my way when I feel it's about time." She did not specify a timeline, adding that it should matter to "no one whether I die at 94 or 96" and that she would "hate to perish in a nursing home."

Psychiatry was consulted to evaluate Ms. A in the ER. On evaluation by the psychiatry resident, Ms. A appeared pleasant, well-spoken, neatly dressed, talked about visiting a local senior center a few times every week. She shared that she had been widowed for the last 15 years. Her score on the Montreal Cognitive Assessment scale [1] was 26/30, ruling out significant cognitive impairment. She did not meet diagnostic criteria for any mood, anxiety, or psychotic disorder. The ER and Psychiatry physicians discussed her thoughts to end her life, which were not imminent, had an undetermined timeframe, but were accompanied by a specific plan. Her thoughts were in stark contrast to her overall good physical health and the absence of overt mental illness. The physicians questioned whether Ms. A was safe

M. Balasubramaniam, M.D., M.P.H. (✉)
Department of Psychiatry, New York University School of Medicine,
One Park Avenue, New York, NY 10016, USA
e-mail: meera.balasubramaniam@nyumc.org

© Springer International Publishing Switzerland 2017
R.E. McCue, M. Balasubramaniam (eds.), *Rational Suicide in the Elderly*,
DOI 10.1007/978-3-319-32672-6_11

to be discharged home. They discussed the need to "take away the weapon," which in this case was the helium hood in her home. Ms. A insisted that her thoughts were "rational" and wished to return home.

Are Ms. A's thoughts to end her life rational? The question of whether suicide in the absence of a diagnosable mental illness can be rational is increasingly being encountered. Does the lack of a diagnostic label to describe the state of mind where suicide appears the best available option reflect a flaw in the existing nosology? Or is this a truly rational phenomenon that we are going to increasingly encounter as life expectancy continues to increase? Many psychiatric illnesses are associated with a high risk for suicide. However, many individuals diagnosed with the very same illnesses never attempt suicide, while others may make multiple attempts. There is clearly a lot more to individuals than their diagnoses alone to distinguish suicide attempters from the nonattempters.

When encountering a patient who wishes to die, it is the clinician's responsibility to explore with curiosity and kindness the meaning of their life and the purpose that the act of self-destruction will serve. To echo Karl Menninger, we as a society are more curious about the motives of murder but willingly and "with astonishing naiveté" accept simplistic explanations for suicide [2]. The wish to commit suicide offers a glimpse into a nuanced human mind, and a clinician should offer the direction and space for it to unfold. The chapter is written with this focus. We first review prominent theories of suicide. Following that, we explore what is known about Ms. A from the perspective of these theories to obtain a deeper understanding of Ms. A's suicidal wishes.

11.2   Theories of Suicide: Freud and Beyond

Freud described suicide as an act of "turning against the self." Aggressive impulses directed at others are unconsciously displaced onto oneself. He believed that the aggressive impulses were originally toward an external object, typically a person with whom the individual has had a conflictual relationship. These externally directed aggressive impulses may not find release for a variety of reasons. These include the external resistance offered by reality, internal resistance in the form of fear and guilt, and a sense of ambivalence due to conflicting positive and negative feelings towards the object. From this ambivalence, the individual identifies with and internalizes the object. Once the hated object is introjected, the separation between the self and the object are lost; the aggressive negative impulses that were originally externally channeled are now displaced toward oneself. The introjected hated person can then be destroyed by destroying oneself by suicide [3].

Menninger believed that for suicide to occur there must be three components: the wish to kill, the wish to be killed, and the wish to die [2]. Each of these has its own conscious and unconscious motives. The *wish to kill* component is similar to Freud's theory of turning against the self, explained above. Menninger described the *wish to be killed* as an extreme form of submission. When one harbors an unconscious wish to destroy an object, it is perceived intrapsychically as actual destruction. Having brought about destruction, the individual feels guilty and is overcome by an intense urge to atone by punishing oneself. He elucidated this concept with reference to familial clustering of suicide. Unconscious death wishes are often felt toward family members, especially those toward whom one may have conflictual feelings. When such a person dies suddenly by suicide, one's unconscious wishes are unexpectedly gratified. The gratification soon gives way to intense guilt which can only be overcome by destroying oneself. The *wish to die* was believed by Menninger to be the realization of the death instinct. He believed that it determined the ultimate success of a suicide attempt.

Hendrick proposed a concept of suicide which differed from that of Freud in terms of identification with an object and how it contributes to suicide. Freud's theory of turning against the self requires that identification with an introjected object take place before aggressive impulses are directed at oneself. To Hendrick, the identification with an object is often the goal of suicide, rather than its mechanism. He described the case of a young woman who had made a suicide attempt by rolling off a bridge with the intention to drown. With psychoanalysis, the patient made associations that revealed several aspects of her suicide attempt mirrored her brother's death. The shade of blue she wore, the town she drove past, her act of driving "in circles" before jumping off the bridge, and her inclination that her body not be discovered for at least 2 months after her death were unconsciously linked to her brother who died in a foreign country in an airplane crash, with the airplane falling "in circles," and his body was discovered a few months later. Hendrick went on to elaborate that the patient's brother formed an early internal representation of a satisfying object relationship for the patient as she had had a troubled relationship with her parents. A severe interpersonal crisis that preceded the suicide attempt led her to disintegrate emotionally, such that identifying herself with her dead brother, by way of suicide, felt as the only option to feel whole again [4].

Winnicott and Kohut conceptualized suicide as a reaction to narcissistic injuries. Winnicott believed that suicide was a defense to protect the true self from annihilation. In the absence of a "good-enough" mother who is attuned to the infant's spontaneous gestures and early needs, the development of the "true self" is hindered. Instead, the infant builds a "false self," one that is molded to fit into the external environment but devoid of the aliveness that characterizes the individual's "true self." When there is an external crisis, it is the "false self" that acts on suicidal urges in the absence of a developed "true self." Suicide can be understood as the escape from a state of being falsely imprisoned ("false self") when the core ("true self") is already dead [5]. Kohut has described that in the absence of the mother's empathic attunement to a child's early needs, the child goes on to develop a fragile sense of self. During life, he is then in perpetual need of external supports to bolster his self-esteem. When external influences fail to meet the individual's narcissistic needs, it results in a profound sense of disintegration and anguish [6, 7] that may lead to suicide. These principles are very relevant to those cases of elderly individuals who have faced multiple losses over a short span of time and across various domains. These losses can include the loss of relationships, retirement from work, ill-health, and the loss of youthful attractiveness. If these have maintained the sense of self through adulthood, a person with a fragile sense of self may react to these losses with intolerable distress from which suicide is an escape.

Maltsberger and Buie [8] proposed that suicide was motivated by the desires for revenge, riddance, and rebirth. *Revenge* was the unconscious wish of an individual to inflict pain and anguish on others by causing one's own death. Such individuals reportedly indulged in daydreams of their own funeral and pictured the grief of those around them. Revenge was also believed to be a part Menninger's concept of the wish to kill, mentioned earlier in this chapter. Menninger's experience with suicidal children suggested that their wish to kill often represented aggression directed at their parents. They harbored a desire to seek revenge on parents by robbing them of their most prized possession, that is, the child. However, they separated the reality of their own finality from this strongly held fantasy of inflicting pain on others [2]. Suicide for *riddance* can occur in individuals with a fragmented sense of self. Their unconscious self-representation consisted of two subdivisions: "me" who is experienced as helpless and the "other," derived from hostile introjects, who is experienced as scornful and alien. In times of crisis, this fragmentation can become so profound that "me" becomes terrified of the "other," seeking to destroy the latter to protect itself. Muskin has described how this split in the experience of oneself may come into play in medically ill individuals [9]. Such individuals may feel overwhelmed by the medical, psychosocial, and emotional needs brought about by their illness and the split may be externally discernible in the form of statements such as "I don't recognize the person I've become." They wish for the "sick" part of themselves to be killed, leaving the healthy self to live. Interestingly, the "me" or "healthy self" seeks to destroy the "other" or "sick self" with the fantasy of a better state of being after getting rid of the "other." However, they lack the awareness that this would result in annihilation of the whole being. Maltsberger and Buie have elaborated on the desire for *rebirth* as a fantasy of fusion with a comfort-giving mother figure. Individuals deprived of early nourishment from caregivers develop a poor sense of agency and difficulty tolerating separation from a comforting object. Such individuals frequently entertain an illusion of death, which appears to them not as terrifying isolation but as blissful fusion with a maternal object.

The psychological understanding of suicide would be incomplete without mentioning the work of Schneidman, the father of contemporary suicidology, although his postulates are not purely psychoanalytic. Schneidman introduced the concept of "psychache" as a necessary condition for suicide [10]. He described it as an unbearable sense of anguish, a profound frustration about the lack of fulfillment of one's vital psychological needs. This leads to a perception of constricted choice, such that suicide appears to be the only way to ameliorate "psychache." He was of the opinion that subjective experiences of anguish are often lost in the quest for diagnostic bracketing and that "suicide is not a psychiatric disorder." All individuals who commit suicide are anguished, but not necessarily diagnosable with a mental illness. He believed that depression does not lead to suicide unless it contributed to "psychache" and stated that the latter should be the target for preventing suicide.

The concept of suicide as an escape from the self was proposed by Baechler [11] and subsequently elucidated by Baumeister [12] as a stepwise phenomenon. The first step is an undesirable situation, resulting from an acute setback, extremely high expectations or both. Internalization of the blame for the event then follows. This self-attribution results in a negative view of oneself as worthless, undesirable, and inadequate. Such intensely negative self-perceptions trigger aversive emotions such as sadness, guilt, and anxiety. The individual seeks to escape from the emotionally aversive state; the first step in this process is the state of "cognitive deconstruction." Baumeister described this state as being relatively numb, concrete, focused on simple immediate tasks, and less capable of nuances in thinking and feeling. While this may succeed in blocking out negative emotions and perceptions, it is marked by numbness and emptiness rather than positive emotions. This deconstructed state is also disinhibiting for it separates meaning from action. One can therefore imagine that an individual who remains focused on the immediate steps of suicide as a means of ending painful emotions, but is unable to evaluate the larger meaning and consequences of death.

11.3 Revisiting the Case of Ms. A

We will now return to Ms. A and, using psychodynamic theories, develop hypotheses to understand her situation at a deeper level.

Ms. A was a 93-year-old lady, a sprightly retired teacher who presented to the Emergency Room. She had been widowed for the last 15 years and attended a senior center regularly.

Even with the minimal demographic information provided about Ms. A, we are aware that she has experienced life changes across various domains. She has aged and experienced at least one significant relational loss. Her role as a teacher has been replaced with spending time with peers of her age group at the senior center. If her sense of self was previously bolstered by her identity as a teacher, a married woman, and being physically healthy, then, from the perspective of Kohut, Ms. A has suffered significant narcissistic injuries [6]. Information regarding her early childhood, the presence or absence of caregivers to soothe her during times of distress, and her sense of self-worth through her adult life would provide useful information to us about how these losses are influencing her wish to die.

From our knowledge of Erikson's stages of psychosocial development [13], we know that Ms. A is probably at the stage when she is reflecting on her life and asking herself "is it ok to have been me?" Her reflection comes at a time when she is bereaved of loved ones she considered close and trusted, when she is no longer performing the role of a teacher, and when she is experiencing physical limitations. The process of reflection at the end of life typically brings to the fore unresolved conflicts from all earlier developmental tasks, namely trust, autonomy, initiative, industry, identity, intimacy, and generativity. Richman [14] described this re-emergence "in full force" of problems in earlier developmental tasks as a factor unique to suicide in the elderly. He believed that the ability of elderly individuals to make rational choices involving life and death is governed by their life review, during which they look back at past experiences, process the present, and take stock of what is required for the future. Ms. A's suicidal wish reflects not only her present circumstances but also her

previous unresolved developmental conflicts. We must support Ms. A in this process
of exploring the deeper, richer aspects of her psyche. Terming her wish as rational or
not based on her immediate circumstances alone is overly simplistic.

*Ms. A presented to the ER complaining of dizziness. She reported with concern that she had
fallen twice within the past month. She uses a walker to ambulate.*

Ms. A has experienced bodily changes by virtue of her advanced age. What did
her physical self and body mean to a younger Ms. A? How has she adapted to the
changes in her physical vitality over the years? These are important points to ponder. Body love and care have been postulated to result from internalization of positive parental attunement and responsiveness of the caregiver to early needs [15–17].
Orbach has extensively written about the relationship between the physical body
and the inner psyche in determining the sense of self-preservation [17]. His work
describes how negative attitudes toward one's body, triggered by early physical
abuse or rejection, result in the development of bodily dissociation as a defense.
This increases pain threshold and creates bodily distancing, such that the individual
feels that they have little to lose by way of bodily pleasures if they were to die. King
and Apter have drawn an association between medical illness and bodily appreciation in the case of children with insulin dependent diabetes who, by way of injecting
themselves daily, go on to develop mixed feelings toward their bodies [18].

The elderly experience changes in their bodies, both aesthetically and function-
ally. This may occur rather precipitously in those who experience a cerebrovascular
stroke, gradually but markedly among those with Parkinson's disease, and more
subtly in the rest. This need for ongoing adaptation to change is superimposed on
pre-existing positive and negative notions of one's body. In a case series of elderly
suicidal men, Lindner discusses the feelings of helplessness, envy, and disappointment that were noted in his sample, as their physical well-being decreased and
dependency increased [19]. These feelings were then projected on to the body with
the desire for annihilation. The same paper describes an elderly man who perceives
his son's inheritance of an eye condition as a personal failure and goes on to experience such intense guilt, that he wishes to destroy not only himself but also his son
who he views intrapsychically as a part of himself.

Ms. A's death wish must be understood in the context of how changes in her life
have been associated with changes in her body. The evolution of her body image
and her attitude toward her aging body must be understood. Is there any split in the
perception of Ms. A's healthy and sick parts of herself? Is the part of the patient who
feels dizzy, falls, and relies on a walker integrated with her overall sense of identity
as a person? If the sick parts of Ms. A are viewed intrapsychically as alien, the wish
for suicide to achieve riddance might be at play [8, 9].

*Ms. A had been widowed for the last 15 years. She said that it should matter to "no one
whether I die at 94 or 6."*

Suicide has been described in several theories as involving an object, with the
unconscious desire for identification, revenge, or rebirth. Schneidman proposed that

suicide is a dyadic event, such that the "suicidal drama" in the mind always involves interplay with another, whether it is a significant other in the preventive phase or a survivor–victim after the suicide [10]. Ms. A's emphasis of the absence of an object ("should matter to no one") paradoxically highlights the need for us to understand the quality of her relationships, including objects of love and hate. We must explore Ms. A's relationship with her husband, the manner of his death, her reactions to his death, and her feelings about outliving him for over a decade. Guilt is a common theme noted among veterans who expressed self-hatred about surviving war when their close friends had not [20, 21]. Although grief and depression are talked about frequently in the context of elderly bereavement, survival guilt is a less well-established but equally vital theme to be looked for. How do elderly individuals such as Ms. A perceive their relationship with dead objects? It is not uncommon for individuals to cherish fantasies of reunion with dead loved ones by way of suicide [20, 22].

Despair has often been the term of choice to indicate the mental state of suicidal patients. It is marked by loneliness, self-hatred, and the inability to view any human connection as being significant [20, 23, 24]. Ms. A's strong statement about her death mattering to no one warrants further discussion on who constitutes "no one" to her. Such a discussion would give us a deeper understanding of the quality of the patient's attachments with objects in their lives, for it is not common to have conflictual or even negative feelings toward close family members. Feelings of jealousy and rage toward physically healthier spouses have been reported [19]. Unconscious motivation for revenge toward surviving family members must be considered, similar to that observed by Menninger in suicidal children who sought revenge against their parents by robbing them of their own presence [2]. Richman emphasized the errors of "treating the patient as a purely biological entity living in a social vacuum" and called not only for deeper understanding of patients' relationships but also for direct involvement of their families as well [14].

Ms. A casually told her nurse about "the helium hood" she had purchased. She explained that she planned to execute the "final exit" someday.

Ms. A shared details of her death wish with the ER nurse who was reviewing her discharge papers. Given that the patient was deemed ready for discharge by her physician, it is unlikely that the nurse specifically inquired about suicidality. Three elements stand out in this interaction (1) the suicidal thought was reported by Ms. A despite not being specifically asked about it, (2) this piece of information was conveyed by an elderly patient to a young provider, and (3) the interaction evoked significant anxiety in the nurse and physicians in the ER. We must remember that the mention of suicidality, although casual, unsolicited, and not imminent as in this case, is nonetheless a cry for help. It could be a real death wish or a proxy for unbearable distress brought forth by stressors in her life. Ms. A is very possibly asking her nurse and physicians to re-affirm the value of her life, one that she is beginning to lose sight of in the face of age and illness. As Siegel recommends, as clinicians we should make efforts to bolster self-esteem, foster acceptance, and preserve attachments, particularly when the patient is compromised by illness or disability [25]. Second, there is the possibility of other unconscious motives that caused Ms. A to report her suicidal thoughts to the much younger nurse, which she knew would evoke intense feelings of anxiety and discomfort in clinical staff. Negative feelings toward younger, healthier individuals are not uncommon among the elderly who are grappling with changes in their own vitality and coming to terms with dependency. Lindner described the case an elderly man who enacted an intense power struggle with his younger therapist evoking anxiety in the latter [19]. Muskin [9] has suggested that patients may experience rage at their providers and harbor fantasies of inflicting harm on them, by way of one's own death. What function was served by Ms. A's sharing of her suicidal wish with the nurse? How did she think the nurse would react? In the case of unconscious motivations such as revenge, Muskin believes that timely and appropriate psychotherapy will help the patient gain an understanding about how their positive and negative feelings are intrapsychic creations, and that suicide is unlikely to have the impact that is unconsciously desired.

> She denied thoughts of wanting to hurt herself at the present time but added that she "will do it my way when I feel it's about time."

It is interesting to note that that while Ms. A verbalizes the availability of suicide as an option, she denies any intention of acting on her suicidal thoughts at the time of her conversation in the ER. What purpose is being served by the option of suicide in this elderly individual with a recent but nonfatal illness? Is the suicidal thought a harbinger of an actual self-injurious attempt? Or is it antithetically a life-sustaining force? These are questions we must carefully explore with Ms. A. The example of Kate Cutrer, a character in "The Moviegoer," who uses suicidal thoughts as a means to soothe herself brings this conundrum to light [26, 27]: *"They all think any minute I'm going to commit suicide. What a joke. The truth of course is the exact opposite: suicide is the only thing that keeps me alive. Whenever everything else fails, all I have to do is consider suicide and in 2 seconds I'm as cheerful as a nitwit."* In the face of distress, an individual is able to cope with crisis by way of internalized object representations of early comforting caregivers. When this fails to provide satisfactory soothing, external measures of comfort in the form of family, friends, or care providers may help reduce one's sense of distress. Many elderly individuals are often bereaved of long-term sources of such external support. We must consider the possibility that under such circumstances, suicidal fantasies by creating the illusion of "a way out" provide a sense of control and mastery, preserve cohesion of the disintegrating ego, and offer comfort. Maltsberger and colleagues describe case histories of individuals who gave up their suicidal reveries only after they were able to acquire, by way of treatment, more adaptive ways of buttressing their self-esteem during moments of crisis [27]. However, while Ms. A could be entertaining suicidal reveries to preserve her sense of mastery in the face of helplessness brought forth by her advanced age and medical problems, we must be mindful of the possibility that this could eventually give way to an actual self-injurious attempt. Affective distress [20, 27], motor agitation [28], and a constricted view of available choices to reduce distress [10] are important factors to look for, even in individuals for whom suicidal fantasies have chronically played a life-sustaining role.

11.4 Conclusion

Suicide is always rational, in the moment, to the person making the choice. But does that truly make it a choice that is well thoughtout, consistent, and devoid of conflicts? Menninger believed that suicidal individuals bring about justifications in their external reality to satiate their unconscious motivations [2]. Our own review of several theories of suicide in this chapter has highlighted examples of individuals who perceived self-harm as appropriate or perhaps even befitting their situation. However, these individuals did so without conscious awareness of what motivated those beliefs and that suicide actually amounted to self-annihilation. In Ms. A's case, the possibility of suicide could have been a defense against living a life that she perceived as suboptimal. Human choices are complex and the act of dichotomizing a choice as either being fully rational or as one stemming from a mental illness would be premature and reductionist. Richman who has extensively worked and written about suicide in the elderly believed that there is opportunity for free choice only after conflicts are resolved, individual wishes are given the opportunity to be processed, and important relationships are cohesive, all of which can be done in an appropriate therapeutic setting [14]. We live in an environment where there is considerable stigma around seeking psychiatric help. While life expectancy has increased, ageism persists. Under these circumstances, dichotomizing suicide as simply rational or pathological would further limit the willingness of an elderly individual who is considering suicide to seek treatment and explore these wishes. We must explore an expression of a death wish with curiosity, compassion, and clinical depth before making premature pronouncements of a psychiatric diagnosis. As our understanding of an individual becomes deeper and richer, the element of rationality, or the lack of it, is likely to clarify itself, not only for the clinician but also to the individual for whom suicide feels like the best available choice.

References

1. Nasreddine ZS, Phillips NA, Bédirian V, et al. The Montreal cognitive assessment, MoCA: a brief screening tool for mild cognitive impairment. J Am Geriatr Soc. 2005;53(4):695–9. doi:10.1111/j.1532-5415.2005.53221.x.
2. Menninger KA. Psychoanalytic aspects of suicide. Int J Psychoanal. 1933;14:376–90.
3. Freud S. Mourning and Melancholia. Standard Edition 14. London: Hogarth; 1917.
4. Hendrick I. Suicide as wish fulfillment. Psychiatry Q. 1940;14:30–42.
5. Winnicott D. The maturational process and the facilitating environment. New York: International Universities Press; 1965.
6. Kohut H. The restoration of the self. New York: International Universities Press; 1977.
7. Huprich SK. Psychodynamic conceptualization and treatment of suicidal patients. J Contemp Psychoanal. 2004;34(1):23–39.
8. Maltsberger JT, Buie DH. The devices of suicide: revenge, riddance, and rebirth. Int Rev Psychoanal. 1980;7:61–72.
9. Muskin PR. The request to die: role for a psychodynamic perspective on physician-assisted suicide. JAMA. 1998;279:323–8.
10. Schneidman ES. Suicide as psychache. J Nerv Ment Dis. 1993;181:147–9.

11. Baechler J. A strategic theory. Suicide Life Threat Behav. 1980;10:70–99.
12. Baumeister RF. Suicide as escape from self. Psychol Rev. 1990;97(1):90–113.
13. Erikson E. Childhood and society. New York: Norton; 1950.
14. Richman J. A rational approach to rational suicide. Suicide Life Threat Behav. 1992;22(1): 130–40.
15. Maltsberger JT. Confusion of the body, the self, and others in suicidal states. In: Leenaars A, Berman AL, Cantor P, Litman RE, Maris RW, editors. Suicidology: Essays in honor of Edward Schneidman. Northvale: Aronson; 1993. p. 148–72.
16. Van der Velde CD. Body image of one's self and of others: developmental and clinical significance. Am J Psychiatry. 1985;142:527–37.
17. Orbach I. Suicide and the suicidal body. Suicide Life Threat Behav. 2003;33(1):1–8.
18. King A, Apter A. Psychoanalytic perspectives on adolescent suicide. Psychoanal Study Child. 1996;51:491–511.
19. Lindner R. Suicidality in the elderly. Dtsch Med Wochenschr. 2012;137(40):2002–4.
20. Hendin H. Psychodynamics of suicide, with particular reference to the young. Am J Psychiatry. 1991;148:1150–8.
21. Hendin H, Haas AP. Suicide and guilt as manifestations of PTSD in Vietnam combat veterans. Am J Psychiatry. 1991;148:586–91.
22. Hendin H. The psychodynamics of suicide. J Nerv Ment Dis. 1963;136:236–44.
23. Maltsberger JT. Suicide risk: the formulation of clinical judgment. New York: New York University Press; 1981.
24. Lifton R. Suicide: the quest for a future. In: Jacobs D, Brown H, editors. Suicide: understanding and responding. Madison: International Universities Press; 1989.
25. Siegel K. Psychosocial aspects of rational suicide. Am J Psychother. 1986;40(3):405–18.
26. Gabbard GO. Miscarriages of psychoanalytic treatment with suicidal patients. Int J Psychoanal. 2003;84:249–61.
27. Maltsberger JT, Ronningstam E, Weinberg I, Schecter M, Goldblatt MJ. Suicide fantasy as a life-sustaining recourse. J Am Acad Psychoanal Dyn Psychiatry. 2010;38(4):611–24.
28. Koukopolous A, Koukopolous A. Agitated depression as a mixed state and the problem of melancholia. Psychiatr Clin N Am. 1999;22:547–64.

Impact of Psychotherapy on Rational Suicide

12

Darryl Etter and Elissa Kolva

12.1 Introduction

Suicidality is one of the most challenging issues in clinical work. Often, it demands greater urgency than other targets of intervention, and it involves more specific legal and ethical obligations. Patient death by suicide is one of the most stressful, distressing occurrences for clinicians, in part because it feels like one has failed one's patient by not taking sufficient clinical or environmental steps to prevent their death [1]. In a profession where attending to and repairing ruptures is a key piece of the work, suicide can represent a substantial rupture, and we do not have an opportunity to repair it. The case of rational suicide is additionally complicated: the burden and challenges of more "traditional" suicidality are present, as well as the ethical challenge of how to best serve a patient for whom continued life may be reasonably considered to be very burdensome while staying true to one's own professional and personal values.

Clinicians typically work to reduce suicidality and prevent suicidal behavior. Clinicians may feel strongly that a hastened death is morally wrong, based on faulty logic, or otherwise something to be prevented. Alternatively, when patients, particularly those who are older, terminally ill, or in significant pain, express a reasonable wish to die, we may feel pulled to join with them and may even feel that hastening their death is the ethical thing to do given difficult current circumstances.

D. Etter, Psy.D.
Department of Primary Care—Mental Health Integration, VA Eastern Colorado Health Care System, 1055 Clermont Street, Denver, CO 80220, USA
e-mail: Darryl.etter@va.gov

E. Kolva, Ph.D. (✉)
Division of Medical Oncology, Department of Medicine, University of Colorado School of Medicine, 12801 E. 17th Avenue, Mail Stop 8117, Research 1, South Aurora, CO 80045, USA
e-mail: elissa.kolva@ucdenver.edu; ekolva@gmail.com

© Springer International Publishing Switzerland 2017
R.E. McCue, M. Balasubramaniam (eds.), *Rational Suicide in the Elderly*,
DOI 10.1007/978-3-319-32672-6_12

In this chapter, we take the view that an individual is responsible for their own life, and that it is valuable to explore a range of alternatives before choosing death because it is irreversible. Cultural, philosophical, and legal views of suicidality influence providers' obligations and approaches to care, and these are often based on a framework that considers hastened death to always be harmful and the provider's responsibility to always be preventing death. However, openly exploring patients' and one's own values around life and death is likely to improve patient outcomes, such as reduced distress and increased existential coherence, and to reduce the emotional burden on providers by emphasizing patients' responsibility for their own lives [2]. Furthermore, clinical discussion of suicidality with patients actually helps to reduce the likelihood of death by suicide [3]. This open, direct approach underpins the clinical approaches reviewed and recommended here.

To be considered rational, the desire for death typically must occur in the context of a predictably unremittingly hopeless situation [4]. This can refer to an individual who is currently in distress with a low likelihood of relief (e.g., end-stage renal disease, chronic pain, treatment-resistant severe persistent mental illness, cerebral palsy), one who expects significant physical or mental decline that would be associated with distress and compromised personal integrity (e.g., early diagnosis of Huntington's disease or dementia), or one diagnosed with a terminal condition (e.g., advanced cancer). The nature of an individual's physical condition has often influenced the terminology used to refer to their wish for death, as has the involvement of a third party. We believe that there is significant conceptual overlap between many of these related terms, including rational suicide, hastened death, physician-assisted death, physician-assisted suicide, euthanasia, preemptive suicide, withdrawal/refusal of treatment, early death, and palliative/terminal sedation. "Rational suicide" can serve as an umbrella term to refer to many of the situations encompassed by these terms; however, we also use "hastened death" and "desire for hastened death" in this chapter. "Hastened death" is useful in that it does not connote a means by which death is caused, reflects the existential truth that all humans die, and does not carry the stigma and medico-legal baggage of "suicide" [4]. Although there are some conceptual differences between all these terms and situations that can affect ethical and legal considerations, the clinical goal and approach remains largely the same.

Psychotherapy with older adults considering rational suicide is still fundamentally psychotherapy and, as such, has a foundation of providing and exploring new perspectives, ideas, and skills. The clinician's goal is to understand what pieces of the individual's life are causing distress, help the individual to understand this in a way that feels actionable, and to help the individual develop strategies for improving the balance between distressing and rewarding aspects of their life. Rational suicidality often represents an effort to relieve distress or to establish some sense of control over an uncertain, potentially prolonged and unpleasant end-of-life process; therefore, clinical intervention can seek to relieve distress, develop patients' tolerance to temporary exacerbations of mood or physical symptoms, coordinate care to reduce logistical burdens, and provide information to reduce uncertainty about prognosis or the dying process [5].

Treatment of depressive symptoms has decreased desire for hastened death and led to individuals expressing a greater preference for life-saving and -sustaining treatments, though depression treatment does not appear to wholly resolve suicidality or to universally lead to a preference for more aggressive treatment [6–8]. This suggests that desire for hastened death is unique from depression, and an individual's experience of pain, hopelessness, and desire to die should be considered as potentially valid, even in the presence of psychiatric symptoms [9]. With all individuals, an assessment of the rationality of suicidality should establish that their current state does not represent an acute exacerbation of distress and that the individual has a good understanding of their current situation, prognosis, treatment and behavior options, and the nature of death.

We agree with Leeman [10] that, having established a rational basis for suicide, providers should not be obligated to interfere with an individual's effort to hasten their own death; however, because death is final, efforts should be made to ameliorate any changeable factors that are influencing the individual's decision to die. We believe the broad goal of clinical work is to maximize positive and minimize negative experiences. In the large majority of cases, we do not think that death best accomplishes this goal, so clinicians should first aim to delay patients' deaths and engage them in a process of finding ways to improve their quality of life.

In this chapter, we discuss a number of therapeutic approaches relevant to addressing rational suicidality in older adults. Where possible, we draw directly from literature addressing rational suicide or related concepts (e.g., desire for hastened death) in older adults; however, research in this area has been relatively limited [11]. We also review and draw recommendations from approaches designed to directly reduce suicidal ideation and behavior, to manage symptoms often associated with suicidality such as depression and anxiety, and to improve quality of life in older adults. Other relevant populations were considered to be individuals with chronic medical conditions, individuals with life-threatening illnesses (e.g., cancer, HIV/AIDS), and individuals at high risk of suicide (e.g., military veterans, individuals with borderline personality disorder). Finally, we also acknowledge the personal toll involved in this work and emphasize the importance of self-care and reflection.

12.2   Motivational Interviewing

We begin with Motivational Interviewing (MI; [12]) because it underpins much of the assessment and intervention techniques described in this chapter. Its foundation is in supporting patients' autonomy and developing motivation to change a behavior by acknowledging and exploring ambivalence around the decision to change. This is important in discussing desire for death because medical and mental health providers often avoid asking patients specific questions about suicidality or acknowledging that suicide is an option out of fear that doing so will increase the patient's likelihood of committing suicide. This belief is not accurate. Talking about suicide with patients does not increase their likelihood of attempting suicide [3]. In fact, the MI model suggests that a therapist providing a rationale for the undesired outcome (death) elicits more change talk from patients in the direction of the desired outcome (life; [13]).

The spirit of motivational interviewing is based on *collaboration* with the patient (rather than confrontation), *evocation* of strategies and motivation for change from the patient (rather than education by the clinician), and support of the patient's *autonomy* (rather than the clinician's authority; see [12]). In early treatment, the emphasis of therapy is on building motivation to change; an individual must feel that the change is important for them, that they are capable of making the change, and that it is currently a priority for them. This is accomplished by *expressing empathy*, particularly around a patient's ambivalence about a change; *developing discrepancy* between their current and desired situations; *rolling with resistance* to change, in which one actively avoids argumentativeness or defensiveness in the face of patients voicing low motivation to change; and *supporting self-efficacy* as patients identify and pursue strategies for change.

The techniques MI uses toward these ends include open-ended questions, affirmations, reflections, and summaries. *Change talk*, or statements made by a patient indicating greater dissatisfaction with their current situation and motivation to change, is often elicited with scaling questions (e.g., "From 0 to 10, how ready are you to change? Why did you choose X and not [a lower number]?"), as well as questions and reflections about extremes (e.g., "What are you most concerned about if you don't change?", "Continuing to live like this is the most important thing to you right now"). Resistance can be more difficult to respond to than change talk, and MI encourages clinicians to avoid the pull to try to "fix" the problem or barrier patients identify. For instance, when a patient states that a suggestion "doesn't work," a clinician could roll with that resistance by saying "Tell me about when you've tried it before," "It's really frustrating to keep trying to make changes and have it not work the way you were hoping," or "Great! We already have data about that. What other ideas would you like to try?"

Motivational Interviewing has been adapted for specific use with individuals expressing suicidal ideation (Motivational Interviewing for Suicidal Ideation; MI-SI; [13]). MI-SI identifies suicidal ideation and behavior as a detrimental health behavior to target. MI can also be specifically applied to restricting means for suicide, with an emphasis not only on identifying reasons for living, but also on reasons to engage in means restriction [14]. Integration of MI with cognitive-behavioral therapy (CBT) for suicide prevention to enhance engagement in treatment has also been proposed given the challenges of attrition from treatment in suicidal populations [15]. MI has additionally been integrated with the CAMS-SSF-III suicide assessment and prevention protocol in an emergency department setting [16], attesting to its usability in acute settings and compatibility with established institutional procedures.

12.2.1 Empirical Research

A small pilot study demonstrated that MI-SI was well tolerated in a psychiatric inpatient population of military veterans, and participants had significant reductions in suicidal ideation both immediately after the very brief (1–2 sessions) intervention and 60 days later [17]. MI-SI was also well tolerated by patients presenting to a psychiatric emergency department and reporting high levels of suicidal ideation, and the clinicians interviewing these patients indicated they found MI-SI to be helpful and feasible with this acute population and brief setting [15].

Motivational Interviewing has been successfully used as a pretreatment or adjunct treatment for anxiety, depression, and other mental health issues to enhance motivation to engage in treatment and to increase treatment efficacy [18, 19]. Meta-analyses have found significant effects of MI on a broad range of health behaviors and improvement in overall well-being, including in primary care and chronic medical condition patients [20–22]. The magnitude of these effects has been small to moderate, consistent with other effective psychological interventions despite usually having a briefer duration [20], often as little as one session [22]. Importantly, MI was found to increase motivation and engagement in treatment, and the effects on behavior and well-being appear to be durable, with effects maintained for at least a year [20].

With older adults, MI has been effectively applied to a number of health behaviors, including diabetes management, physical activity, and smoking cessation [23]. There is some indication that older adults may even benefit more from MI than younger individuals [20]. This may be due to the open, patient-centered nature of MI, which could appeal to older adults, who often are reluctant to engage with mental health services. Along with acknowledging this reluctance, clinicians using MI with older adults should incorporate adaptations used with other therapies in older adults, including flexibility in logistics, collaboration with healthcare providers and other helpers, slower pace, and reiteration of material to aid in encoding [24].

12.2.2 Application to Rational Suicide

Applied to rational suicide, it is important to note that even if the clinician has an opinion on what the outcome should be for the patient (e.g., psychiatric hospitalization to reduce risk of death by suicide, more aggressive medical treatment to prolong life), an MI-adherent approach would still emphasize the patient being the agent of decision-making and implementation of any plans. With rational suicide, this could entail empathizing with decreased or anticipated declines in physical functioning, and ongoing physical or emotional distress. The clinician could help the patient to clarify values and explore benefits and costs of choosing to live or die to develop discrepancy. Individuals who have lost some autonomy due to physical limitations and requirements of medical care may resist change in an effort to maintain autonomy; it would be important that clinicians roll with this resistance—acknowledging the validity of reluctance to change and avoiding "fixing" responses—to reassure the patient that the choice and the change are their own. For many patients experiencing rational suicidality, a significant concern is the loss of self-efficacy in later and end-of-life phases. Emphasizing the patient's self-efficacy in making a choice about living or dying could be very therapeutic and enhance the patient's confidence about being able to lead a life worth living and, therefore, their motivation to do so.

Rational suicidality differs from "traditional" suicidality primarily in the context in which the thoughts occur (e.g., shorter expected lifespan, greater debility), and it is in elucidating these complex factors influencing an individual's motivations to live and to die that MI seems especially applicable. Furthermore, rational suicide involves personal and cultural values, and a MI stance can assist clinicians in remaining curious and validating of the patient's values, even when they may differ from the clinician's. With early empirical support for the applicability of MI to suicide prevention and evidence that MI can facilitate health behavior change in older adults, it seems reasonable that clinicians apply the spirit and some of the techniques of MI to their work with older adults expressing rational suicidality, at least as a pretreatment or adjunct to other strategies.

12.3   Safety Planning

One of the first tasks working with an older adult expressing a desire to die is to collaboratively develop a robust safety plan. Such a plan typically aims to reduce access to means for suicide; identifies triggers to increased suicidal ideation; and plans for how to how to adjust environmental, behavioral, and cognitive circumstances to reduce the likelihood of a suicide attempt (e.g., [25]). This can increase patient safety and essentially buy time for further psychotherapy interventions. A safety plan should not be confused with a no-suicide contract, in which a patient is asked to verbally or in writing commit to not attempting suicide. These contracts are generally not effective at preventing suicidal behavior, can be detrimental to clinical dynamics and future risk assessment, and can place clinicians in a murky area with regard to their legal and ethical obligations to an individual they believe is at risk of harm to themselves [26, 27].

Whereas a no-suicide contract is focused on what *not* to do, a safety plan provides patients with information about what *to* do in a crisis [28]. This ensures patients feel they have the resources to successfully assume responsibility for their life. Safety plans are often presented as a component of a broader therapeutic approach but have also been described as stand-alone approaches to risk and crisis management [25, 29]. Safety planning identifies triggers to suicidal ideation and behavior, internal coping strategies, social circumstances (specific people or places) that can serve as distractions and improve mood, and individuals who can be appropriately supportive when the patient discloses they are having suicidal thoughts. Professional resources, such as therapists, crisis hotlines, and emergency rooms, are also identified. Finally, the clinician and patient plan for restricting access to potential means for suicide, especially more lethal means such as firearms. This process should be collaborative and involve preemptive problem solving to ensure that the strategies and resources identified can reasonably be accessed at a time of crisis. Documenting this process can demonstrate that clinicians have met the standard of care for individuals expressing suicidal ideation [26, 29].

12.3.1 Empirical Research

Research on safety planning itself is limited, but broader interventions incorporating safety planning have demonstrated efficacy at reducing suicidal ideation and behavior. Specifically, Cognitive Behavior Therapy-Suicide Prevention (CBT-SP; [30]) and Dialectical Behavior Therapy (DBT; [31]) use safety planning as part of their protocol, and they will be discussed further later in this chapter. Means restriction is also an important part of safety planning. At a population level, means restriction is especially useful with common and very lethal means of committing suicide, such as firearms in the United States, and are considered part of best practices for suicide prevention [32, 33].

12.3.2 Application to Rational Suicide

Applied to rational suicide in older adults, safety planning would maintain its core features. In identifying triggers to greater desire to die, clinicians should particularly attend to potential changes in physical functioning, medical status, and social dynamics. Development of internal coping strategies can draw from the therapeutic approaches discussed in this chapter. In older adults, especially those dealing with the physical and logistical burdens of significant medical issues, identifying sources of social support that can be readily accessed at a time of crisis can be challenging. Creativity and acceptance of less-than-ideal solutions is important. Role playing with patients around disclosure of their desire to die to their social supports can also help older patients navigate changing relationships, such as needing their adult child to function more as a peer to provide support. Coordination with home care and medical providers is critical to ensure that multiple sources of information about an older adult's functioning are available and that the individual is able to access crisis services at all times and in all settings. Collaboration with medical providers is also important to restricting means for suicide; specifically, it is important to determine how adherent the patient has been to their prescriptions and whether they may have a surplus of available medications.

Safety planning is an important part of basic clinical care and represents a component of clinicians' medicolegal duties. That suicidal ideation may seem rational does not necessarily absolve clinicians of these responsibilities. Collaboratively implemented, safety planning can begin the process of establishing a sound therapeutic alliance and important targets for therapy to improve patients' quality of life.

12.4 Cognitive-Behavioral Therapy

Many of the strategies identified in safety planning processes are drawn from cognitive-behavioral therapy (CBT), and many of the other approaches to addressing rational suicidality in older adults discussed here have their foundations in CBT. There are a number of approaches to CBT (e.g., [34]) that share a worldview that formulates human experience in terms of the interaction between one's cognitions, behaviors, emotions, and physical state. Cognitive and behavioral domains are seen as the most modifiable and are most often targeted in therapy. Although it is more directive than traditional insight- or dynamic-oriented therapies, CBT is best used flexibly and should be based on a patient's own experience, reflecting the context in which the patient finds themselves, including personal history, relationship dynamics, and life goals. It focuses on developing concrete skills through homework patients complete between sessions. Many of the skills are also used in other therapies, so we briefly review these interventions here.

Behavioral interventions seek to identify behaviors associated with mood states and to increase patients' engagement in rewarding activities relative to activities associated with low mood. Depending on patients' complaints, *relaxation strategies*, sleep hygiene, physical activity, diet, and adherence to medical recommendations may also be targets for reducing physical vulnerabilities to unhelpful cognitive and behavioral patterns.

The cognitive strategies in CBT largely rely on use of thought records, in which patients record a situation that triggered a notable emotional response for them (usually depressive or anxious mood), the thoughts associated with that situation (especially those relating to their sense of self), and their emotional response. The clinician then collaborates with the patient to identify patterns of distorted thinking (e.g., catastrophizing, all-or-none, "shoulds") that may be leading to more distress or maladaptive behavior. These distorted thoughts are then challenged by examining the evidence for and against the thought, viewing the situation in a different context (e.g., if it had happened to a friend instead of yourself), and evaluating the helpfulness of the thought. A more realistic, proportionate, balanced alternative thought is generated, and the patient evaluates how this new thought impacts their emotional experience. With practice, patients are able to internalize this process and note their tendencies so they can choose to think more adaptive alternative thoughts in the moment without having to write out this whole process.

12.4.1 Empirical Research

Meta-analyses have found CBT for older adults efficacious at reducing depression and anxiety, with generally moderate-to-large effect sizes that were larger than other treatments [35–37]. The effectiveness of CBT has also been demonstrated with older adults of minority ethnicities in nonstandard delivery environments [38], especially when patients are able to increase their satisfaction with their social support [39]. Older adults with cognitive deficits have also benefitted from CBT in terms of improvements in mood and disability [40, 41]. Importantly for individuals facing a significant stressor such as a terminal medical condition, CBT has shown some efficacy in facilitating meaning-making among highly educated depressed older adults [42]. In individuals with cancer, CBT interventions have been found to be beneficial for both psychological well-being and physical health, including longer cancer-free survival following treatment and longer duration of life [43]. Among individuals who had attempted suicide necessitating hospitalization, a course of cognitive therapy reduced the likelihood of subsequent suicide attempt over 18 months by approximately 50 % compared to treatment as usual [44].

12.4.2 Application to Rational Suicide

Adaptations of CBT to reduce depression and suicidality in older adults have incorporated behavioral activation, cognitive restructuring, increased social engagement, and safety planning that includes identification of protective factors [45], and these approaches are likely applicable to older adults expressing rational suicidality. In this population, it is especially important to be creative in developing behavioral strategies to reflect any physical limitations. Finding modified versions of pleasant activities (e.g., watching a movie at home instead of in the theater, calling a friend instead of driving to visit them, walking for 5 min rather than an hour) and relaxation strategies can foster self-efficacy and hope in individuals who may have become discouraged because they have been unable to fully engage in desired activities [46]. Clinicians may also be more successful emphasizing evaluating the helpfulness of automatic thoughts rather than their accuracy. Because these individuals may, indeed, have a shorter time remaining or impending debility, their concerns about death, declines in physical functioning and autonomy, and unresolved relationship and existential issues may be realistic. Coordination with medical providers is important to appropriately differentiate between realistic and unrealistic worries [46].

Cognitive and behavioral strategies dovetail well with the pragmatic, skills-oriented nature of foundational safety planning recommended here for work with older adults expressing rational suicidality. Furthermore, there is broad evidence that CBT can reduce suicidality and predisposing mood states in older adults, suggesting that it would help individuals improve their quality of life, avoid impulsive behavior to hasten death, and better understand the potential for distress to respond to intervention. It is effective with diverse patient populations, which is important when working with a group as heterogeneous as older adults. It may also be valuable for clinicians to approach work with older adults as requiring specific cultural competence to appropriately respond to generational and cohort effects [47].

12.5 Dialectical Behavior Therapy

Dialectical Behavior Therapy (DBT; [31]) was originally developed to reduce self-directed violence in individuals with borderline personality disorder by developing emotional awareness, emotion regulation skills, and adaptive interpersonal skills. The dialectical approach seeks to acknowledge and balance the complex, changing, and sometimes even contradictory nature of existence. In this view, seemingly mutually exclusive things can be simultaneously true; an individual can be kind and mean, the world can be random and predictable, and a relationship can be supportive and maladaptive. In session, DBT therapists tolerate this tension and help patients to apply such an approach to their lives. Patients are seen as both doing their best and able to do better; they are stuck and always changing; the therapist understands the patient's experience and can learn more. In understanding truth as always changing and amenable to exploration, patients are able to find hope rather than feel discouraged or desperate in the face of immutable truths, buffer themselves from impulsive or habitual behavior, take an active and mindful role in life choices, and develop of an integrated sense of self.

In its traditional application, DBT entails individual therapy focused first on addressing self-harm and other therapy-interfering behaviors, then on developing this integrated sense of self and more adaptive interactions with the world by using coping skills. Therapists are available on call 24/7 to help patients manage crises, often by reinforcing use of coping skills. These skills are taught in structured group classes and are what many practitioners think of as "DBT." DBT skills are focused on developing the capacity for improved emotion regulation—which DBT conceptualizes as the core deficit underlying borderline personality disorder and its characteristic self-harm behavior—and interpersonal functioning.

Core Mindfulness skills taught include taking an *observational* stance toward experiences, often by *describing* that experience; *participating* fully in an experience and engaging in one experience at a time (*one-mindfully*); remaining *nonjudgmental* toward experiences and actions; and choosing behaviors based on their *effectiveness* rather than on value judgments (e.g., fair, deserved, right, good). *Interpersonal Effectiveness* skills include communication strategies for making requests and expressing wants; declining requests and maintaining self-respect; and maintaining relationships with empathetic, nontransactional interactions. *Emotion Regulation* skills include developing emotional awareness and understanding of the function of emotions, nonjudgmental acceptance of emotions, and intentional engagement in activities that prompt more positive emotions or do not perpetuate maladaptive cycles, as by engaging in *opposite action* (e.g., scheduling an activity with a friend when feeling like staying home by oneself). *Distress Tolerance* skills include distraction with behavioral activation; grounding focused on use of pleasant stimuli; use of relaxation and imagery; mindful engagement in activities; and focusing on values, goals, and spirituality to understand the distress and one's choice to tolerate it as part of a larger whole, as validation of one's values, and as motivation to move toward a life more worth living.

12.5.1 Empirical Research

DBT has produced significant reductions in suicidal behavior in randomized clinical trials [48], and these effects have led to its dissemination and adaptation for a number of populations and settings outside of borderline personality disorder and specialty mental health services. Of particular note, DBT has demonstrated efficacy in reducing depressive symptoms in older adults beyond the effect of antidepressant medication alone [49, 50]. Standard DBT is a very intensive treatment, involving multiple therapeutic contacts per week and lasting for at least 1 year. However, even a single DBT skills session has led to decreased suicidal ideation 1 month later [51]. The skills component of DBT appears to be especially effective at reducing depressive symptoms and reducing use of self-directed violence [52].

12.5.2 Application to Rational Suicide

One of the assumptions of DBT is that patients' lives are currently unbearable as they are being lived; essentially, it posits that suicidality is a rational response to current distress, but that it also represents an irrational understanding of one's current situation as unchanging and unchangeable. Clearly, this has direct application to an older adult population expressing rational suicidality in the face of a real or anticipated shortened lifespan, decreased physical functioning, and physical and mental pain. In this population, mindfulness skills facilitate patients engaging more fully in activities, especially those that are meaningful to them, and practicing non-judgmental acceptance of life circumstances. Dialectical Behavior Therapy has shown unique effectiveness in reducing suicidal behavior in individuals known for being treatment-resistant and to be at high risk of suicide and has been successfully applied very briefly and with older adults. The dialectical approach is also well suited to work with rational suicide. It acknowledges the challenges facing individuals with a shortened lifespan, pain, and physical limitations while also giving voice to the individual's goals, values, and beliefs that can be bases for developing a more enjoyable life. Older adults expressing rational suicidality are not likely to be able to engage in the full DBT program, which is long and intensive, so the brief use of some of its component parts, including mindfulness and emotion regulation skills and DBT-oriented individual therapy, will likely be more feasible.

12.6 Mindfulness and Acceptance

Along with DBT, other therapies hold mindfulness skills as important to limiting the effect of distress on one's experience and facilitating values-based, adaptive behavior. The most researched of these therapies are Mindfulness-Based Stress Reduction (MBSR; [53]), Mindfulness-Based Cognitive Therapy (MBCT; [54]), and Acceptance and Commitment Therapy (ACT; [55]). These approaches teach skills to selectively attend to certain aspects of experience and, in so doing, understand them as merely parts of our experience, as modifiable, and as not inherently meaningful. Distress, therefore, does not define all of our experience, can be selectively ignored, and does not even necessarily have to be distressing. For instance, one may feel sad some of the time or even concurrently with more pleasant feelings; one can give more attention to those more pleasant experiences; and one can reframe the experience of sadness to imply resilience to difficult circumstances, evidence of strongly valuing something not immediately present, or even as a natural ebb and flow after a period of happiness.

Mindfulness is taught in MBSR and MBCT; primarily through mindfulness meditation and gentle yoga [53, 54]. These meditation practices involve both concentrative and receptive meditation, in which one intentionally draws attention to a particular experience (e.g., breath) or maintains nonjudgmental awareness of experiences (e.g., thoughts, emotions, sounds), respectively [56]. Techniques used include body scans, guided imagery, multisensory exploration of a stimulus (e.g., a raisin), and seated and walking meditation. Both therapies entail 8 weeks of 2–3 h group sessions and one full-day retreat, with MBCT differentiated from MBSR by its focus on negative mood states and inclusion of psychoeducation on typical patterns of cognitive distortions.

Acceptance and Commitment Therapy uses a combination of cognitive, behavioral, and mindfulness approaches in furtherance of values-based actions. Patients come to decrease associations between their internal experiences and their identities, allowing them greater flexibility in how they define themselves and pursue their values. From an ACT perspective, the socially-driven use of inherently judgmental language (e.g., "negative" emotions) contributes to individuals struggling, and inevitably failing, to avoid internal states. This struggle and failure leads to suffering, which cyclically perpetuates *experiential avoidance*, decreased engagement in valued activities, and distress. Along with meditation, ACT uses metaphors and imagery to develop an observational stance toward internal experience, exercises such as repeating a word over and over until its meaning is separated from its sound for the patient, thought records, values clarification, and goal setting [55].

Suicidality can be conceptualized as the ultimate expression of experiential avoidance, and mindfulness-based therapy can serve to reduce this avoidance by fostering increased *contact with the present, psychological acceptance, cognitive diffusion*, and understanding of the *self as context*. Those in contact with the present are less likely to ruminate on past hurts and to engage with a vision of the future based on an unending extrapolation of current distress. Greater acceptance of current distress allows one to refocus energy on pursuit of longer term, values-based goals rather than on short-term avoidance of pain. By taking an observational stance toward internal states, thoughts, emotions, and behavior are less fused and one can begin to understand oneself as being a self separate from the content of temporary circumstances [57]. Mindfulness is proposed to help manage suicidality by teaching the skill of purposefully attending to the present moment, rather than following a mindless "autopilot" mode; that leaves one susceptible to over-interpreting external and internal stimuli as indicating that one's circumstance is unbearable and unchangeable [58]. Outside of frank suicidality, mindfulness-based therapy has been put forward as a therapeutic framework that can address the depressive, anxious, existential, and spiritual concerns associated with advanced cancer to improve quality of life for individuals with potentially short remaining lifespans [59].

12.6.1 Empirical Research

Meta-analyses have found that MBSR has a small, potentially underestimated effect on depression, anxiety, and overall psychological well-being among individuals with chronic medical conditions [60] and a moderate effect on mental and physical health outcomes, including depression and pain, in broader participant pools [61, 62]. Additionally, development of mindfulness skills has been associated with increased spirituality and posttraumatic growth among cancer patients [63]. Mindfulness-based therapy has generally been found to be feasible with and acceptable to older adults, and it has produced improvements in a number of domains, including mood, anxiety, and pain; however, it is not clear that mindfulness-based approaches are significantly more effective than other active therapies [64]. In contrast, Wetherell and colleagues [65] found that older adults were more likely to have reductions in pain with ACT than with CBT, the opposite pattern of younger adults, suggesting that mindfulness-based approaches may be especially well suited to older adults.

Clinical trials of MBCT have produced decreases in suicidal ideation, greater memory specificity for past suicidal crises, and increased specificity about life goals [66–69]. These effects all reduce risk of suicidal behavior, including by allowing individuals to better recognize suicidal prodromes and be more effective in problem solving during future crises. Similarly, a large effectiveness evaluation found that ACT was effective at reducing depressive symptoms and suicidal ideation among veterans in outpatient therapy and specifically implicated mindfulness and experiential acceptance in these improvements [70]. Patients who received mindfulness training in a randomized controlled trial of MBCT were less susceptible to suicidality; in the face of increased depressive symptoms [71]. The emphasis in mindfulness on remaining in contact with distressing emotions and developing skills to remain present and grounded may be uniquely helpful compared to strictly cognitive interventions for individuals whose personal histories are associated with dissociative or avoidant stress responses [72]. Though this finding was related to childhood abuse experiences, older adults experiencing a trauma that could result in dissociation and avoidance, such as diagnosis of a life-limiting illness, might similarly benefit from these skills.

12.6.2 Application to Rational Suicide

Applying mindfulness-based therapy to rational suicide would likely need little adaptation other than the modifications described for older adults generally, such as decreasing the duration of sessions and use of body positions that are more comfortable for older adults (e.g., sitting rather than lying meditation). For individuals with medical conditions that are limiting physical functionality and life duration, the emphasis of mindfulness-based therapies on nonjudgmental acceptance rather than "fixing" would likely fit well, and the development of specific skills could increase their usefulness in a more medicalized setting. Clinicians should note that it is likely unrealistic to expect older adults with a desire for hastened death to complete the full 30+ hours of training involved in MBSR or MBCT; however, this does not suggest that these patients cannot benefit from briefer mindfulness training. Mindfulness and acceptance-based approaches are also consistent with theories of successful aging that encourage dynamic reprioritization of activities and values to reflect current circumstances and abilities [47].

Older adults expressing rational suicidality could benefit from such an approach, wherein more valued experiences can be selectively attended to and pursued despite circumstances that may shorten one's life or otherwise change one's worldview or ability to pursue activities.

12.7 Existential Therapies

Existential therapies aim to develop individuals' sense of meaning, dignity, spiritual engagement, and perceived ability to cope with the existential distress, especially around "boundary" situations such as end-of-life processes. In particular, they consider existential issues including loss of autonomy and dignity, feeling burdensome to others, loss of meaning, regret about life experiences and relationships, and hopelessness [73]. Experiences that challenge our assumptions that the world is fair, understandable, and controllable and that we are generally safe and essentially immortal produce existential distress. Avoidant, rigid coping with these experiences leads to greater distress and psychopathology, whereas flexible, accepting coping allows one to more fully pursue one's values. Existential therapies share many techniques with other approaches, such as use of genuine empathy and reflection on the therapy process, but are set apart by their explicit discussion of the hard existential truths that cause existential distress, such as mortality, responsibility, and uncontrollability [74].

12.7.1 Empirical Research

Meaning-Centered Group Psychotherapy [75] is centered around exploring the work of Viktor Frankl [76] with patients to identify sources of meaning in the context of a life-limiting or -threatening illness. The intervention is time limited and can be applied in group or individual [77, 78] formats. In contrast to many other existential therapies, such as Supportive-Expressive Group Therapy (SEGT; [79]), MCGP is considered a structured, educational intervention. A meta analysis has found MCGP to have moderate-to-large effect sizes on psychological well-being, sense of purpose in life, and self-efficacy and found that MCGP tended to be more effective than supportive expressive and other existential therapies [80]. A recent randomized controlled trial confirmed the results of the meta-analysis. Compared to an active support group for cancer, MCGP had a moderate effect on a range of psychosocial variables, including decreased desire for hastened death, decreased depression, increased quality of life, and increased spiritual well-being [81].

Dignity Therapy [82] is a brief narrative intervention consisting of an interview with the patient about their life, values, relationships, and wishes for their death. This interview is transcribed by the therapist and presented to the patient as a generativity document, usually with the intention of the patient sharing it with family or others close to them. Research has been mixed with regard to the effects of Dignity Therapy on distress and other symptom measures. Some studies have found it to be associated with reductions in depression and anxiety [82, 83], whereas others have found no effect on outcomes such as distress, depression, hopefulness, or quality of life [84–88].

Reminiscence and life review, which take a similar narrative approach to exploring important life events and themes, have been found to have moderate effects on psychological well-being in older adults [89]. These effects seem to be maintained, at least to some extent, for 3 years following the intervention [90]. Notably, it also seems feasible to incorporate existential or spiritual content into other therapy approaches. For instance, Psycho-Spiritual Integrative Therapy (PSIT) uses a small group modality to teach mindfulness, acceptance, and other cognitive coping skills and integrates broad, individual sources of spiritual support and values clarification to guide values-oriented behavior to increase quality of life and adjustment to life changes, including cancer diagnosis and treatment [91].

12.7.2   Application to Rational Suicide

Existential therapy directly addresses one of the factors associated with rational suicidality: existential distress. However, existential therapies are generally concerned with individuals who do not want to die, and in fact may have a strong fear of death, so some modifications may need to be made to address the desire for hastened death in older adults. To begin with, it is important to engage in risk assessment and safety planning, as well as to validate the individual's feelings of hopelessness, helplessness, and purposelessness rather than too quickly focusing on meaning-making. The subsequent emphasis on meaning-making in existential therapy can make the idea of acceptance of difficult circumstances more palatable. Though many of the manualized existential therapies involve many hours of clinical contact, they provide specific prompts (e.g., "What are your most important accomplishments, and what do you feel most proud of?") that can be helpful for clinicians to begin to incorporate existential themes into their work when a full course of a specific therapy is not indicated due to the patient's physical or logistical limitations.

Existential distress is often a core component of why we might consider suicidality to be rational. Essentially, when a person is no longer able to live in a way that gives pleasure or purpose the way they have experienced them before, we consider it reasonable that they would no longer want to live at all. Existential therapy names this distress, normalizes it, and seeks to mobilize patients to find value in continued existence. An approach drawing from MCGP, which has directly shown decreased desire for hastened death in older adults, is likely to be beneficial.

12.8 Psychodynamic Therapy

Modern psychodynamic therapies retain some aspects of psychoanalytic therapy but tend to be more time-limited and focused on specific presenting issues. They share a view of pathology as based in interpersonal relationship patterns and emphasize within-session change to a greater extent than the more skills- and homework-oriented CBT-based interventions. Psychodynamic therapies have been less manualized than CBT-based treatment, which has made research on these approaches more difficult, but some manualized approaches include Time-Limited Dynamic Psychotherapy (TLDP; [92, 93]), Interpersonal Therapy (IPT; [94]), Supportive-Expressive Psychotherapy [95], and Pragmatic Psychodynamic Psychotherapy [96]. We should note that the developers of IPT do not consider it a psychodynamic approach; however, its focus on interpersonal dynamics and role transitions, as well as the lower level of directiveness involved in its practice, closely align with a psychodynamic approach for the purposes of this review.

Generally, these approaches formulate cases as involving cyclical patterns of maladaptive behavior, expectations of others, experiences, and internalized views of the self [97]. Therapy involves interventions that exist on a spectrum from *supportive* of the patient and focused on developing rapport to *expressive* of the therapist's interpretations and challenges to the patient to adopt a new perspective or change behavior. Because interpersonal patterns are assumed to be reflected in the patient's relationship with the therapist, the therapeutic relationship is used to develop the patient's insight into these patterns; provide opportunities to practice new interaction styles; and to give novel, therapeutic interpersonal experiences.

12.8.1 Empirical Research

Short-term psychodynamic psychotherapy has been shown to be effective in treating depression, including in older adults [98–100]. Efficacy has also been demonstrated in medical populations, with TLDP producing significant decreases in distress in a sample of HIV+ men who have sex with men [101]. Large multisite, randomized controlled trials have used IPT in primary care settings and found that it, with or without concurrent antidepressant medication use, was effective at reducing depression and suicidal ideation in older adults [102, 103]. Those older adults receiving IPT and/or antidepressant medication were also less likely to die over the course of 5 years [104]. A small, 16-session, trial of an adapted form of IPT for older adults at risk of suicide showed reductions in suicidal ideation and depressive symptoms. These adaptations entailed focusing exploration of interpersonal processes on those interactions that involved suicidal thoughts or behavior, along with the addition of pragmatic safety planning for imminent suicide risk and increased access to the therapist, as in DBT [105].

12.8.2 Application to Rational Suicide

The relational focus of psychodynamic approaches is applicable for addressing rational suicidality, targeting issues such as feeling like a burden to family members, seeking resolution to relationship problems, and managing life and role transitions (i.e., receiving care from others, taking a "patient" role, dying). In practice, dynamic therapy for rational suicidality would develop a conceptualization of how the desire for hastened death is precipitated and perpetuated by interpersonal interactions. The clinician would work with the patient to provide corrective experiences in and out of therapy. Our experiences suggest that patient-therapy match is especially important with psychodynamic approaches. Although many patients appreciate exploration of personal history and a relational focus, others find such approaches to be too "touchy-feely," for them to successfully engage with treatment. Therefore, we encourage clinicians to present the conceptualization and treatment model they propose to use to check for patient agreement.

12.9 Interdisciplinary Collaboration

Most older adults expressing a rational suicidality are involved with a number of medical providers to address physical issues and community and government agencies to address tangible resource deficits. They may also have family, friends, and caregivers significantly involved in their care and their day-to-day lives. For interventions to be maximally effective, clinicians will need to not only understand the complexity of these systems and challenges for patients in navigating the systems and coordinating between all involved, but also to collaborate with patients' providers and caregivers to work toward psychosocial treatment goals.

Collaboration with patients' other providers is important, first, to provide clinicians with accurate information about the patients' physical status, experience through treatment, and likely prognosis. Lacking this information increases the burden on the patient to inform the clinician about their medical course and reduces the time available for psychosocial intervention. Collaborating with other providers also provides the opportunity to open lines of communication that may have been closed due to medical providers and patients' shared discomfort addressing end-of-life issues. For instance, interviews with older dialysis patients and dialysis providers indicated that there is often inadequate communication about goals and expectations for treatment and a tendency to defer to patients' passive assent to ongoing treatment rather than fostering active choice of treatment [106]. Coordinating with patients' multiple providers may also alleviate a contributor to desire for hastened death: frustration with perceived unresponsiveness of the health-care system and difficulty navigating it [5].

An interdisciplinary approach to treatment of suicidality in older adults not only produces a more patient-specific treatment plan but also increases available psychosocial resources. A systematic review of intervention studies to reduce suicide in older adults found that depression-focused care coordination in primary care, community depression screening and education, and telephonic and in-person counseling reduced depressive symptoms, reduced suicidality, and improved overall functioning [107]. Interventions to increase patients' level of social support, such as engagement in community activities, are recommended as means to improve psychological well-being in older adults with life-limiting illness [108].

12.10 Practice Guidelines

In many ways, this discussion of the effect of psychotherapy on rational suicidality falls into the same "Dodo Bird problem" as much research on psychotherapy effectiveness: it is difficult to demonstrate that one approach to therapy is especially more effective than others. However, we believe some recommendations can be made.

12.10.1 Prevent Impulsive Behavior

Clinicians have an obligation to prevent impulsive suicidal behavior; this is true with "traditional" suicidality and with rational suicide. This is best accomplished through thoughtful assessment of the factors contributing to an individual's desire for hastened death, factors associated with a motivation to continue living, and the immediacy of the risk that the individual might harm themselves. Such an assessment lays the foundation for collaborating with the patient to develop a safety plan, usually involving use of internal coping strategies, distraction, environmental situations that reduce vulnerability to suicidal behavior, a range of types of social support, and professional and crisis supports as needed. This process is well described and manualized as the standalone Safety Planning Intervention [25]. The desire for hastened death tends to fluctuate [109], and useable safety planning can help patients avoid impulsive, irreversible behavior at a time of acutely exacerbated suicidality.

12.10.2 Nonjudgmentally Explore Suicidality and Values

Providers are often uncomfortable engaging in discussions of suicidality as an option for coping with distress for fear that doing so will increase the likelihood that a patient will engage in suicidal behavior. When providers encounter older adults expressing a rational desire for hastened death, they are often part of the individual's medical treatment team, making it even more difficult to validate what could be seen as the patient "quitting" on treatment that could extend their life. However, it is possible to validate the distress underlying this suicidality without necessarily agreeing that a hastened death is a good solution. This reflects a Motivational Interviewing [12] approach. In fact, by speaking to the desire for a hastened death, clinicians may elicit more endorsement of a desire to live from patients, and this approach will have the dual benefit of also increasing patients' sense of being understood by the provider.

12.10.3 Cognitive-Behavioral and Mindfulness Skills Can Be Helpful

Among older adults, CBT and mindfulness-based approaches have been shown to be effective at reducing depression, anxiety, pain, and suicidality. Broadly, these approaches seem to work by increasing individuals' meta-awareness, facilitating more intentional thought and behavior rather than reinforcing patterns associated with distress and debility, and clarifying life goals and values. Furthermore, by fostering specific skills, these approaches can increase older adults' sense of self-efficacy and demonstrate the possibility of change, providing evidence against the hopelessness and helplessness often associated with desire for hastened death. Though many of the studies described earlier involved relatively intensive treatment (i.e., at least weekly for at least 60 min for several weeks), there is also evidence that these approaches can be successfully adapted into shorter sessions and briefer (even single) session formats, which increase their feasibility working with older adults who may have physical, logistical, or motivational limitations on their ability to engage in more in-depth therapy.

12.10.4 Existential Concerns are Important

Rational suicide is often differentiated from "traditional" suicide by the circumstances in which an individual finds themselves—usually with a significant change in current or expected functioning. This external stressor, be it a terminal medical condition, amputation, or brain disease, comes with a challenge to one's identity and, therefore, an existential pressure to change who we are. Suicide represents a change in terms of one's biological state, whereas many of the options that might follow from psychotherapy are changes in one's psychological, behavioral, or social state. The most direct research on the effect of psychotherapy on rational suicidality involves a therapy specifically aimed at addressing existential issues–Meaning-Centered Group Psychotherapy [75]. It has found that working with patients expressing a desire for hastened death to clarify and redefine their sense of meaning in life decreased suicidality. These existential themes can be incorporated into other therapeutic approaches and will likely be important for clinicians seeking to connect with aspects of a patient's distress outside of just symptomatology.

12.10.5   Collaboration with Patients' Systems Is Critical

Without good communication with a patient's medical team, clinicians cannot adequately understand the rationality of expressed suicidality, the feasibility of behavioral strategies, the reasonableness of distressing cognitions, or the nature of existential challenges facing a patient. For older adults with physical or cognitive limitations, strategies to improve mood and manage risk will also be much more likely to be implemented if clinicians involve patients' family, caregivers, friends, neighbors, and other sources of support. Coordination with other providers and increased interpersonal contact in and of itself may be an effective intervention to reduce rational suicidality, based on findings in primary care practices [102, 110].

12.10.6   Some Things Are Not Recommended

As mentioned earlier, no-suicide contracts are *not* recommended due to the lack of demonstrated efficacy and their potential negative clinical and medicolegal implications. Additionally, interventions that have not yet shown efficacy for reduction of suicidality or desire for hastened death, such as Dignity Therapy, Supportive-Expressive Group Therapy, or Time-Limited Dynamic Psychotherapy, are not recommended as stand-alone treatments, especially with acutely suicidal individuals. These and other approaches may be helpful in addressing existential concerns and mood disturbance when an individual is more psychologically stable, ultimately reducing the incidence or severity of suicidality; however, clinicians should be prepared to use treatments that more directly address the contributors to suicidal ideation and develop older adults' capacity to manage this distress if their suicidality becomes more prominent.

12.10.7   Be Mindful of Own Values

End-of-life situations elicit responses from clinicians based on our own values and health beliefs, and self-awareness around those biases will help clinicians work within the patient's perspective and engage in appropriate self-care. Even in the case of arguably strictly rational suicide, one may feel that there is something wrong or mistaken about an individual's decision to die, such that it is very difficult to identify a plausible scenario in which suicide feels truly rational, particularly outside the context of a clear terminal condition and old age [111]. However, many patients considering hastened death do not consider actions toward that end, such as withdrawal of hemodialysis, to be suicide [112], emphasizing the importance of clinicians questioning their assumptions and judgments placed on patients' decisions.

Importantly, our own cultural judgments likely play a role in this evaluation of a patient making a "mistake." Such cultural influences might include shame about having failed as a society to provide sufficiently rewarding circumstances for the individual to continue living or fear at the idea that, in fact, we are mistaken in our appraisal that our own life is worth continuing. Clinicians may have values, including those based in religious tradition, that reflect the idea that hastened death is always morally wrong. We may have had personal experiences with individuals choosing to prolong or shorten life that influence our sense of what the "right" decision is for a patient. As clinicians, our desire to be effective in our work, even in the context of a terminal illness or other difficult situation, may lead us to direct therapy in a certain direction.

We do not advocate for clinicians being opinionless in therapy with adults expressing rational suicidality, nor for clinicians to disregard their values. Rather, we encourage clinicians to reflect on their values and responses to patients both in and out of session. Seek consultation when necessary. Be genuine, and embrace the opportunity to explore a challenging but necessary aspect of existence. In our experience, patients appreciate the opportunity to discuss their thoughts about death and to receive frank opinions from an informed provider. Actively engaging in a reflective process will also help clinicians engage in appropriate self-care and prevent burnout.

12.11 Conclusions

Desire for hastened death is a common but not universal experience in the context of existentially challenging situations, such as life-limiting illness or anticipated physical decline. This suicidality can be seen as rational given the physical and logistical burdens associated with such conditions, and it is not necessarily the product of mood disturbance. However, rational suicidality often responds to treatment for depression, including psychotherapy. A number of psychotherapeutic approaches show promise for reducing rational suicidality, with direct evidence currently available for Meaning-Centered Group Psychotherapy [75]. Clinicians working with patients expressing the desire for hastened death should use risk assessment and safety planning approaches similar to those used in "traditional" suicide, and subsequent interventions should take a nonjudgmental stance, such as that in Motivational Interviewing. Skills-based therapy approaches can be especially helpful in reducing more acute suicidality, and approaches that incorporate mindfulness and acceptance skills can help reduce the risk of recurrence of suicidality. Acknowledgement and exploration of existential issues is valuable in demonstrating empathy, finding meaning in a difficult situation, and helping clinicians remain cognizant of the personal and professional challenges involved in this work.

References

1. Ellis TE, Patel AB. Client suicide: what now? Cogn Behav Pract. 2012;19(2):277–87. doi:10.1016/j.cbpra.2010.12.004.
2. Ho AO. Suicide: rationality and responsibility for life. Can J Psychiatr. 2014;59(3):141–7.

3. Dazzi T, Gribble R, Wessely S, Fear NT. Does asking about suicide and related behaviours induce suicidal ideation? What is the evidence? Psychol Med. 2014;44(16):3361–3. doi:10.1017/S0033291714001299.
4. Werth JL, Holdwick DJ. A primer on rational suicide and other forms of hastened death. Couns Psychol. 2000;28(4):511–39.
5. Nissim R, Gagliese L, Rodin G. The desire for hastened death in individuals with advanced cancer: a longitudinal qualitative study. Soc Sci Med. 2009;69(2):165–71. doi:10.1016/j.socscimed.2009.04.021.
6. Breitbart W, Rosenfeld B, Gibson C, Kramer M, Li Y, Tomarken A, Nelson C, Pessin H, Esch J, Galietta M, Garcia N, Brechtl J, Schuster M. Impact of treatment for depression on desire for hastened death in patients with advanced AIDS. Psychosomatics. 2010;51(2):98–105.
7. Eggar R, Spencer A, Anderson D, Hiller L. Views of elderly patients on cardiopulmonary resuscitation before and after treatment for depression. Int J Geriatr Psychiatry. 2002;17(2): 170–4. doi:10.1002/gps.523.
8. Reinke LF, Slatore CG, Udris EM, Moss BR, Johnson EA, Au DH. The association of depression and preferences for life-sustaining treatments in veterans with chronic obstructive pulmonary disease. J Pain Symptom Manag. 2011;41(2):402–11. doi:10.1016/j.jpainsymman.2010.05.012.
9. Hewitt J. Why are people with mental illness excluded from the rational suicide debate? Int J Law Psychiatry. 2013;36(5–6):358–65. doi:10.1016/j.ijlp.2013.06.006.
10. Leeman CP. Distinguishing among irrational suicide and other forms of hastened death: implications for clinical practice. Psychosomatics. 2009;50(3):185–91. doi:10.1176/appi.psy.50.3.185.
11. Hudson PL, Kristjanson LJ, Ashby M, Kelly B, Schofield P, Hudson R, Aranda S, O'Connor M, Street A. Desire for hastened death in patients with advanced disease and the evidence base of clinical guidelines: a systematic review. Palliat Med. 2006;20(7):693–701. doi:10.1177/0269216306071799.
12. Miller WR, Rollnick S. Motivational interviewing: helping people change. New York: Guilford; 2012.
13. Britton PC, Williams GC, Conner KR. Self-determination theory, motivational interviewing, and the treatment of clients with acute suicidal ideation. J Clin Psychol. 2008;64(1):52–66. doi:10.1002/jclp.20430.
14. Britton PC, Bryan CJ, Valenstein M. Motivational interviewing for means restriction counseling with patients at risk for suicide. Cogn Behav Pract. 2014;23:51–61. doi:10.1016/j.cbpra.2014.09.004.
15. Britton PC, Patrick H, Wenzel A, Williams GC. Integrating motivational interviewing and self-determination theory with cognitive behavioral therapy to prevent suicide. Cogn Behav Pract. 2011;18(1):16–27. doi:10.1016/j.cbpra.2009.06.004.
16. Zerler H. Motivational interviewing in the assessment and management of suicidality. J Clin Psychol. 2009;65(11):1207–17. doi:10.1002/jclp.20643.
17. Britton PC, Conner KR, Maisto SA. An open trial of motivational interviewing to address suicidal ideation with hospitalized veterans. J Consult Clin Psychol. 2012;68(9):961–71. doi:10.1002/jclp.21885.
18. Romano M, Peters L. Evaluating the mechanisms of change in motivational interviewing in the treatment of mental health problems: a review and meta-analysis. Clin Psychol Rev. 2015;38:1–12. doi:10.1016/j.cpr.2015.02.008.
19. Westra HA, Aviram A, Doell FK. Extending motivational interviewing to the treatment of major mental health problems: current directions and evidence. Can J Psychiatry. 2011;56(11):643–50.
20. Lundahl BW, Kunz C, Brownell C, Tollefson D, Burke BL. A meta-analysis of motivational interviewing: twenty-five years of empirical studies. Res Soc Work Pract. 2010;20(2):137–60. doi:10.1177/1049731509347850.
21. O'Halloran PD, Blackstock F, Shields N, Holland A, Iles R, Kingsley M, Bernhardt J, Lannin N, Morris ME, Taylor NF. Motivational interviewing to increase physical activity in people

with chronic health conditions: a systematic review and meta-analysis. Clin Rehabil. 2014;28(12):1159–71. doi:10.1177/0269215514536210.

22. VanBuskirk KA, Wetherell JL. Motivational interviewing with primary care populations: a systematic review and meta-analysis. J Behav Med. 2014;37(4):768–80. doi:10.1007/s10865-013-9527-4.

23. Cummings SM, Cooper RL, Cassie KM. Motivational interviewing to affect behavioral change in older adults. Res Soc Work Pract. 2009;19(2):195–204. doi:10.1177/1049731508320216.

24. Bugelli T, Crowther TR. Motivational interviewing and the older population in psychiatry. Psychiatr Bull. 2008;32(1):23–5. doi:10.1192/pb.bp.106.010405.

25. Stanley B, Brown GK. Safety planning intervention: a brief intervention to mitigate suicide risk. Cogn Behav Pract. 2012;19(2):256–64. doi:10.1016/j.cbpra.2011.01.001.

26. Lee JB, Bartlett ML. Suicide prevention: critical elements for managing suicidal clients and counselor liability without the use of a no-suicide contract. Death Stud. 2005;29(9):847–65. doi:10.1080/07481180500236776.

27. Rudd MD, Mandrusiak M, Joiner TJ. The case against no-suicide contracts: the commitment to treatment statement as a practice alternative. J Clin Psychol. 2006;62(2):243–51. doi:10.1002/jclp.20227.

28. Matarazzo BB, Homaifar BY, Wortzel HS. Therapeutic risk management of the suicidal patient: safety planning. J Psychiatr Pract. 2014;20(3):220–4. doi:10.1097/01.pra.0000450321.06612.7a.

29. Linehan MM, Comtois KA, Ward-Ciesielski EF. Assessing and managing risk with suicidal individuals. Cogn Behav Pract. 2012;19(2):218–32. doi:10.1016/j.cbpra.2010.11.008.

30. Stanley B, Brown G, Brent DA, Wells K, Poling K, Curry J, Kennard BD, Wagner A, Cwik MF, Klomek AB, Goldstein T, Vitiello B, Barnett S, Daniel S, Hughes J. Cognitive-behavioral therapy for suicide prevention (CBT-SP): treatment model, feasibility, and acceptability. J Am Acad Child Adolesc Psychiatry. 2009;48(10):1005–13.

31. Linehan MM. DBT® skills training manual. New York: Guilford; 2014.

32. van der Feltz-Cornelis CM, Sarchiapone M, Postuvan V, Volker D, Roskar S, Grum AT, Carli V, McDaid D, O'Connor R, Maxwell M, Ibelshäuser A, Van Audenhove C, Scheerder G, Sisask M, Gusmão R, Hegerl U. Best practice elements of multilevel suicide prevention strategies: a review of systematic reviews. Crisis. 2011;32(6):319–33. doi:10.1027/0227-5910/a000109.

33. Yip PF, Caine E, Yousuf S, Chang S, Chien-Chang Wu K, Chen Y. Means restriction for suicide prevention. Lancet. 2012;379(9834):2393–9. doi:10.1016/S0140-6736(12)60521-2.

34. Beck JS. Cognitive behavior therapy: basics and beyond. New York: Guilford; 2011.

35. Gould RL, Coulson MC, Howard RJ. Cognitive behavioral therapy for depression in older people: a meta-analysis and meta-regression of randomized controlled trials. J Am Geriatr Soc. 2012;60(10):1817–30. doi:10.1111/j.1532-5415.2012.04166.x.

36. Gould RL, Coulson MC, Howard RJ. Efficacy of cognitive behavioral therapy for anxiety disorders in older people: a meta-analysis and meta-regression of randomized controlled trials. J Am Geriatr Soc. 2012;60(2):218–29. doi:10.1111/j.1532-5415.2011.03824.x.

37. Pinquart M, Duberstein PR, Lyness JM. Effects of psychotherapy and other behavioral interventions on clinically depressed older adults: a meta-analysis. Aging Ment Health. 2007;11(6):645–57. doi:10.1080/13607860701529635.

38. Scogin FR, Moss K, Harris GM, Presnell AH. Treatment of depressive symptoms in diverse, rural, and vulnerable older adults. Int J Geriatr Psychiatry. 2014;29(3):310–6. doi:10.1002/gps.4009.

39. LaRocca MA, Scogin FR. The effect of social support on quality of life in older adults receiving cognitive behavioral therapy. Clin Gerontol. 2015;38(2):131–48. doi:10.1080/07317115.2014.990598.

40. Goodkind MS, Gallagher-Thompson D, Thompson LW, Kesler SR, Anker L, Flournoy J, Berman MP, Holland JM, O'Hara RM. The impact of executive function on response to cognitive behavioral therapy in late-life depression. Int J Geriatr Psychiatry. 2015;31(4):334–9. doi:10.1002/gps.4325.

41. Simon SS, Cordás TA, Bottino CC. Cognitive behavioral therapies in older adults with depression and cognitive deficits: a systematic review. Int J Geriatr Psychiatry. 2015;30(3): 223–33. doi:10.1002/gps.4239.
42. Holland JM, Chong G, Currier JM, O'Hara R, Gallagher-Thompson D. Does cognitive-behavioural therapy promote meaning making? A preliminary test in the context of geriatric depression. Psychol Psychother Theory Res Pract. 2015;88(1):120–4. doi:10.1111/papt.12030.
43. Antoni MH. Psychosocial intervention effects on adaptation, disease course and biobehavioral processes in cancer. Brain Behav Immun. 2013;30(Suppl):S88–98. doi:10.1016/j.bbi.2012.05.009.
44. Brown GK, Ten Have T, Henriques GR, Xie SX, Hollander JE, Beck AT. Cognitive therapy for the prevention of suicide attempts: a randomized controlled trial. JAMA. 2005;294(5):563–70. doi:10.1001/jama.294.5.563.
45. Bhar SS, Brown GK. Treatment of depression and suicide in older adults. Cogn Behav Pract. 2012;19(1):116–25. doi:10.1016/j.cbpra.2010.12.005.
46. Greer JA, Park ER, Prigerson HG, Safren SA. Tailoring cognitive-behavioral therapy to treat anxiety comorbid with advanced cancer. J Cogn Psychother. 2010;24(4):294–313. doi:10.1891/0889-8391.24.4.294.
47. Laidlaw K, Kishita N. Age-appropriate augmented cognitive behavior therapy to enhance treatment outcome for late-life depression and anxiety disorders. Geropsych. 2015;28(2):57–66. doi:10.1024/1662-9647/a000128.
48. Kliem S, Kroger C, Kosfelder J. Dialectical behavior therapy for borderline personality disorder: a meta-analysis using mixed-effects modeling. J Consult Clin Psychol. 2010;78(6):936–51. doi:10.1037/a0021015.
49. Lynch TR, Cheavens JS, Cukrowicz KC, Thorp SR, Bronner L, Beyer J. Treatment of older adults with co-morbid personality disorder and depression: a dialectical behavior therapy approach. Int J Geriatr Psychiatry. 2007;22(2):131–43. doi:10.1002/gps.1703.
50. Lynch TR. Treatment of elderly depression with personality disorder comorbidity using dialectical behavior therapy. Cogn Behav Pract. 2000;7(4):468–77. doi:10.1016/S1077-7229(00)80058-9.
51. Ward-Ciesielski EF. An open pilot feasibility study of a brief dialectical behavior therapy skills–based intervention for suicidal individuals. Suicide Life Threat Behav. 2013;43(3):324–35. doi:10.1111/sltb.12019.
52. Linehan MM, Korslund KE, Harned MS, Gallop RJ, Lungu A, Neacsiu AD, McDavid J, Comtois KA, Murray-Gregory AM. Dialectical behavior therapy for high suicide risk in individuals with borderline personality disorder: a randomized clinical trial and component analysis. JAMA Psychiatry. 2015;72(5):475–82. doi:10.1001/jamapsychiatry.2014.3039.
53. Kabat-Zinn J. Full catastrophe living (revised edition): using the wisdom of your body and mind to face stress, pain, and illness. New York: Bantam Books; 2013.
54. Segal ZV, Williams JMG, Teasdale JD. Mindfulness-based cognitive therapy for depression: a new approach to preventing relapse. New York: Guilford; 2002.
55. Hayes SC, Strosahl KD, Wilson KG. Acceptance and commitment therapy: an experiential approach to behavior change. New York: Guilford; 1999.
56. Lutz A, Slagter HA, Dunne JD, Davidson RJ. Attention regulation and monitoring in meditation. Trends Cogn Sci. 2008;12(4):163–9. doi:10.1016/j.tics.2008.01.005.
57. Luoma JB, Villatte JL. Mindfulness in the treatment of suicidal individuals. Cogn Behav Pract. 2012;19(2):265–76. doi:10.1016/j.cbpra.2010.12.003.
58. Williams JG, Swales M. The use of mindfulness-based approaches for suicidal patients. Arch Suicide Res. 2004;8(4):315–29. doi:10.1080/13811110490476671.
59. Angiola JE, Bowen AM. Quality of life in advanced cancer: an acceptance and commitment therapy view. Couns Psychol. 2013;41(2):313–35. doi:10.1177/0011000012461955.
60. Bohlmeijer E, Prenger R, Taal E, Cuijpers P. The effects of mindfulness-based stress reduction therapy on mental health of adults with a chronic medical disease: a meta-analysis. J Psychosom Res. 2010;68(6):539–44. doi:10.1016/j.jpsychores.2009.10.005.

61. Grossman P, Niemann L, Schmidt S, Walach H. Mindfulness-based stress reduction and health benefits: a meta-analysis. J Psychosom Res. 2004;57(1):35–43. doi:10.1016/S0022-3999(03)00573-7.

62. Khoury B, Lecomte T, Fortin G, Masse M, Therien P, Bouchard V, Chapleau MA, Paquin K, Hofmann SG. Mindfulness-based therapy: a comprehensive meta-analysis. Clin Psychol Rev. 2013;33(6):763-71. doi: 10.1016/j.cpr.2013.05.005.

63. Labelle LE, Lawlor-Savage L, Campbell TS, Faris P, Carlson LE. Does self-report Mindfulness-Based Stress Reduction (MBSR) on spirituality and posttraumatic growth in cancer patients? J Posit Psychol. 2015;10(2):153–66. doi:10.1080/17439760.2014.927902.

64. Geiger PJ, Boggero IA, Brake CA, Caldera CA, Combs HL, Peters JR, Baer RA. Mindfulness-based interventions for older adults: a review of the effects on physical and emotional well-being. Mindfulness. 2015;7:296–307. doi:10.1007/s12671-015-0444-1.

65. Wetherell JL, Petkus AJ, Alonso-Fernandez M, Bower ES, Steiner AW, Afari N. Age moderates response to acceptance and commitment therapy vs cognitive behavioral therapy for chronic pain. Int J Geriatr Psychiatry. 2015;31:302–8. doi:10.1002/gps.4330.

66. Chesin MS, Sonmez CC, Benjamin-Phillips CA, Beeler B, Brodsky BS, Stanley B. Preliminary effectiveness of adjunct mindfulness-based cognitive therapy to prevent suicidal behavior in outpatients who are at elevated suicide risk. Mindfulness. 2015;6:1345–55. doi:10.1007/s12671-015-0405-8.

67. Crane C, Winder R, Hargus E, Amarasinghe M, Barnhofer T. Effects of mindfulness-based cognitive therapy on specificity of life goals. Cogn Ther Res. 2012;36(3):182–9. doi:10.1007/s10608-010-9349-4.

68. Forkmann T, Wichers M, Geschwind N, Peeters F, van Os J, Mainz V, Collip D. Effects of mindfulness-based cognitive therapy on self-reported suicidal ideation: results from a randomised controlled trial in patients with residual depressive symptoms. Compr Psychiatry. 2014;55(8):1883–90. doi:10.1016/j.comppsych.2014.08.043.

69. Hargus E, Crane C, Barnhofer T, Williams JG. Effects of mindfulness on meta-awareness and specificity of describing prodromal symptoms in suicidal depression. Emotion. 2010;10(1):34–42. doi:10.1037/a0016825.

70. Walser RD, Garvert DW, Karlin BE, Trockel M, Ryu DM, Taylor CB. Effectiveness of acceptance and commitment therapy in treating depression and suicidal ideation in veterans. Behav Res Ther. 2015;74:25–31. doi:10.1016/j.brat.2015.08.012.

71. Barnhofer T, Crane C, Brennan K, Duggan DS, Crane RS, Eames C, Radford S, Silverton S, Fennell MJ, Williams JM. Mindfulness-based cognitive therapy (MBCT) reduces the association between depressive symptoms and suicidal cognitions in patients with a history of suicidal depression. J Consult Clin Psychol. 2015;83(6):1013–20. doi:10.1037/ccp0000027.

72. Williams JG, Crane C, Barnhofer T, Brennan K, Duggan DS, Fennell MV, Hackmann A, Krusche A, Muse K, Von Rohr IR, Shah D, Crane RS, Eames C, Jones M, Radford S, Silverton S, Sun Y, Weatherley-Jones E, Whitaker CJ, Russell D, Russell IT. Mindfulness-based cognitive therapy for preventing relapse in recurrent depression: a randomized dismantling trial. J Consult Clin Psychol. 2014;82(2):275–86. doi:10.1037/a0035036.

73. LeMay K, Wilson KG. Treatment of existential distress in life threatening illness: a review of manualized interventions. Clin Psychol Rev. 2008;28(3):472–93. doi:10.1016/j.cpr.2007.07.013.

74. Vos J, Cooper M, Correia E, Craig M. Existential therapies: a review of their scientific foundations and efficacy. J Soc Existent Anal. 2015;26(1):49–69.

75. Breitbart W, Poppito S. Meaning-centered group psychotherapy for patients with advanced cancer: a treatment manual. Oxford: New York; 2014.

76. Frankl VF. Man's search for meaning. Boston: Beacon Press; 1959/1992.

77. Henry M, Cohen SR, Lee V, Sauthier P, Provencher D, Drouin P, Gauthier P, Gotlieb W, Lau S, Drummond N, Gilbert L, Stanimir G, Sturgeon J, Chasen M, Mitchell J, Huang LN, Ferland MK, Mayo N. The meaning-making intervention (MMi) appears to increase meaning in life in advanced ovarian cancer: a randomized controlled pilot study. Psychooncology. 2010;19(12):1340–7. doi:10.1002/pon.1764.

78. Lee V, Cohen SR, Edgar L, Laizner AM, Gagnon AJ. Meaning-making intervention during breast or colorectal cancer treatment improves self-esteem, optimism, and self-efficacy. Soc Sci Med. 2006;62(12):3133–45. doi:10.1016/j.socscimed.2005.11.041.
79. Spiegel D, Spira J. Supportive-expressive group therapy: a treatment manual of psychosocial intervention for women with recurrent breast cancer. Palo Alto: Stanford University School of Medicine, Department of Psychiatry and Behavioral Sciences, Psychosocial Treatment Laboratory; 1991.
80. Vos J, Craig M, Cooper M. Existential therapies: a meta-analysis of their effects on psychological outcomes. J Consult Clin Psychol. 2015;83(1):115–28. doi:10.1037/a0037167.
81. Breitbart W, Rosenfeld B, Pessin H, Applebaum A, Kulikowski J, Lichtenthal WG. Meaning-centered group psychotherapy: an effective intervention for improving psychological well-being in patients with advanced cancer. J Clin Oncol. 2015;33:749–54. doi:10.1200/JCO.2014.57.2198.
82. Chochinov HM, Hack T, Hassard T, Kristjanson LJ, Clement S, Harlos M. Dignity therapy: a novel psychotherapeutic intervention for patients near the end of life. J Clin Oncol. 2005;23:5520–5. doi:10.1200/JCO.2005.08.391.
83. Julião M, Oliveira F, Nunes B, Vaz Carneiro A, Barbosa A. Efficacy of dignity therapy on depression and anxiety in Portuguese terminally ill patients: a phase II randomized controlled trial. J Palliat Med. 2014;17(6):688–95. doi:10.1089/jpm.2013.0567.
84. Aoun SM, Chochinov HM, Kristjanson LJ. Dignity therapy for people with motor neuron disease and their family caregivers: a feasibility study. J Palliat Med. 2015;18(1):31–7. doi:10.1089/jpm.2014.0213.
85. Chochinov HM, Kristjanson LJ, Breitbart W, McClement S, Hack TF, Hassard T, Harlos M. The effect of dignity therapy on distress and end-of-life experience in terminally ill patients: a randomised controlled trial. Lancet Oncol. 2011;12(8):753–62. doi:10.1016/S1470-2045(11)70153-X.
86. Hall S, Goddard C, Opio D, Speck P, Higginson IJ. Feasibility, acceptability and potential effectiveness of dignity therapy for older people in care homes: a phase II randomized controlled trial of a brief palliative care psychotherapy. Palliat Med. 2012;26(5):703–12. doi:10.1177/0269216311418145.
87. Houmann LJ, Chochinov HM, Kristjanson LJ, Petersen MA, Groenvold M. A prospective evaluation of dignity therapy in advanced cancer patients admitted to palliative care. Palliat Med. 2014;28(5):448–58. doi:10.1177/0269216313514883.
88. Bentley B, O'Connor M, Kane R, Breen LJ. Feasibility, acceptability, and potential effectiveness of dignity therapy for people with motor neurone disease. PLoS One. 2014;9(5), e96888. doi:10.1371/journal.pone.0096888.
89. Bohlmeijer E, Roemer M, Cuijpers P, Smit F. The effects of reminiscence on psychological well-being in order adults: a meta-analysis. Aging Ment Health. 2007;11(3):291–300. doi:10.1080/13607860600963547.
90. Haight BK, Michel Y, Hendrix S. The extended effects of the life review in nursing home residents. Int J Aging Hum Dev. 2000;50(2):151–68. doi:10.2190/QU66-E8UV-NYMR-Y99E.
91. Corwin D, Wall K, Koopman C. Psycho-spiritual integrative therapy: psychological intervention for women with breast cancer. J Spec Group Work. 2012;37(3):252–73. doi:10.1080/01933922.2012.686961.
92. Levenson H. Time-limited dynamic psychotherapy: a guide to clinical practice. New York: Basic Books; 1995.
93. Strupp HH, Binder JL. Psychotherapy in a new key: a guide to time-limited dynamic psychotherapy. New York: Basic Books; 1984.
94. Weissman MM, Markowitz JC, Klerman GL. Comprehensive guide to interpersonal psychotherapy New York: Basic Books; 2000.
95. Luborsky L. Principles of psychoanalytic psychotherapy: a manual for supportive-expressive treatment. New York: Basic Books; 1984.
96. Summers RF, Barber JP. Psychodynamic therapy a guide to evidence-based practice. New York: Guilford; 2010.

97. Vinnars B, Frydman Dixon S, Barber JP. Pragmatic psychodynamic psychotherapy—Bridging contemporary psychoanalytic clinical practice and evidence-based psychodynamic practice. Psychoanal Inq. 2013;33(6):567–83. doi:10.1080/07351690.2013.835159.
98. de Mello MF, de Jesus Mari J, Bacaltchuk J, Verdeli H, Neugebauer R. A systematic review of research findings on the efficacy of interpersonal therapy for depressive disorders. Eur Arch Psychiatry Clin Neurosci. 2005;255(2):75–82. doi:10.1007/s00406-004-0542-x.
99. Driessen E, Cuijpers P, de Maat SM, Abbass AA, de Jonghe F, Dekker JM. The efficacy of short-term psychodynamic psychotherapy for depression: a meta-analysis. Clin Psychol Rev. 2010;30(1):25–36. doi:10.1016/j.cpr.2009.08.010.
100. Tolin DF. Is cognitive–behavioral therapy more effective than other therapies? A meta-analytic review. Clin Psychol Rev. 2010;30(6):710–20. doi:10.1016/j.cpr.2010.05.003.
101. Pobuda T, Crothers L, Goldblum P, Dilley JW, Koopman C. Effects of time-limited dynamic psychotherapy on distress among HIV-seropositive men who have sex with men. AIDS Patient Care Stds. 2008;22(7):1–7. doi:10.1089/apc.2007.0250.
102. Alexopoulos GS, Reynolds CI, Bruce ML, Katz IR, Raue PJ, Mulsant BH, Ten Have T. Reducing suicidal ideation and depression in older primary care patients: 24-month outcomes of the PROSPECT study. Am J Psychiatry. 2009;166(8):882–90. doi:10.1176/appi.ajp.2009.08121779.
103. Bruce ML, Ten Have TR, Reynolds CF, Katz II, Schulberg HC, Mulsant BH, Brown GK, McAvay GJ, Pearson JL, Alexopoulos GS. Reducing suicidal ideation and depressive symptoms in depressed older primary care patients: a randomized controlled trial. JAMA. 2004;291(9):1081–91. doi:10.1001/jama.291.9.1081.
104. Gallo JJ, Bogner HR, Morales KH, Post EP, Lin JY, Bruce ML. The effect of a primary care practice-based depression intervention on mortality in older adults: a randomized trial. Ann Intern Med. 2007;146(10):689–98.
105. Heisel MJ, Talbot NL, King DA, Tu XM, Duberstein PR. Adapting interpersonal psychotherapy for older adults at risk for suicide. Am J Geriatr Psychiatry. 2015;23(1):87–98. doi:10.1016/j.jagp.2014.03.010.
106. Russ AJ, Shim JK, Kaufman SR. The value of 'life at any cost': talk about stopping kidney dialysis. Soc Sci Med. 2007;64(11):2236–47. doi:10.1016/j.socscimed.2007.02.016.
107. Lapierre S, Erlangsen A, Waern M, De Leo D, Oyama H, Scocco P, Gallo J, Szanto K, Conwell Y, Draper B, Quinnett P, International Research Group for Suicide among the Elderly. A systematic review of elderly suicide prevention programs. Crisis. 2011;32(2):88–98. doi:10.1027/0227-5910/a000076.
108. Applebaum AJ, Stein EM, Lord-Bessen J, Pessin H, Rosenfeld B, Breitbart W. Optimism, social support, and mental health outcomes in patients with advanced cancer. Psychooncology. 2014;23(3):299–306. doi:10.1002/pon.3418.
109. Rosenfeld B, Pessin H, Marziliano A, Jacobson C, Sorger B, Abbey J, Olden M, Brescia R, Breitbart W. Does desire for hastened death change in terminally ill cancer patients? Soc Sci Med. 2014;111:35–40. doi:10.1016/j.socscimed.2014.03.027.
110. Unützer J, Tang L, Oishi S, Katon W, Williams JJ, Hunkeler E, Hendrie H, Lin EH, Levine S, Grypma L, Steffens DC, Fields J, Langston C, IMPACT Investigators. Reducing suicidal ideation in depressed older primary care patients. J Am Geriatr Soc. 2006;54(10):1550–6. doi:10.1111/j.1532-5415.2006.00882.x.
111. Pilpel A, Amsel L. What is wrong with rational suicide. Philosophia. 2011;39:111–23. doi:10.1007/s11406-010-9253-x.
112. Cohen LM, Dobschka SK, Halis KC, Pekow PS, Chochinov HM. Depression and suicidal ideation in patients who discontinue the life-support treatment of dialysis. Psychosom Med. 2002;64:889–96. doi:10.1097/01.PSY.0000028828.64279.84t.

Spirituality, Religion, and Rational Suicide

13

Joshua Briscoe and Warren Kinghorn

13.1 Introduction

Grade 4 glioblastoma is a diagnosis that no one ever wants to receive. It is an aggressive malignancy that portends seizures, cognitive deficits, and likely death. Beyond its physical sequelae, however, people with terminal brain cancer may face loneliness, role transition and loss, and increasing dependence on others. Loss of control of bodily functions, dependence on others for basic care, and loss of autonomy are often described in our culture as a loss of dignity. During an interview before her death, one of several that made her famous as an advocate for physician-assisted death, Brittany Maynard explained, "The worst thing that could happen to me is that I wait too long because I'm trying to seize each day but that I somehow have the autonomy taken away from me because of my disease" [1]. Faced with such prospects, Maynard moved from California to Oregon, where assisted suicide was legal at the time, and died in November 2014 after ingesting a lethal dose of barbiturates.

Brittany Maynard's strong desire to avoid further debility was evident in her articulate defense of her desire for assisted suicide. She was already experiencing troubling seizures and other neurologic deficits, but her fear that her autonomy would be "taken away from me because of my disease" was for her an even greater concern. This aligns with the findings of studies reporting that autonomy, functional

J. Briscoe, M.D.
Department of Internal Medicine and Department of Psychiatry and Behavioral Sciences,
Duke University Medical Center, Durham, NC 27708, USA

W. Kinghorn, M.D., Th.D. (✉)
Department of Psychiatry and Behavioral Sciences, Duke University Medical Center,
Duke Divinity School, 407 Chapel Drive, Box 90968, Durham, NC 27708, USA
e-mail: warren.kinghorn@duke.edu

© Springer International Publishing Switzerland 2017
R.E. McCue, M. Balasubramaniam (eds.), *Rational Suicide in the Elderly*,
DOI 10.1007/978-3-319-32672-6_13

status, burdensomeness to others, "pointless suffering," and loss of dignity provide significant motivation for patients to seek assisted suicide, sometimes to a greater degree than physical pain itself [2, 3].

The concepts of autonomy, dignity, rationality, and suffering inevitably accompany any discussion of assisted suicide, and are well debated in the literature of medicine and bioethics. But these are not uniquely medical concepts; they are rather concepts that touch on the deepest questions about what it means to be a human being, and to live well. They reach to the core of the meaning of human life, and as such, they are concepts that are engaged by religious and spiritual traditions as well as by clinicians and bioethicists. In this chapter, we will reflect on the influence that religion and spirituality might have on decisions about rational suicide. To illustrate how clinicians might engage patients in conversations about religion and spirituality, we start by introducing a well-known instrument for spiritual assessment in the clinical setting, the FICA Spiritual History Tool [4]. We then review evidence that religious belief and practice may affect patient decision-making related to rational suicide, and offer an extended engagement of assisted suicide from within the context of Christianity, which remains the self-identified religious tradition of over 70 % of the American population. We then conclude with brief recommendations for clinicians around engaging patients in conversations about religion and spirituality in relation to rational suicide.

13.2 Engaging Religion and Spirituality: The FICA Spiritual History Tool

Although there are multiple ways that clinicians might approach conversations about religion and spirituality, the FICA Spiritual History Tool, developed by Christina Puchalski at George Washington University, offers a straightforward and reasonable form of engagement [4]. The FICA Spiritual History Tool is designed not as a closed-ended checklist but as a framework within which to invite patients into deeper conversation about religion and spirituality as it relates to their health and medical care. Further resources related to the tool, including an online training module, can be found at www.gwish.org. The tool consists of questions in four categories [4]:

1. *F*aith, Belief, and Meaning. Clinicians might begin a conversation by asking broad questions such as, "Do you consider yourself spiritual or religious? Do you have spiritual beliefs, values, or practices that help you cope with stress? What gives your life meaning?"
2. *I*mportance and Influence. Clinicians might follow these first questions by asking, "What importance does your faith or belief have in your life? Have your beliefs influenced you in how you handle stress? Do you have specific beliefs that might influence your health care decisions? If so, are you willing to share those with your health care team?"

3. *Community.* Depending on answers to the first items, clinicians might ask, "Are you part of a spiritual or religious community? Is this of support to you and how? Is there a group of people you really love or who are important to you?"
4. *Address/Action in Care.* Clinicians might then ask, "How should I address these issues in your health care?"

13.3 Religion, Spirituality, and Rational Suicide, with Focus on Christianity

There is some evidence for an inverse correlation between spirituality and religiosity and the desire for rational suicide. For instance, in a study comparing 55 Oregonians requesting physician-assisted death with 39 other individuals with advanced disease, Smith et al. documented that low self-reported spirituality was the strongest predictor of pursuit of physician-assisted death [5]. In a 1994 survey of 500 residents in Detroit, self-identification as black and "very religious" were both associated with lower odds of supporting euthanasia or physician-assisted suicide, as well as diminished interest in personally pursuing those options [6]. In another study of 893 caregivers of terminally ill patients, self-identification as "very religious" was associated with a lower odds of supporting euthanasia or physician-assisted suicide [7]. Burdette et al. suggest that religious service attendance may be more predictive of opposition to physician-assisted suicide than self-reported religious affiliation [8]. In a survey of U.S. physicians, Curlin et al. documented that physicians who reported high levels of intrinsic religiosity were 4.2 times more likely to object to physician-assisted suicide than physicians who reported low levels of intrinsic religiosity [9].

Consistent with these empirical findings, many but not all major religious traditions discourage suicide and, in some cases, actively oppose physician-assisted suicide. Curlin et al. [9] documented that Jewish physicians were less likely to object to physician-assisted suicide and terminal sedation than Catholic, Protestant, and Muslim physicians, and Hindu physicians were more likely to object to terminal sedation. Although attitudes of individual Jews toward assisted suicide is variable, most Jewish rabbis and teachers oppose assisted suicide [10]. Among the three Abrahamic traditions, Islam maintains perhaps the strongest and most consistent objection to suicide; unlike either the Hebrew Bible or the Christian New Testament, the Qur'an explicitly prohibits suicide (Qur'an, sura 4, ayat 29). And this discouragement of assisted suicide is common to most, but not all, Christian traditions.

Sociologically speaking, there is no single "Christian tradition"; within the United States, rather, there exists a wide diversity of Christian communities that agree on some things and disagree, sometimes unpredictably and contentiously, on many others. Some Americans who identify as Christian support the legalization of assisted suicide, and many others do not. Despite this, however, there is remarkable consistency in the official teachings of Christian churches and communities in the United States that assisted suicide is inconsistent with faithful Christian life. At the time of this writing, among prominent Christian bodies in the United States, only the Unitarian Universalist Association has unequivocally endorsed support for the legalization of assisted suicide [11]. In order to assist clinicians working with self-identified Christian patients to understand their context, therefore, we will focus most of our attention on two ways that people speaking from a Christian theological viewpoint seek to challenge the increasingly prevalent narrative about rational suicide that emerges from organizations such as Compassion and Choices and that was exemplified in the public discussion about Brittany Maynard's death. First, we will describe work that argues that "rationality" is itself a contested concept that carries with it particular philosophical and theological presuppositions; it is not clear, in the view of some Christian thinkers, that any act that results in one's own death can be "rational." Second, we will show that this philosophical debate about rationality reflects only a small part of historical Christian reflection on suicide. A more fully theological Christian response to assisted suicide would focus not on rationality per se but on how humans belong to and with each other in community, and how humans belong to God. In this account, the most important thing about humans is not that humans are "rational" but that humans are loved and claimed by God, belonging to God and to God's people, and that vulnerability is not an exception but is the norm and rule of human life. The proper response to vulnerability, in this account, is not the assertion of autonomy nor or technological escape, but rather a community of solidarity, support, and hope.

13.4 Historical Christian Perspectives on Suicide

Christian opinion on suicide has not been unanimous, either today or in ages past. The lack of consensus proceeds, in part, from the fact that neither the Hebrew Bible/Old Testament nor the New Testament explicitly condemn the act of suicide. Some texts in the New Testament—particularly Paul's comment in his letter to the Philippians that "for me, living is Christ and dying is gain" and that "my desire is to depart and to be with Christ, for that is far better" (Phil. 1:21,23, NRSV) even suggest that Christians might welcome death as a gateway to union with God (though in this text, Paul indicates his desire to remain alive for the sake of his followers). This, coupled with sporadic Roman imperial persecution of early Christians, blurred the line between martyrdom and suicide, particularly when martyrs chose death over a forced recantation or violation of their faith.

Despite this lack of overt condemnation in Christian scripture, early Christian writers condemned suicide as incompatible with Christian teaching, in contrast to contemporary Stoic figures like Seneca (~4 BCE-65 CE) who were generally supportive of suicide as a way to avoid the dependence and vulnerability of illness and old age [12]. Clement of Alexandria, writing in the second century CE, viewed suicide with disdain (in contrast with martyrdom, of which he approved) [13]. Christian prohibition of suicide in any form, particularly in the Latin West, hardened as a result of the influential work of Augustine of Hippo (354–430 CE), who equated suicide with killing and denounced suicide as part of a broader Christian (and Jewish) commandment not to kill an innocent person who belongs to God [14].

In the medieval period, drawing on Augustine's teaching, the Church systematically condemned suicide and at times condoned regrettable practices that contributed to the stigmatization of suicide, such as refusing to allow persons who completed suicide to be buried within city walls [13].

Even before the modern era, Christian condemnation of suicide was not uniform. In his treatise *Biathanatos* (1608), for example, Anglican priest and poet John Donne (1572–1631) defended suicide on the grounds that Jesus's self-giving death on the cross was suicide. If Jesus committed suicide, Donne argued, then it could not be a condemnable act [15]. Such overt Christian defenses of suicide were rare until the modern era. But just as it is possible to trace the influence of Christian thought in modern arguments against rational suicide, it is also possible to trace the influence of Christian thought in modern arguments *for* assisted suicide, in ways that were not clearly foreseen. For instance, theologian Gerald McKenny has argued that the Protestant Reformation, and particularly the thought of Reformation-era British polymath Francis Bacon (1561–1626), led to a powerful conception of the role of technology in relation to the body that continues to influence modern approaches to biomedicine. Early Protestant thinkers, in McKenny's account, understood the material world—including the material of the human body—not as static "creation" to be contemplated but rather as manipulable nature to be used for human ends and purposes. Furthermore, early Protestants insisted that the highest good of Christian life was not monastic contemplation but, rather, the love of one's neighbor, as evidenced by the reduction of his or her suffering. These two affirmations—that "nature" is given to humans for use and that relief of suffering is a foremost good—gave rise to what McKenny terms the "Baconian project" to use science "to relieve the human condition of subjection to the whims of fortune or the bonds of natural necessity" [16]. This commitment to use technology to relieve suffering continues to be felt powerfully within modern biomedicine, and perhaps especially in modern defenses of assisted suicide.

13.5 Contemporary Christian Perspectives on Suicide

The rare Christian bodies that have officially endorsed the legalization of assisted suicide have generally grounded this in compassion for those who suffer, and respect for the individual as an autonomous moral agent [17]. But even among Christian bodies that continue to condemn suicide, most attempt to balance this teaching with compassion for individuals who struggle with suicidal thoughts, with support for bereaved families, and with acknowledgement of the complex mental health challenges that many people face. The *Catechism of the Catholic Church*, for example, forbids suicide, holding that it is contrary to love of self, love of others, and love of God [18]. Cooperation with suicide is also forbidden. However, psychological disturbances (as well as "grave fear of hardship, suffering, or torture") may reduce one's moral culpability. The Catholic Church now provides encouragement to those that would despair of the salvation of persons who have committed suicide, as "God can provide the opportunity for salutary repentance." The Greek and Russian

Orthodox Churches also condemn suicide but make similar allowances for those who may have had impaired agency at the time of their death.

With the earlier noted exceptions, most Protestant bodies—including the Evangelical Lutheran Church in America, the Episcopal Church, the Southern Baptist Convention, the United Methodist Church, the Presbyterian Church in America, and the Assemblies of God—stand against the permissibility of suicide and assisted suicide [17, 19]. Their reasons for opposition vary. For example, while the Southern Baptist Convention views suicide as murder (following Augustine), the United Methodist Church only recognizes that "suicide is not the way life should end," but avoids outright condemnation of the one who commits suicide [20].

As noted earlier, however, official church teaching only imperfectly reflects the attitudes of these churches' adherents. A 2013 Pew Research Center survey revealed that 61% of white mainline Protestants, 55% of white Catholics, 33% of Hispanic Catholics, 30% of white evangelical Protestants, and 22% of black Protestants approved of "laws to allow doctor-assisted suicide for terminally ill patients" [21]. The survey determined that this support was qualified: a right to suicide garnered the most support when respondents considered a patient who was in great pain with no hope of recovery, while being an "extremely heavy burden on family" received the least support for warranting that right. Clearly, many oppose the official doctrines of their own denominations in these matters, which is important information for clinicians to keep in mind as these issues are addressed with patients.

13.6 Two Affirmations Behind Modern Christian Objections to Rational Suicide

Why do most Christian bodies continue to object to rational suicide? To be sure, not all Christian opposition to assisted suicide is driven by theory: many Christians no doubt carry forward unarticulated stigma against suicide that has accrued over centuries of Western history. Others affirm Augustine's simple and juridical teaching that suicide is a form of murder. But here we consider two affirmations that underlie many modern Christian arguments against assisted suicide: first, that "autonomy" and "rationality" are modern constructions that are unsustainable apart from a theological context; and second, that individuals belong not to themselves alone, but to God and to the community of which they are a part.

13.6.1 Affirmation 1: "Autonomy" and "Rationality" Are Modern Constructions

Modern bioethics is dominated by individualist, intellectualist, and procedural accounts of rationality and autonomy. An individual (it is nearly always, in contemporary discussion, an individual) is "rational" if his or her convictions, desires, or actions are well justified [22]. "Autonomy," furthermore, is a presumptive good that is to be accorded to every "rational" individual. Autonomy and rationality are symbiotic with each other: rationality names the *potential* of an individual to deliberatively guide his or her action, and autonomy confers the right to *actually* direct one's action in this way.

The affirmation of the truth-discerning capacity of the human intellect and the right of self-determination according to the dictates of conscience are woven deeply into Christian history and teaching. But this teaching was historically framed within a larger theological context: for thirteenth-century theologian Thomas Aquinas (~1225–1274), for example, one was "rational" to the extent that one aligned one's mind and one's life according to God's *ratio* or ordering of the world, and the individual could reliably direct his or her action only insofar as this alignment with God's *ratio* was maintained ([23], IaIIae q. 91 a. 2 *resp.*). When the intellect conforms to the divine *ratio*, the intellect is a reliable discerner of truth, and can discern what forms of action are good and appropriate. Over time, the individual becomes able to discern what is good, even apart from the command of external rule or law; in this way, individuals habituated in virtue can become autonomous ("self-ruling"), in that they can discern what is good apart from the constraint of external law [24]. On the other hand, when the intellect departs from the contours of this divine *ratio*, it errs and becomes unreliable and "irrational," and the capacity for autonomy, even if one's action is guided by deliberation and "reason," is eroded.

"Autonomy" as a norm in medical decision-making has received much scrutiny and criticism. Safranek has recognized that an act cannot be said to be good (or bad) by merely understanding it to be autonomous [25]. He argues that while autonomy may be necessary to discern the moral nature of a given act, it is not sufficient. Some other criteria must be used to condemn or commend the act. If such criteria are required, then once articulated and enforced, these criteria would ultimately subvert the autonomy of those individuals with a competing understanding of the good. If this is the case, though, autonomy alone cannot provide substantive grounding for normative claims about the permissibility of rational suicide. Though Safranek is not writing within a theological context, his argument resonates within Christian reflection on moral agency: in Christian thought, the fact that an action is self-directed does not mean that it is morally salutary. Though not limited to Protestant Christianity, this sentiment is clearly expressed by the sixteenth-century Protestant reformer John Calvin (1509–1564):

> The pagans say that true glory consists in an upright conscience. Now, this is true, but it is not the whole truth. Since all men are blinded by too much self- love, we are not to be satisfied with our own judgment of our deeds. We must keep in mind what Paul says elsewhere: that even though he is not aware of anything [wrong] in him, he is not therefore justified [26].

13.6.2 Affirmation 2: Vulnerability Is Normative, and Christians Belong to God and to Each Other

The second Christian objection to assisted suicide goes beyond abstract consideration of the concepts of rationality and autonomy, and toward an account of human dignity that is conferred by God and centered in community and belonging, and not in capacities. In modern debates about rational suicide, "dignity" often connotes autonomy and control, such that to preserve one's "dignity" or to live or die with "dignity" entails that one remains capable of directing the course of one's life and managing bodily vulnerability. Terminal, degenerative illness inevitably threatens dignity conceived in this way. This conception of dignity as the capacity for self-regulation and self-control resonates with ancient Stoic philosophy [12]. But Christian (and Jewish and Islamic) tradition offers a different account of human dignity that has historically stood alongside, and sometimes in the place of, capacity-based accounts of dignity. Within Christianity, humans possess incomparable dignity because humans were created by God, in God's image (Gen. 1:27); because God loves humans; and furthermore (and specific to Christianity), because God united Godself to human nature in the person of Jesus in order to invite all of humanity into God's life. Human dignity is conferred by God in creation, and is in no way dependent on capacities or enacted excellences. It was this new conception of dignity that allowed Christians in the late Roman empire to look at people who were sick, poor, and ostracized—those rendered invisible within the capacity-based valuations of Roman culture—and to see them as humans bearing God's image, worthy of care and concern [27].

By grounding human dignity in God's love rather than on capacities for self-determination and self-control, early Christians were able to understand vulnerability in a new way, relative to the dominant values of ancient Rome. Vulnerability and finitude were not threats to dignity, but rather simply the norm of human life, proof that humans are finite creatures and not themselves gods. The apostle Paul, arguably the most important biblical writer for the subsequent development of Christian thought, seemed to celebrate his own limitations of body, his "thorn in the flesh," by writing, "I will boast all the more gladly of my weaknesses, so that the power of Christ may dwell in me. Therefore I am content with weaknesses, insults, hardships, persecutions, and calamities for the sake of Christ; for whenever I am weak, then I am strong" (2 Cor 12:9, NRSV).

Neither the New Testament nor subsequent Christian teaching generally celebrates illness as a positive good: Christians are repeatedly commanded to pray for healing (James 5:16) and to seek appropriate medical treatment [27]. But physical illness and vulnerability is regarded as an opportunity to be reminded of one's dependence on God and—importantly—on others. Paul tells early Christians that they are united in an interdependent body: "you are the body of Christ and individually members of it" (1 Cor 12:27, NRSV). Individual members of the body, Paul states, are to bear with those that are weak, to suffer together with other members who suffer, and to "clothe with greater honor" those members that seem less honorable. To be a Christian, in other words, is not to be self-sufficient and autonomous, but rather to be loved and claimed by God, and to belong to God and to the body of Christ, the church. Moral agency is valued, but not for its own sake; instead, it is to be used to love God and one's neighbor. Individuals do not belong to themselves, but rather to God and to each other [28]. Joel Shuman and Brian Volck, writing about Christian engagement with modern medicine, draw upon this Christian celebration of community and interdependence when they note that if Christians were to understand themselves as part of a gathered people (i.e., the Church), they would realize they "never go to the doctor alone" [29]. Nor are medical decisions simply a matter of autonomous personal values, but are rather a matter for collective, communal discernment.

Christians who have been formed to affirm vulnerability, dependence, and mutual belonging will resist the conclusion that if one loses significant agency and independence, life may become not worth living. Contrary to modern arguments that dependence may create a duty to die in order to keep from being a burden on others [30], Christian teaching recognizes that we are, all of us, already burdens to those who love us (Gal. 6:2). For that matter, Christians are told not only to be burdened by friends and family, but even by strangers and enemies, for Christians are called to love all (Matt. 5:44), and love encompasses the bearing of burdens. In this light, many Christians may object to any cultural milieu that devalues or vilifies dependence.

13.7 Two Christian Objections to Rational Suicide

How might these two Christian affirmations, one about the nature and role of "rationality" and the other about the ground of human dignity and the normativity of dependence and vulnerability, affect deliberation about the ethics of rational suicide? These affirmations, we suggest, lead to the specific critiques that suicide (1) addresses suffering by eliminating the sufferer, thereby reflecting an inadequate imagination for how suffering might be borne and (2) diminishes the role of community in bearing the burdens, and vulnerability, of those who suffer.

13.7.1 Objection 1. Suicide Addresses Suffering by Eliminating the Sufferer

Suffering has been variably conceived by different sources. Eric Cassell, the most prominent theorist of suffering within modern bioethics, has claimed that suffering occurs when an "impending destruction of the person is perceived" [31]. Cassell argues that suffering is not synonymous with mere physical pain: persons are most fully understood as more than biological, and have mental, spiritual, and social dimensions. Writing from a Catholic Christian perspective, Daniel Sulmasy agrees with Cassell that suffering is linked with the nature of being human, and reflects that suffering is linked with the universal human experience of finitude [32]. In the view of these two writers and many others, suffering should not be reduced to pain, and suffering requires more than technical medical intervention to relieve.

Relief of unbearable suffering is often cited as a common reason for pursuing physician-assisted suicide [33]. Rational suicide, in the view of some defenders, is an appropriate response not only to unremitting pain but also to existential threats such as loss of autonomy. Underlying this view, however, is the assumption that suffering is such a threat to human flourishing and dignity that it should be ameliorated by any course of action that is freely chosen by the sufferer.

Christian tradition is quite varied about the meaning and role of suffering in human life. Many biblical texts seem to support a connection between personal suffering and sin, either of an individual (1 Sam. 12) or of a people (Jer. 11), though Jesus warned his disciples not to make this a general rule, insisting that in the case of a man blind from birth, "Neither this man nor his parents sinned; he was born blind so that God's works might be revealed in him" (Jn. 9:3, NRSV). More notable than consistent *explanation* for suffering, however, is the frequency and intensity with which suffering is engaged in the Bible. Suffering appears in nearly every biblical book, and several biblical texts, including the books of Job, Jeremiah, Lamentations, and many of the Psalms, can be read as extended commentaries on suffering, emerging from the context of significant trauma and political violence. The Psalmist, for example, laments to God that "all day long my disgrace is before me, and shame has covered my face" (Ps. 44:15), asks God how long God will wait before bringing justice (Ps. 13; Ps. 74:10–11), and remarks mournfully upon the transience of human life (Ps. 90:3–6). Job, afflicted with the loss of social status, family, health, and livelihood, laments, "let the day perish in which I was born, … let gloom and deep darkness claim it … because it did not shut the doors of my mother's womb and hide trouble from my eyes" (Job 3:1,5,10). The prophet Jeremiah, anticipating and witnessing the destruction of Jerusalem and its holy places, cries, "My joy is gone, grief is upon me, my heart is sick" (Jer. 8:18). These raw biblical portraits of suffering refuse to paint over suffering with trite maxims or seemingly easy solutions. There is no attempt to hide suffering, to pretend that God has already done something that God clearly has not yet done, or to forcefully reconcile God's benevolence with the existence of suffering.

The Christian New Testament both continues and develops the biblical lament tradition. Jesus claims and carries forward the form of Jewish lament by reciting Psalm 22 from the cross: "My God, my God, why have you forsaken me?" (Matt. 27:46), and in so doing, "makes the human cry of lament his own cry" [34]. Reflecting on the crucifixion, death, and resurrection of Jesus, early Christian teachers encouraged Christians to locate their own suffering within Christ's suffering, and in so doing, to know both that God was present to them in their suffering (2 Cor. 1:3–7) and that God, while not necessarily the author of suffering, could use suffering for God's glory (2 Cor. 12:6–10, 1 Pt. 4:12–16). Furthermore, early Christians were taught that suffering is to be borne not individually, but in the community of the Church, which is Christ's body (1 Cor. 12:26) and which shares in Christ's sufferings. The relief of suffering after the foundation of the Church occurs always in community with God and with others.

Present-day Christian teachers and theologians adopt a wide variety of approaches to suffering. Some, like the late Pope John Paul II, encourage Christians to locate their suffering within Christ's suffering, and thereby to experience their own suffering as redemptive [35]. Others, aware of the way that portraying suffering as a good has coincided with the infliction of suffering on others, strongly reject any doctrine of redemptive suffering and instead focus on God's presence and solidarity with the sufferer as she resists evil [36]. Others emphasize the ongoing relevance of the biblical lament tradition [34]. But all of these approaches regard suffering, however unjust and unwanted, as an invitation into more meaningful relationship with God and with community, as God—working in and through community—cares for the sufferer, shares the pain of the sufferer, and grants courage and grace for the bearing of suffering.

This understanding of suffering as an opportunity for solidarity and for more meaningful relationship with God and community contrasts starkly with any response to suffering that encourages suicide in the name of "care." There may be no easy solution for the one who suffers, just as there was no easy solution for Jesus as he prayed to avoid his own suffering (Lk. 22:42), but that does not mean that the one who suffers will be abandoned. The goal of Christian response to suffering is not to eliminate suffering by eliminating the sufferer, but rather to respect the dignity of a sufferer as a good and interdependent creature, loved by God and joined to a community, whose suffering should never be borne alone; as physician and theologian Margaret Mohrmann comments, "to acknowledge a sufferer in all her anguish is to begin the process of restoring her to full personhood" [37]. Suicide, because it leads to complete alienation from community, renders this sort of communal care impossible.

13.7.2 Objection 2. Suicide Diminishes the Role of Community in Bearing the Burdens, and Vulnerability, of Those Who Suffer

This concern about responding to suffering by eliminating the sufferer is closely tied to a second objection grounded in the character of human community relative to the individual. In order to grasp this distinction, let us briefly consider two types of commonly-encountered communities in modern western culture. The first type we may call "instrumental communities." Instrumental communities are primarily voluntary associations of individuals who cooperate in the pursuit of shared goods. Corporations and universities are examples of instrumental communities. Instrumental communities survive as long as they deliver value to their individual members. If this is the case, then withdrawing from a community when it no longer serves one's purposes—or, conversely, shunning a member of the community who no longer contributes to the good of the whole—is defensible.

Conversely, within "noninstrumental communities," individuals are related to their communities not primarily as contributors or beneficiaries, but simply as *members* who belong to the community, and who need not justify this membership by any indicator of utility. Noninstrumental communities exist even in liberal western societies that privilege instrumental communities, but are often considered "private" rather than "public." Families—at least many families—are examples of noninstrumental communities. There is no threat, in noninstrumental communities, that nonproductive or vulnerable individuals will be expelled, because their relationship to the community is not predicated on ability or productivity but simply on belonging, as members, to the whole. In these sorts of communities, suicide is not a relief (of the burden of a nonproductive member), but rather a deep loss of a member who belongs to the whole, and whose absence diminishes the whole. It is this communitarian logic that led Thomas Aquinas, following Aristotle, to argue that "every part, as such, belongs to the whole. Now every man is part of the community, and so, as such, he belongs to the community. Hence by killing himself he injures the community" ([23]. IIaIIae q. 64 a. 5 *resp.*).

We may then ask the question: is human community itself—not this-or-that organization, but rather humanity as a whole—best understood as an instrumental or as a noninstrumental community? Is it appropriate for an individual to separate permanently from human community when it no longer serves one's purposes? Conversely, is it appropriate for society as a whole to cast off nonproductive members, in order to better serve the good of the whole? If humanity is regarded as an instrumental community, the answer would be "yes." But Christian teachers have traditionally answered "no."

Because Christian tradition grounds human dignity in God's creative love and not in capacities, and because Christians are knit together not only in human community but in the community of the church, Christian tradition is suspicious of any account of human community that forces its members to justify their existence instrumentally, or that measures the worth of members by any metric of productivity or capacity. Such accounts frequently, even if unintentionally, devalue persons with disability, as do Sinnott-Armstrong and Miller, who in their analysis of what makes killing wrong, argue that it is not the explicit loss of life that constitutes moral harm, but rather universal and irreversible disability [38]. In this view, if someone is universally and irreversibly disabled (e.g., in a persistent vegetative state), no further harm can be done to them by killing them.

Proponents of assisted suicide may argue that freely available assisted suicide does not force anyone to justify their ongoing existence, and in no way threatens those who are vulnerable and/or who live with disability, because assisted suicide does not *restrict* choice but rather *expands* it. For someone who is suffering, or who is worried about being a burden on their loved ones in the context of a prolonged illness, assisted suicide provides an additional alternative that can be declined, for religious or other reasons. But there is a burden associated with this new "choice." If one of us were invited by the dean of our medical school to join her for dinner, we would have newfound "choice" to share a meal with her—but because of her invitation, we would no longer have the freedom to pursue alternative dinner plans without informing our dean that we had done so, or at least that we were unable to join her [34, 39]. Analogously, the widespread legal availability of amniocentesis and abortion has given expecting parents the freedom to avoid the birth of children with trisomy 21 (Down syndrome) in almost all circumstances—and indeed over 90 % of fetuses with Down syndrome are terminated prior to birth. But this new choice means that all expecting parents must now justify to themselves (and perhaps to others also) why they would bring a child with Down syndrome to term, given the significant emotional, financial, and lifestyle implications of this decision. Many Christians (and disability advocates) believe that over time, legalized assisted suicide will have the same effect with respect to certain forms of disability and end-of-life suffering. Trained over a lifetime to fear suffering and to avoid "being a burden," individuals facing disability and decline will increasingly be forced to justify to themselves (and perhaps to others also) why they would remain burdens to their communities.

Because Christians recognize that humans are valuable not because of any particular ability or capacity they may have, because Christians affirm that God has created humans for belonging, and because Christians are taught to pay special attention to the needs of those who are weak and vulnerable, traditional Christian teaching rejects any social practice, including assisted suicide, that requires people who are vulnerable to justify their ongoing existence. Rather, Christians are encouraged to regard disability and vulnerability as an opportunity for a community to provide care, support, and encouragement, even when simple solutions are unavailable. This alternative vision of community emerged in press coverage related to Brittany Maynard's death in the voice of Kara Tippetts, who spoke of her own experience with life-threatening breast cancer from a specifically Christian perspective. Tippetts, who died in 2015 after multiple failed cancer treatments, became well-known through her book in which she reflected upon her suffering, as well as through a letter she wrote to Brittany Maynard imploring her to reconsider the decision to pursue assisted suicide [40]. Tippetts' account was not only of her own experience; she also documented the experiences of her children, husband, and church, testifying to the fact that her life was inseparable from theirs. However, it was not only the experience of grief that they shared. Meditating upon the fact that she could no longer muster the strength to drive a car, she wrote, "All the driving my body can no longer do will now be captured by my community, my loves, my people. And there will be other strengths that will languish, and my people will press into love and provide us the needed strength and support to manage that new edge" [41].

Kara Tippetts' story of how her faith (shared with her family and local community) interacts with her diagnosis, prognosis, and dying is tightly interwoven with her Christian identity. Christians are taught that the church exists in part to provide opportunities to serve and be served, helping and loving each person therein, recognizing that each member possesses unique qualities that are suited to serve others (1 Cor. 12:14–27). Suicide, even in the context of great suffering, alienates the sufferer from this organic community, depriving each other of the opportunity to walk together through "the valley of the shadow of death" (Ps. 23:4, KJV), that feared valley in which lifetimes of aspiration and pretense dissolve, and in which human fear, vulnerability, and beauty is starkly exposed. Christians are taught not to seek this valley but neither to avoid or to fear it, for they are not alone: God is there with them, as are others. And God will carry them through that valley, into a life that is beyond death.

13.8   Conclusions: Practical Recommendations for Clinicians

In this chapter we have presented the FICA Spiritual History Tool as a way to engage patients regarding religion and spirituality, have briefly reviewed evidence suggesting that religion and spirituality affects patient decision-making regarding rational suicide, and then have presented an extensive engagement of rational suicide from the perspective of Christian tradition. We conclude with four recommendations for how clinicians might engage patients in conversation about how religion and spirituality affect patient decisions around rational suicide. These recommendations apply to patients from all religious traditions and none (i.e., not just Christians).

1. *Explore religion and spirituality in an open-ended way.* In a diverse and pluralistic world, even religious leaders and scholars may not be aware of the many forms of spiritual and religious expression in any community. Open-ended FICA questions like "Do you have spiritual beliefs, values, or practices that help you cope with stress?" invite patients to describe their religious commitments and affiliations on their own terms.
2. *Explore patients' relationship to their formative religious traditions, and how this relationship affects their judgments about assisted suicide.* Knowing about patients' spirituality and religious affiliation is helpful, but more relevant for discussions of assisted suicide or "death with dignity" is the quality of patients' relationship with these formative traditions. A self-identified Catholic Christian who attends mass twice yearly and who is deeply angry with the Catholic Church over sexual abuse by priests may approach church teaching about assisted suicide very differently than a self-identified Catholic Christian who finds deep peace and joy in Catholic teaching and practice. Clinicians, perhaps with assistance from healthcare chaplains and clergy, can explore these relationships in detail, even when a patient's dominant account of these relationships is one of estrangement and disaffection.
3. *Explore the role of religious and spiritual practices.* Many religious traditions offer practices, rituals, and resources that can be of great support to those who are suffering. For Christians, for example, practices such as praying the psalms of lament (e.g., Psalm 13, Psalm 88), receiving the (Catholic) Sacrament of the Sick, praying the rosary, and participation in liturgies of healing can be sustaining in times of prolonged illness and vulnerability.
4. *Explore the role of community, and connect patients to their communities if appropriate.* As described in detail earlier, "religion" (as opposed to "spirituality") is rarely done alone; highly religious individuals may be embedded in communities capable of offering substantial physical and emotional support in times of vulnerability and need. For patients who are amenable, encouraging connection with these communities can be deeply healing and may well reduce the perceived isolation and fear of "being a burden" that lies behind many decisions for assisted suicide. Encouraging patients to be in contact with religious leaders, if appropriate, can facilitate communal connection and support.

References

1. Cohen S. Brittany Maynard: new face of right to die. The big story. Associated Press. 2014. http://bigstory.ap.org/article/30a58a58a06046cab8f894ddcc2828e8/young-terminal-new-face-right-die. Accessed 23 Dec 2015.
2. Wilson K, et al. Desire for euthanasia or physician-assisted suicide in palliative cancer care. Health Psychol. 2007;26(3):314–23.
3. Jansen-van der Weide M, et al. Granted, undecided, withdrawn, and refused requests for euthanasia and physician-assisted suicide. Arch Intern Med. 2005;165:1698–704.
4. Puchalski C. The FICA spiritual history tool #274. J Palliat Med. 2014;17:105–6.
5. Smith K, et al. Predictors of pursuit of physician-assisted death. J Pain Symptom Manage. 2015;49(3):555–61.
6. Lichtenstein R, et al. Black/white differences in attitudes toward physician-assisted suicide. J Natl Med Assoc. 1997;89(2):125–33.
7. Emanuel E, et al. Attitudes and desires related to euthanasia and physician-assisted suicide among terminally ill patients and their caregivers. JAMA. 2000;284(19):2460–8.
8. Burdette A, et al. Religion and attitudes toward physician-assisted suicide and terminal palliative care. J Sci Study Relig. 2005;44(1):79–93.
9. Curlin F, et al. To die, to sleep: US physicians' religious and other objections to physician-assisted suicide, terminal sedation, and withdrawal of life support. Am J Hosp Palliat Med. 2008;25(2):112–20.
10. Dorff E. Matters of life and death: a Jewish approach to modern medical ethics. Philadelphia: Jewish Publication Society; 1988. p. 180–6.
11. Unitarian Universalist Association. The right to die with dignity: 1988 general resolution. http://www.uua.org/statements/right-die-dignity. Accessed 5 Jan 2016.
12. Seneca. *Episulae morales ad Lucilium [Moral Epistles to Lucilius]*, ep. 70, 77.
13. Droge A. "Suicide." The Anchor Bible dictionary, vol. 6. New York: Doubleday; 1992. p. 225–31.
14. Retterstøl N, Ekeberg O. Christianity and suicide. In: Wasserman D, Wasserman C, editors. Suicidology and suicide prevention. New York: Oxford University Press; 2009.
15. Donne J. Biathanatos. New York: Garland; 1982.
16. McKenny G. To relieve the human condition: bioethics, technology, and the body. Albany: State University of New York Press; 1997. p. 2.
17. Pew Research Forum. Religious groups' views on end-of-life issues. 2013. http://www.pewforum.org/2013/11/21/religious-groups-views-on-end-of-life-issues/. Accessed 23 Oct 2015
18. Vatican City: Libreria Editrice Vaticana. 1993. Catechism of the Catholic Church. http://www.vatican.va/archive/ENG0015/__P7Z.HTM. Accessed 17 Aug 2015.
19. Presbyterian Church in America. PCA digest: position papers. 1988. http://pcahistory.org/pca/2-378.html. Accessed 31 Aug 2015.
20. United Methodist Church. The book of discipline of the United Methodist Church. "Suicide." 2004. http://archives.umc.org/interior.asp?mid=1735. Accessed 17 Aug 2015.
21. Pew Research Forum. Views on end-of-life medical treatments. 2013. http://www.pewforum.org/2013/11/21/views-on-end-of-life-medical-treatments/. Accessed 23 Dec 2015
22. Wittwer H. The problem of the possible rationality of suicide and the ethics of physician-assisted suicide. Int J Law Psychiatry. 2013;36:419–26.
23. Thomas Aquinas. Summa theologica. 5 vols. Trans. by Fathers of the English Dominican Province. Notre Dame: Christian Classics; 1980.
24. Pinckaers S. The sources of Christian ethics. Trans. Sr. Mary Thomas Noble. Washington, DC: Catholic University of America Press; 1995.
25. Safranek J. Autonomy and assisted suicide: the execution of freedom. Hastings Cent Rep. 1998;28(4):32–6.
26. Cherry M. Why physician-assisted suicide perpetuates the idolatry of medicine. Christ Bioeth. 2003;9(2–3):245–71.

27. Ferngren G. Medicine and health care in early Christianity. Baltimore: Johns Hopkins University Press; 2009.
28. The Heidelberg Catechism. www.ccel.org/creeds/heidelberg-cat-ext.txt. Accessed 9 Sept 2015.
29. Shuman J, Volck B. Reclaiming the body: Christians and the faithful use of modern medicine. Brazos: Grand Rapids; 2006.
30. Hardwig J. Is there a duty to die? Hastings Cent Rep. 1997;2:34–42.
31. Cassell E. The nature of suffering and the goals of medicine. N Engl J Med. 1982;306(11): 639–45.
32. Sulmasy D. The healer's calling: a spirituality for physicians and other healthcare professionals. New York: Paulist; 1997.
33. Varelius J. Voluntary euthanasia, physician-assisted suicide, and the goals of medicine. J Med Philos. 2006;31:121–37.
34. Verhey A. Reading the Bible in the strange world of medicine. Grand Rapids: Eerdmans; 2003. p. 134.
35. John Paul II. Salvifici doloris, Apostolic exhortation. 1984. http://w2.vatican.va/content/john-paul-ii/en/apost_letters/1984/documents/hf_jp-ii_apl_11021984_salvifici-doloris.html. Accessed: 5 Jan 2016.
36. Williams D. Sisters in the wilderness: the challenge of womanist god-talk. 2nd ed. Orbis: Maryknoll; 2013.
37. Mohrmann M. Medicine as ministry: reflections on suffering, ethics, and hope. Pilgrim: Cleveland; 1995.
38. Sinnott-Armstrong W, Miller F. What makes killing wrong? J Med Ethics. 2013;39(1):3–7.
39. Velleman D. Against the right to die. J Med Philos. 1992;17:665–81.
40. Tippetts K. Dear Brittany: why we don't have to be so afraid of dying and suffering that we choose suicide. Blog. A Holy experience. 2014. http://www.aholyexperience.com/2014/10/dear-brittany-why-we-dont-have-to-be-so-afraid-of-dying-suffering-that-we-choose-suicide/. Accessed 4 Sept 2015.
41. Tippetts K. By degrees—living and dying. Blog. Mundane faithfulness. 2014. http://www.mundanefaithfulness.com/2014/12/29/by-degrees-living-and-dying/. Accessed 4 Sept 2015.

Classic Psychedelics and Rational Suicide in the Elderly: Exploring the Potential Utility of a Reemerging Treatment Paradigm

14

Peter S. Hendricks and Charles S. Grob

14.1 Introduction

Whether suicide might be considered rational in any circumstance is a matter of debate and beyond the scope of the present chapter. It is acknowledged, however, that some individuals may express the desire to end their lives in the absence of obvious and diagnosable mental health conditions. Such "rational" suicidality may be concentrated among the elderly and driven by a sense of hopelessness about a future that promises little beyond pain, isolation, decline, and ultimate demise (as discussed in this text). The purpose of this chapter is to explore the potential utility of classic psychedelics in reversing this view of a future marked by suffering and devoid of meaning.

14.2 Sociopolitical History of Classic Psychedelics

Classic psychedelics, also known as classic hallucinogens and entheogens, can occasion mystical-type experiences and primarily act as agonists on serotonin 2A ($5HT_{2A}$) brain receptors [1]. Among the most notable of these substances are dimethyltryptamine (DMT), widespread in the plant kingdom and the chief psychoactive component of the South American admixture known as *ayahuasca*; lysergic

P.S. Hendricks, Ph.D. (✉)
Department of Health Behavior, School of Public Health, University of Alabama at Birmingham, 1665 University Boulevard, Birmingham, AL 35233, USA
e-mail: phendricks@uab.edu

C.S. Grob, M.D.
Department of Psychiatry, David Geffen School of Medicine at UCLA,
University of California Los Angeles School of Medicine,
10833 Le Conte Avenue, Los Angeles, CA 90095, USA
e-mail: cgrob@labiomed.org

© Springer International Publishing Switzerland 2017
R.E. McCue, M. Balasubramaniam (eds.), *Rational Suicide in the Elderly*,
DOI 10.1007/978-3-319-32672-6_14

acid diethylamide (LSD), derived from the ergot fungus; psilocybin, the primary psychoactive constituent of *Psilocybe* and other mushroom genera; and mescaline, the primary psychoactive constituent of peyote and other cacti. Classic psychedelics have been used across multiple cultures for millennia, typically in highly ritualized sacramental and healing contexts, and may be among the first psychoactive substances used by human beings [2–6]. Indeed, classic psychedelic use within ritualized settings in prehistoric cultures was often regarded as a means of communication with the afterworld. From the indigenous use in many regions of the Americas of various mescaline-containing cacti, to indigenous Central American sacramental employment of psilocybin mushrooms, to the Amazonian plant decoction ayahuasca, the name of which is derived from the Quechua language of the Central Andes of South America and translates as "Vine of the Soul" or "Vine of the Dead," these powerful psychoactive substances allowed the native peoples from distant times and distant lands to address the great existential challenges of death and dying. Whereas much of this ancient knowledge has been lost over time with the relentless and worldwide extinction of native cultures, the potential value of these sacramental medicines has attracted growing interest among modern anthropologists, ethnobotanists, natural product chemists, and medical scientists.

Following the discovery of LSD by Albert Hofmann in 1943, the scientific community of the 1950s through the early 1970s responded prolifically, producing thousands of manuscripts that suggested classic psychedelics might potentiate psychotherapeutic effectiveness for a range of clinical conditions [3, 4, 7, 8]. Also during this time, the United States Army and Central Intelligence Agency explored the possibility of weaponizing classic psychedelics, administering the substances to persons without their knowledge or consent, but met with limited success [9]. Burgeoning recreational use of classic psychedelics attracted significant sensationalized media coverage, as did the reckless advocacy of former Harvard University professor Timothy Leary. Such coverage contributed to the concern that classic psychedelics were fueling the countercultural revolution of the late 1960s, which was viewed as a serious threat to the national security by then-president Richard Nixon [9, 10]. Accordingly, a series of regulatory barriers including placing the most prominent classic psychedelics into Schedule I of the Controlled Substances Act of 1970 (designated as having a high potential for abuse, no currently accepted medical use, and a lack of accepted safety under medical supervision) and the withdrawal of federal funding rendered human research with classic psychedelics essentially defunct.

The moratorium on classic psychedelic research appears to have been sociopolitically motivated, but was it empirically justified? Gable [11, 12], in two extensive reviews of the literature, concluded that LSD and psilocybin—along with cannabis—carry the lowest risks of dependence and lethality among 20 abused substances. In a report published in *The Lancet*, Nutt et al. [13] instructed an expert panel to score 20 abused substances according to the harms they pose to the individual and others, with a maximum total score of 100 points. Alcohol (score=72), heroin (score=55), and crack cocaine (score=54) were deemed most harmful, whereas LSD (score=7) and psilocybin (score=6) were deemed least harmful.

Thus, the medical or scientific rationale for the de facto ban on classic psychedelics appears to have been poorly informed. This conclusion is made more obvious bearing in mind that virtually every other major class of abused substance has therapeutic applications (e.g., opiates as analgesics, cocaine as a local anesthetic, depressants as anxiolytics). Professor David Nutt, former Chair of the United Kingdom's Advisory Council on the Misuse of Drugs, commented that the justification for banning classic psychedelics was "unquestionably one of the most effective pieces of disinformation in the history of mankind" [14].

14.3   Empirical Findings with Classic Psychedelics: Implications for Rational Suicide

Where does this leave us today? Despite the passage of time, the older data on the potential utility of classic psychedelics remains persuasive. Scientific interest in these substances has persisted, and as a consequence classic psychedelic research has experienced a modest renaissance over the past two and a half decades. This research is preliminary in nature, but suggests classic psychedelics could mitigate rational suicide risk in the elderly. In a milestone study marking the return of human experimental research with classic psychedelics, Griffiths et al. [15] evaluated the acute and longer term effects of a single dose of psilocybin relative to methylphenidate among 36 healthy adult hallucinogen-naïve volunteers using a double-blind between-group crossover design. Results confirmed that psilocybin can occasion mystical-type experiences characterized by a sense of unity/oneness, transcendence of time and space, bliss, sacredness, and introspection/insight. No serious adverse events were reported. Two months after psilocybin administration, 12 % of volunteers rated their psilocybin experience as the single most meaningful personal experience of their lives (including experiences such as the birth of a child) with 55 % rating their psilocybin experience among the top five most meaningful personal experiences. In addition, 33 % of volunteers rated their psilocybin experience as the single most meaningful spiritual experience of their lives, with 38 % rating their psilocybin experience among the top five most meaningful spiritual experiences. Psilocybin also produced significant self-reported improvements in positive attitudes about life and/or self, positive mood, altruistic/social effects, and positive behavior corroborated by community observers. These effects were sustained at 14-month follow-up [16] and overall findings were replicated in a subsequent study of dose-related effects [17]. It is possible, therefore, that a single administration of a classic psychedelic such as psilocybin may promote the enduring view that life is worth living. Significantly, these studies have demonstrated that the optimal utilization of a classic psychedelic treatment model may reliably and predictably facilitate psychospiritual experiences. The implications of these findings are promising, particularly given the observations of early researchers in the 1960s who identified that terminal cancer patients administered a classic psychedelic in a research setting were more likely to achieve sustained reductions in anxiety, improved mood, and enhanced overall quality of life in the future if during the course of what was often their only treatment session they experienced a psychospiritual epiphany or mystical level of consciousness [18, 19].

Additional research with obvious relevance to rational suicide in the elderly has been conducted among individuals with end-of-life distress. This represented one of more promising lines of work during the initial wave of classic psychedelic research, with findings suggesting profound and sustained improvements in existential anxiety, despair, isolation, and the management of pain (e.g., [20, 21]). More recently, Grob et al. [22] tested the potential efficacy of a single moderate dose of psilocybin among 12 adults with advanced-stage cancer and reactive anxiety using a double-blind placebo-controlled crossover design. Psilocybin was associated with significantly reduced anxiety 1 and 3 months posttreatment and significantly reduced depression 6 months posttreatment. In a similar study, Gasser et al. [23] evaluated the potential efficacy of a single dose of LSD among 12 individuals with anxiety associated with life-threatening disease using an open-label crossover design. LSD produced significant reductions in anxiety that were sustained at 12-month follow-up. In both studies, no serious adverse events were reported. These results suggest that a single administration under optimal conditions of a classic psychedelic may alleviate feelings of desolation that may underlie rational suicide in the elderly.

Although substance misuse may not be linked with rational suicide in the elderly per se, it is otherwise robustly associated with suicide in general [24]. For this reason, the antiaddictive effects of classic psychedelics are briefly discussed here (for reviews, see [25, 26]). A meta-analysis of six randomized controlled trials of treatment for alcohol dependence conducted between 1966 and 1970 found that a single dose of LSD reduced the likelihood of alcohol misuse relative to comparison conditions (OR = 1.96; [27]). A recent single-arm trial of smoking cessation (N = 15) involving as many as three administrations of psilocybin yielded abstinence rates of 80 %, compared with abstinence rates of 25 % or less for the most intensive of typical smoking cessation treatments [28]. Furthermore, a recent single-arm trial of treatment for alcohol dependence (N = 10) involving up to two administrations of psilocybin produced robust reductions in drinking sustained through 9-month follow-up [29]. An observational study of ayahuasca-assisted therapy for addiction among 12 individuals found that participating in up to 2 ayahuasca retreats was associated with reductions in alcohol, tobacco, and cocaine use [30]. As in the aforementioned studies on healthy volunteers and individuals with end-of-life distress, no serious adverse events were reported in these contemporary investigations of addiction treatment. Finally, naturalistic hallucinogen use, which is likely accounted for primarily by the use of classic psychedelics, predicted a reduced likelihood of recidivism among over 25,000 individuals under community corrections supervision with a history of problematic substance use behavior [31]. Considering that the antiaddictive effects of classic psychedelics may be mediated by improved regulation of negative affect (e.g., [26]), these findings may relate to rational suicide in the elderly insofar that rational suicide in the elderly involves at least some affective disturbance.

A number of additional findings warrant brief review here. In two recent open-label trials of ayahuasca among hospitalized in patients with recurrent Major Depressive Disorder, a single administration of ayahuasca was associated with rapid and enduring reductions in depressive symptoms [32, 33]. These findings may have relevance to rational suicide in the elderly to the extent that rational suicide in the elderly may be characterized by depressive symptoms including hopelessness and anhedonia. Classic psychedelics may boost spirituality [26], which can be defined as "the experience of transcendent dimension that gives meaning to existence, and the capacity to experience the sacred" [34]. Spirituality has been shown to protect against suicidality in general, and may also protect against rational suicide in the elderly via religious coping, social support, or other mechanisms [35–37]. In addition, the use of classic psychedelics is associated with increased mindfulness, or moment-to-moment awareness (e.g., [30, 38]), which may be a key determinant of flourishing, or optimal mental health (e.g., [39]). It may be that classic psychedelics protect against rational suicide in the elderly by fostering the perception that every moment is a gift. Finally, the default mode network (DMN), a network of brain regions most active during rest, shows aberrant connectivity (e.g., hyperactivity and hyperconnectivity) among those with psychopathology, which may undergird the cognitive fixedness (i.e., rumination and rigid pessimism) characteristic of several mental health conditions [40, 41]. Classic psychedelics may ultimately normalize the DMN, producing the subjective experience of "mind expansion" commonly espoused by those who have used classic psychedelics (e.g., [40]). Consistent with this notion, a single dose of psilocybin increased personality openness 14 months after administration [42]. Openness may protect against suicide in general among the elderly [43], and may protect against rational suicide specifically in this population through openness to alternative or creative problem-solving. In other words, classic psychedelics may open one's mind to nonsuicide solutions to the problem of suffering.

Only one study has directly examined whether classic psychedelics might prevent suicide. Hendricks et al. [44] tested the relationships of classic psychedelic use with suicidal ideation, suicidal planning, and suicide attempt among over 190,000 adult respondents pooled from years 2008 through 2012 of the National Survey on Drug Use and Health, an annual survey of the United States Department of Health and Human Services. Controlling for a range of potential confounding factors, the authors found that having ever used a classic psychedelic was associated with a 14 % reduced likelihood of past year suicidal thinking, a 29 % reduced likelihood of past year suicidal planning, and a 36 % reduced likelihood of suicide attempt. Consistent with the literature on suicide risk factors, lifetime illicit use of other drugs was by and large associated with an increased likelihood of these outcomes. Whether these results generalize to rational suicide in the elderly is not known, but the extraordinarily large sample suggests generality to the population of those at risk for any suicidality. Hence, for reasons described earlier, classic psychedelics may protect against rational suicide in the elderly.

14.4 Conclusion

Dating back to the 1960s, and corroborated with recent studies, the controlled administration of classic psychedelics to carefully selected subjects approaching the end of life has been demonstrated to evoke a renewed sense of purpose and meaning, leading to higher quality of life and reduced psychopathology in their remaining time [45]. While the advent of the modern hospice movement and field of palliative medicine have made notable advances in ameliorating physical suffering, effectively addressing the existential crises of alienation, isolation, and meaninglessness in the dying has remained a more intransigent problem. In the state of Oregon, where assisted suicide has been legal for most of the last two decades, nonphysical causes of suffering, including persistent existential suffering, have been identified as critical factors in terminally ill people who choose to end their lives [46]. Similar issues are faced by the elderly, even in the absence of imminent life threatening illness. With the growing years and cumulative loss, particularly the inevitable erosion of the sense of self identified with a more vibrant stage of life, the elderly often lose their capacity to retain an ongoing sense of meaning and purpose. The administration of classic psychedelics only one or two times under carefully monitored conditions appears to offer a safe and nontoxic treatment model that may potentially facilitate the experience of profound altered states of consciousness that have the capacity to imbue the individual with greater clarity, expanded worldview, and renewed perspective on life remaining. This sustained amelioration of existential suffering persists long after the direct pharmacologic action of the drug [17, 22]. Finally, the development of such an existential medicine model and its application for individuals in our society approaching the end of life, whether they be elderly or not, may achieve a salutary effect on those (and in the end all) of us preparing to make the inevitable passage at the end of life, as well as to the world left behind.

Of course, whether classic psychedelics do in fact prevent rational suicidality in the elderly is an empirical question that merits future study. Although research with classic psychedelics remains a challenge (see [47]), scientific interest in this long-neglected field continues to grow, and psilocybin may soon be a candidate for approved medical use in the United States [48]. Interested scientists are therefore encouraged to familiarize themselves with published safety guidelines [49]. With time, the broader clinical applications of classic psychedelics will be illuminated. It is hoped that these substances will contribute to the alleviation of suffering associated with the range of mental health conditions, and perhaps for the aging, a peaceful reconciliation with their mortality.

References

1. Vollenweider FX, Kometer M. The neurobiology of psychedelic drugs: implications for the treatment of mood disorders. Nature Rev Neurosci. 2010;11:642–51.
2. El-Seedi HR, De Smet PA, Beck O, et al. Prehistoric peyote use: alkaloid analysis and radio-carbon dating of archaeological specimens of Lophophora from Texas. J Ethnopharmacol. 2005;101:238–42.

3. Grinspoon L, Bakalar JB. Psychedelic drugs reconsidered. New York: Basic Books; 1979.
4. Nichols DE. Hallucinogens. Pharmacol Ther. 2004;101:131–81.
5. Schultes RE. Hallucinogens of plant origin. Science. 1969;163:245–54.
6. Schultes RE, Hoffman A, Rätsch C. Plants of the gods: their sacred, healing, and hallucinogenic powers. Rev. edn. Rochester: Healing Arts Press; 2001.
7. Grob CS, Greer GR, Mangini M. Hallucinogens at the turn of the century: an introduction. J Psychoactive Drugs. 1998;30:315–9.
8. Masters REL, Houston J. The varieties of psychedelic experience. New York: Holt, Rinehart & Winston; 1966.
9. Lee MA, Shlain B. Acid dreams: the complete social history of LSD—The CIA, the Sixties, and Beyond. Rev. edn. New York: Grove Press; 1992.
10. Stevens J. Storming heaven: LSD and the American dream. New York: The Atlantic Monthly Press; 1987.
11. Gable RS. Toward a comparative overview of dependence potential and acute toxicity of psychoactive substances used nonmedically. Am J Drug Alcohol Abuse. 1993;19:263–81.
12. Gable RS. Comparison of acute lethal toxicity of commonly abused psychoactive substances. Addiction. 2004;99:686–96.
13. Nutt DJ, King LA, Phillips LD. Drug harms in the UK: a multicriteria decision analysis. Lancet. 2010;376:1558–65.
14. Derbyshire D. Healing trip: how psychedelic drugs could help treat depression. The Guardian. 2014. http://www.theguardian.com/society/2014/oct/05/healing-trip-psychedelic-drugs-treat--depression. Accessed 10 Jan 2016.
15. Griffiths RR, Richards WA, McCann U, et al. Psilocybin can occasion mystical-type experiences having substantial and sustained personal meaning and spiritual significance. Psychopharmacology (Berl). 2006;187:268–83.
16. Griffiths RR, Richards WA, Johnson MW, et al. Mystical-type experiences occasioned by psilocybin mediate the attribution of personal meaning and spiritual significance 14 months later. J Psychopharmacol. 2008;22:621–32.
17. Griffiths RR, Johnson MW, Richards WA, et al. Psilocybin occasioned mystical-type experiences: immediate and persisting dose-related effects. Psychopharmacology (Berl). 2011;218:649–55.
18. Grof S, Goodman LE, Richards WA, et al. LSD-assisted psychotherapy in patients with terminal cancer. Int Pharmacopsychiatry. 1973;8:129–44.
19. Pahnke WN. The psychedelic mystical experience in the human encounter with death. Harv Theol Rev. 1969;62:1–21.
20. Kast E. Attenuation of anticipation: a therapeutic use of lysergic acid diethylamide. Psychiatr Q. 1967;41:646–57.
21. Kast EC, Collins VJ. Study of lysergic acid diethylamide as an analgesic agent. Anesth Analg. 1964;43:285–91.
22. Grob CS, Danforth AL, Chopra GS, et al. Pilot study of psilocybin treatment for anxiety in patients with advanced-stage cancer. Arch Gen Psychiatry. 2011;68:71–8.
23. Gasser P, Holstein D, Michel Y, et al. Safety and efficacy of lysergic acid diethylamide-assisted psychotherapy for anxiety associated with life-threatening diseases. J Nerv Ment Dis. 2014;202:513–20.
24. Hawton K, van Heeringen K. Suicide. Lancet. 2009;373:1372–81.
25. Bogenschutz MP, Johnson MW. Classic hallucinogens in the treatment of addictions. Prog Neuropsychopharmacol Biol Psychiatry. 2016;64:250–8.
26. Bogenschutz MP, Pommy JM. Therapeutic mechanisms of classic hallucinogens in the treatment of addictions: from indirect evidence to testable hypotheses. Drug Test Anal. 2012;4:543–55.
27. Krebs TS, Johansen PØ. Lysergic acid diethylamide (LSD) for alcoholism: meta-analysis of randomized controlled trials. J Psychopharmacol. 2012;26:994–1002.
28. Johnson MW, Garcia-Romeu A, Cosimano MP, et al. Pilot study of the 5-HT2AR agonist psilocybin in the treatment of tobacco addiction. J Psychopharmacol. 2014;28:983–92.

29. Bogenschutz MP, Forcehimes AA, Pommy JA, et al. Psilocybin-assisted treatment for alcohol dependence: a proof-of-concept study. J Psychopharmacol. 2015;29:289–99.
30. Thomas G, Lucas P, Capler NR, et al. Ayahuasca-assisted therapy for addiction: results from a preliminary observational study in Canada. Curr Drug Abuse Rev. 2013;6:30–42.
31. Hendricks PS, Clark CB, Johnson MW, et al. Hallucinogen use predicts reduced recidivism among substance-involved offenders under community corrections supervision. J Psychopharmacol. 2014;28:62–6.
32. Osório Fde L, Sanches RF, Macedo LR, et al. Antidepressant effects of a single dose of aya- huasca in patients with recurrent depression: a preliminary report. Rev Bras Psiquiatr. 2015;37:13–20.
33. Sanches RF, de Lima OF, Dos Santos RG, et al. Antidepressant effects of a single dose of ayahuasca in patients with recurrent depression: a SPECT study. J Clin Psychopharmacol. 2016;36:77–81.
34. van Dierendonck D. Spirituality as an essential determinant for the good life, its importance relative to self-determinant psychological needs. J Happiness Stud. 2012;13:685–700.
35. Rasic DT, Belik SL, Elias B, et al. Spirituality, religion and suicidal behavior in a nationally representative sample. J Affect Disord. 2009;114:32–40.
36. Rasic D, Robinson JA, Bolton J, et al. Longitudinal relationships of religious worship atten- dance and spirituality with major depression, anxiety disorders, and suicidal ideation and attempts: findings from the Baltimore epidemiologic catchment area study. J Psychiatr Res. 2011;45:848–54.
37. Weber SR, Pargament KI. The role of religion and spirituality in mental health. Curr Opin Psychiatry. 2014;27:358–63.
38. Soler J, Elices M, Franquesa A, et al. Exploring the therapeutic potential of ayahuasca: acute intake increases mindfulness-related capacities. Psychopharmacology (Berl). 2016;233(5):823–9.
39. Catalino LI, Fredrickson BL. A Tuesday in the life of a flourisher: the role of positive emo- tional reactivity in optimal mental health. Emotion. 2011;11:938–50.
40. Carhart-Harris RL, Leech R, Hellyer PJ, et al. The entropic brain: a theory of conscious states informed by neuroimaging research with psychedelic drugs. Front Hum Neurosci. 2014;8:20.
41. Whitfield-Gabrieli S, Ford JM. Default mode network activity and connectivity in psychopa- thology. Annu Rev Clin Psychol. 2012;8:49–76.
42. MacLean KA, Johnson MW, Griffiths RR. Mystical experiences occasioned by the hallucino- gen psilocybin lead to increases in the personality domain of openness. J Psychopharmacol. 2011;25:1453–61.
43. Segal DL, Marty MA, Meyer WJ, et al. Personality, suicidal ideation, and reasons for living among older adults. J Gerontol B Psychol Sci Soc Sci. 2012;67:159–66.
44. Hendricks PS, Thorne CB, Clark CB, et al. Classic psychedelic use is associated with reduced psychological distress and suicidality in the United States adult population. J Psychopharmacol. 2015;29:280–8.
45. Grob CS, Bossis AP, Griffiths RR. Use of the classic hallucinogen psilocybin for treatment of existential distress associated with cancer. In: Carr BI, Steel J, editors. Psychological aspects of cancer. New York: Springer; 2013.
46. Byock I. Evidence-based therapies for persistent suffering. Psychol. 2014;27:677–8.
47. Nutt DJ, King LA, Nichols DE. Effects of schedule I drug laws on neuroscience research and treatment innovation. Nature Rev Neurosci. 2013;14:577–85.
48. Hendricks PS, Johnson MW, Griffiths RR. Psilocybin, psychological distress, and suicidality. J Psychopharmacol. 2015;29:1041–3.
49. Johnson MW, Richards WA, Griffiths RR. Human hallucinogen research: guidelines for safety. J Psychopharmacol. 2008;22:603–20.

Epilogue

15

Anthony M. Daniels

The first question raised by the idea of rational suicide in the elderly is whether the mere fact of advanced age places such suicide in a different category from all or any other rational suicide. It is true that those factors which, *prima facie*, appear to render suicide *rational*, such as painful, intractable, and incurable illness that destroys the quality of life, may be more common in old age than in other period of life, but there is no such factor that occurs *only* in old age. Respiratory failure, for example, often occurs much earlier in life than in old age and entails a horrible and long-drawn-out death that precludes any activity that makes life pleasurable or worthwhile. Loneliness and loss are more frequent in old age than at other ages no doubt, but are certainly not confined to it. Rational suicide in the elderly, then, is not so much a matter of nosology as of epidemiology.

We must also decide who the elderly are. This has changed in my clinical lifetime, in the course of which geriatricians have come to treat older and older age groups. Patients are now referred to geriatricians 10 or even 15 years later in their life than when I qualified (in 1974). This is for at least two reasons. First, the number of persons aged 65 or over has increased both absolutely and relatively in all Western societies. In Britain, the number of people aged 65 or more increased by 47% between 1974 and 2014, and proportionately from just under 13% of the total population to just under 18%.[1] In British hospitals, 68% of all emergency bed days are now taken by those over the age of 65.[2]

---

[1] http://www.ons.gov.uk/ons/rel/pop-estimate/population-estimates-for-ukDOUBLEHYPHENengland-and-walesDOUBLEHYPHENscotland-and-northern-ireland/mid-2014/sty-ageing-of-the-uk-population.html

[2] http://www.kingsfund.org.uk/sites/files/kf/field/field_publication_file/older-people-and-emergency-bed-use-aug-2012.pdf

A.M. Daniels, M.R.C.Psych. (✉)
Retired Consultant, City Hospital, Birmingham, UK
e-mail: anthonymalcolmdaniels@gmail.com

© Springer International Publishing Switzerland 2017
R.E. McCue, M. Balasubramaniam (eds.), *Rational Suicide in the Elderly*,
DOI 10.1007/978-3-319-32672-6_15

In addition, the process of ageing seems to have slowed. The other day I was doing some research on a minor writer called Max Plowman who died in 1941 aged 57. In his last letter, sent four days before his death, he wrote in reference to his lack of energy (and the peptic ulcer from which he had suffered grievously for at least 14 years, itself something almost inconceivable nowadays), 'the machine is not designed to be kept speeded up as one nears 60.'[3] Clearly he considered 60 to be old age.

The Young Visiters, which Daisy Ashford wrote when she was 9 years old, begins with the memorable words, 'Mr Salteena was an elderly man of 42…'[4] (At the time, male life expectancy at birth was 52.5 years, though it was considerably higher at age 42). It is a matter of common experience that, when one looks at photographs of people of bygone years, those who would now be considered middle-aged look aged and wore out.

My father referred to his next-door neighbour, aged 79, as 'the old man', when he himself was 81, and would have been horrified himself to be considered old. Dr McCue has alerted us to the existence of what might be called the first generation of geriatric adolescents, of people who would once have been considered elderly but who refuse to acknowledge that they are no longer young and who continue to live as if they were still young: a development that has both positive and negative aspects or effects. Their refusal to acknowledge the depredations of time preserves an active attitude to life, to the benefit of both physical health and mental well-being; but the denial of inevitable decline magnifies its personal significance when it comes. If one of the causes of supposedly rational suicide in the elderly is the loss of meaning in life, as is suggested by Prof Varelius, we may expect more such suicide among the elderly, even as their situation, considered 'objectively' improves, since such meaning consists more and more the maintenance of a youthful way of life.

Whether the increase in life expectancy over the last century and a quarter will continue is a matter of speculation; obesity and the consequent type II diabetes have been advanced as reasons why life expectancy may lessen in the near future. If life expectancy *does* continue to rise, however, those whom we now consider elderly will not be considered elderly in years to come. But, like suffering, old age cannot be evaded forever. However it may be defined, very few of us will avoid it. At least some among us will have to face the horrible question of whether we would be better off dead.

If suicide is ever rational, it can be so only as an instance of rational action in general. But when is action rational? Hume maintained that 'reason is, and ought only to be, the slave of the passions, and can never pretend to any other office than to serve and obey them'[5]: that is to say the kingdom of ends is beyond the reach of reason. You cannot argue me out of, or refute, my professed purpose in living by pointing to any facts, though it is possible to point out contradictions between my actual behaviour and my professed reasons for living. Motives and ends are not so much rational or irrational, on Hume's view, as *arational*: for what cannot be ratio-

---

[3] *Bridge into the Future: Letters of Max Plowman*, Andrew Dakers, 1944, p.770.

[4] It was first published in 1919.

[5] David Hume, *A Treatise of Human Nature*. There is a slight contradiction, or at least redundancy, in this passage. If reason *can only* be the slave of the passions, there is no sense in which it *ought* to be so, since moral judgements attach only to what might be different as a result of choice.

nal cannot be irrational. A motive is only irrational on his account if it conflicts with another motive higher up in the hierarchy of motives, there being an ultimate motive (for otherwise there would be an infinite regress of motives).

From the psychiatrist's point of view, this is inadequate for a number of reasons. People may genuinely desire six impossible things before breakfast—or, indeed, for the duration of their lives. I may make the heavyweight boxing championship of the world the purpose of my existence, but it is impossible for a number of reasons: I am 66 years of age, I have never boxed in my life, and I am not a heavyweight. It surely would not be stretching the normal sense of the word 'rational' to claim that my ambition did not fulfil the criteria of its application. And yet the impossible pursuit may be perfectly consistent with a happy and fulfilled life.

We all know, moreover, that motives (passions) are not fixed, are often in contradiction to one another while simultaneously and sincerely held, and can be opaque to the person who has them. It is not necessary to believe in the full panoply of Freudian constructs to know that the human mind is not a mechanism for grinding out the logical conclusions to syllogisms, or endowed with invariable self-knowledge. To take only one example, from literature: Shakespeare's *King Lear*. Lear says to Gloucester:

Thou rascal beadle, hold thy bloody hand!
Why dost thou lash that whore? Strip thine own back.
Thou hotly lusts to use her in that kind.
For which thou whip'st her.

And Shakespeare must have assumed that the audience would understand and recognise the phenomenon here described: that motives are often complex and opaque to those who have them.

Anyone who examines his own life will surely find that what gives and gave it meaning changes. The things that seemed all-important at one time—the *sine qua non* of meaningful existence—no longer seem so 20 years on. I had a taste for dangerous adventure in exotic parts when I was young that I no longer have. The prospect of a journey that would once have filled me with excited anticipation now fills me with gloom.

This is one of the ethical difficulties of advanced directives: one cannot know how one will feel in certain circumstances until one is actually in them. Many people suppose that tetraplegia would sap the will to live completely and give rise, almost automatically, to a desire to die; but 'refusal or request for removal of life-sustaining treatment [of tetraplegics]... is, fortunately, an infrequent occurrence...'[6] In the original concept of the Quality-Adjusted Life-Years, the life of the tetraplegic was regarded as having a negative or minus value: in the opinion of those who developed the instrument, he would have been better off dead.

The mutability of our passions is recognised by everyone. Even the most fervent advocates of euthanasia or physician-assisted suicide believe that the desire to die should be constant and durable for some defined period before it is complied with, and not just a matter of whim or petulant reaction to current circumstances. But it is not always irrational to satisfy short-lived or fleeting desires: when one is thirsty one

---

[6] Subharwal, Sunil, *Essentials of Spinal Cord Medicine*, Demos Medicine, 2014, p. 396.

drinks and when hungry one eats. These desires can become overpowering and their satisfaction more important, for a time, than all other considerations whatsoever, and it is not irrational that they should do so, for their satisfaction is the precondition of all other possible desires, of life itself.

There is usually not one thing alone that gives meaning to life, or makes life pleasurable. Some very real pleasures are nevertheless dispensable: for example (and I speak only for myself), while I like good food and take great pleasure from it, I would not be unduly disturbed if I were told that I could never eat anything again but cheese sandwiches. However, an inability to read or write would, I suspect (though, in the light of the example of tetraplegics cited above, I cannot be certain), severely sap my desire to live. Everyone is different in what he would find intolerable and what would render his life meaningless.

Nevertheless, we have an intuitive grasp of a condition so terrible that many people, at least, would not wish to continue to live with it. Such a condition would render all possible sources of pleasure or meaning impossible; though even here it important to remember that religious faith, if sufficiently strong, can make all experience meaningful and even bearable. Once reads with astonishment the account of Philip II of Spain's appalling and painful last illness, probably worse than any death experienced today except by wilful torture, and the equanimity with which he accepted it because of his certainty of salvation in the after-life.[7]

If a rational action is one which brings about a desired end and which is founded on a true appreciation of the facts of the sublunary situation, for example that one is terminally ill, that there is no possibility of cure and that there is a likelihood of continued or increased suffering (as against, for example, a nihilistic delusion), then suicide can surely be a rational act. Indeed, this is implicitly recognised by those who have investigated the prevalence of pre-existing mental disorder among complete suicide by, for example, the method of psychological autopsy. None of them has found a disorder rate of 100% among suicides; they have found that a percentage of healthy or sane people who have committed suicide, albeit a small percentage of the total of suicides. For example, a famous study found that 93% of 100 successive completed suicides were psychiatrically ill, but seven per cent were not.[8] It is surely likely that some or most of these seven per cent were both sane and rational (though, since sanity and rationality are not the same thing, it is possible that there were some sane but irrational suicides).[9] From the philosophical point of view—whether rational suicide is possible—it is sufficient to prove that there is, or has ever been, a single case.

It has been argued philosophically that suicide is never, and can never be, rational. This is because death is an evil incommensurable with any other, the evil of evils, as it were; and also because, for suicide to be rational, the state of being alive

---

[7] See *From Madrid to Purgatory*, Carlos M. N. Eire, Cambridge University Press, 1995.

[8] A Hundred Cases of Suicide: Clinical Aspects, Barraclough B., Bunch J., Nelson B., Sainsbury P., Brit J. Psych., 1974, 125, 335–73.

[9] Nor does it follow that the suicide of someone who is mentally unwell is necessarily irrational. He may be correctly informed as to his prognosis and the likelihood of his continuing unassuageable suffering.

must be compared with that of being dead. Since we know only the state of being alive, and nothing of the state of being dead, we can never make a valid comparison, and therefore suicide can never be rational.[10]

There are, as always, philosophical objections to this philosophical objection. It is true that when I say that 'I would be better off dead', I seem to imply that I will continue to have a ghostly existence after my death that I will deem to be preferable to my existence before it: that I will continue to have a personal identity. But death (assuming there to be no after-life) is the extinction of personal identity, not its continuation in attenuated form.[11] And from the purely intuitive point of view, it is surely plausible that there are states of existence so horrible than non-existence would be preferable to them. It would be a person of very firm principle but very limited imagination who would tax the inmate of a Nazi extermination camp with irrationality for having run into the electrified fence to kill himself on the grounds that death is an evil incommensurable with any other.

One of the reasons, I suspect, that we have been so keen to medicalise suicide and reduce rational suicide to a minimum, if admitting its existence at all, is that we have a strong prejudice that we ought to prevent suicide wherever we find it. To make suicide the product of illness gives us both the *locus standi* and the duty to do so. Once the person who is ill is made well, he will no longer want to kill himself; indeed, loss of suicide ideation is one of the criteria of his recovery. We therefore subconsciously make use of a false syllogism:

We cannot stand by and watch a person kill himself.

We have a right to prevent him only if his desire to kill himself is the product of illness.

Therefore, his desire to kill himself is the product of illness.

When, however, we turn to the reasons why the elderly do want to kill themselves, or be assisted to die, we find that medical reasons, while present, are not sufficient reasons. There is no simple correlation between illness and the desire to die, no one-to-one relationship with any medical cause of suffering and the wish for death. The analogy with chronic pain stands out in which suffering is more proportional to psychosocial factors than to the presence of physical lesions.[12] Over time pain intensity becomes linked less with nociception and more with emotional and psychosocial factors. Suffering may be as related to the meaning of pain as to its intensity.

As Dr Cheung makes clear in this volume, the decision by the elderly to request either physician-assisted suicide or euthanasia (where such is permitted by the law) is not the result of having followed a simple algorithm that is valid for all people in all places at all times. Where comparable surveys have been done, the results have

---

[10] See, for example, Philip E Devine, *The Ethics of Homicide*, Cornell University Press, Ithaca, 1978.

[11] In my experience of parasuicides, many imagine attending their own funerals by a kind of disembodied hovering above them, watching with pleasure the guilt and grief of those who drove them to it.

[12] Ballantyne J and Sullivan M, Intensity of chronic pain—the wrong metric, N Engl J Med 373;22, 2098–9, 2015.

been different, in part perhaps because of national differences. How are we to interpret the fact that euthanasia is up to 29 times as common in the Netherlands as is physician-assisted suicide in the states of Oregon, Washington, and Montana? Is unbearability of life up to 29 times more frequent in the Netherlands than in those states, and if so why? Does it mean that palliative care in the Netherlands is poor and moreover is given no incentive to improve, or that the elderly are more despised there than in the three states? Does it take more courage to ask for death at the hands of a doctor than to ask simply for the means to kill oneself? Having asked for the means to kill themselves, do people pull back at the last minute, as those who survive having thrown themselves from high places are said to regret having done so halfway down? Is it that euthanasia having been available for longer in the Netherlands than has physician-assisted suicide been available in the three states, it is more present in the minds of the population as a possibility, and therefore more commonly asked for? Does the supply create the demand, and if so does it represent a moral advance or a retrogression, given that the conditions in which a person's life may become meaningless can easily be produced by those around him?[13]

If it is the case that the desire for suicide at the end (or any other time) of life is powerfully influenced by social and psychological factors, even once the more obvious forms of psychiatric disturbance have been ruled out, how is the doctor to take them into account in his assessment of whether the patient's desire for suicide is rational or not, and whether he should try to prevent, ignore, or assist that suicide?

Again, as Dr Cheung's article makes clear, there are no dilemmas unique to the treatment of elderly patients that may not arise in patients of other ages. If one reads the Dutch criteria for the legal granting of euthanasia, namely that:

1. The patient's request should be voluntary and well considered.
2. The patient's suffering should be unbearable and without prospect of improvement.
3. The patient should be informed about his situation and prospects.
4. There are no reasonable alternatives.
5. Another, independent physician should be consulted.
6. The termination of life should be performed with due medical care and attention.

It is obvious that there is no reference whatsoever to the age of the applicant. However, the dilemmas of rational suicide, caused by among other things the irreducible subjectivity of unbearability, are more likely, for obvious empirical reasons, to occur in the practice of geriatricians.

Even if we accept that rational suicide exists, the question remains whether it is morally right or permissible. It is well known that the motives for suicide are often

---

[13] I was once on a train in Germany with a German doctor in her 60s as my fellow-passenger in the compartment. The subject of euthanasia came up. 'What would the world say', she asked me, 'if what was going on in the Netherlands was going on in Germany?' Although not an argument in logic, it was certainly a powerful rhetorical question. It brought home the importance not only of considering individual cases, but the historical context in which they occur.

mixed, and include revenge. They can also be altruistic, though sometimes mistakenly so. A person may consider himself a burden to his loved ones, though not considered by them to be such; it is certainly not irrational for him to consider himself a burden, however, because it is true that they have much to do in order to look after him. His suicide, intended altruistically, will then be a cause of lasting grief and guilt.

In his essay on suicide, Hume[14] dismissed one of the common arguments against the permissibility of suicide, namely that it was against natural law. Suicide, argued Hume, could only be committed in accordance with the laws that governed the universe; therefore, it could not be counted an act against natural law. This, it seems to me, is an argument that does not work, or works too well; for if accepted, it means that any possible act, rapine and murder for example, cannot be against natural law.

Another argument in favour of the permissibility of suicide is that humans may dispose of their lives as they see fit; it is their right to do so. By proponents of this argument, men's lives are seen as their property, but this argument fails on two grounds: first that their life is not their property, for they are not distinguishable from their lives; and second, even if their lives were their property, their possession would not necessarily confer unlimited sovereignty over them. I, and no one else, am the owner of my house; but I may not burn it down.

We are social creatures, unless we are long-term anchorites in the desert, and therefore we owe a duty to our fellow-beings; we cannot, in morality, refer only to our own desires in making our decisions. But Hume disposed of this argument in his *Essay*. The benefit society derives from our continued existence may be trivial by comparison with our continued suffering. We cannot demand huge sacrifices of individuals in order to produce trifling benefits to ourselves. Besides, on the utilitarian argument, suicide may not only be permissible, but obligatory, inasmuch as our continued existence may actually detract from or lessen the sum of human well-being. In an ever-richer world of simultaneously rationed resources, it is important to mention this: old people may easily be bullied into believing that their own deaths are ethically desirable.

In practice, physicians of the elderly are more likely to encounter the argument that an easeful death is a human right, and to encounter old people who claim that right for themselves. Personally, I do not think that this argument holds because it entails a duty of someone to comply with it, and I do not think there can be a medical duty to kill on request. But a right that can never be enforced is not a right.

That does not end the matter; however, it merely demonstrates that ethical questions cannot be reduced to a matter of competing rights and duties. It seems to me obvious that it is sometimes better—kinder, more decent, dignified, compassionate—to bring an end to human suffering than to let it continue. It is difficult, though, to legislate for such matters as kindness and decency, or to lay down precise rules as to when such clemency can, or cannot, be exercised. We are forever trying to catch the mists of human existence in the butterfly nets of our concepts; we demand categorical answers where there are only matters of degree. Nowhere is this more in evidence than in the anxiety-generating question of rational suicide in the elderly.

---

[14] David Hume, *On Suicide*.

Index

A
ABCB1 gene, 51
Abetting, 35
Ageism
  adoption of material monism, 69
  ageist attitudes, 64
  attitudes toward suicide, 70
  consciousness, 69
  contemporary society, 72
  deep source, 72
  Descartes' epistemological method, 69
  dystopia, 64
  elders, 64
  elder suicide, 69–72
  fear of death, 66–67
  hindrances, 69
  historical context, 64
  hold prejudice, 63
  interconnected relationships, 72
  lens of social gerontology, 65
  linear perspective vision, 68
  metaphysical assumption, 69
  natural rhythms of life, 72
  in perception, 67–68
  psychological history, 66–69
  racists and sexists, 63
  scientific materialist, 69
  vitalism, 69
  Western civilization, 63
Aid to Capacity Evaluation (ACE), 135
Aiding, 35
Ambivalence, 28, 30
American Association for Geriatric Psychiatry
  (AAGP) 2015 Annual Meeting, 76
American Psychiatric Association, 131
Antiaging skin products, 102
Antisocial personality disorders, 40
Assisted suicide, 188, 190, 192, 193, 198

Assisting suicide, 34–36
Autonomous suicide—suicide, 78
Autonomy value, 75, 77, 81, 82
Ayahuasca, 203, 204, 206, 207

B
Baby boomers
  chronic illnesses, 105–106
  and death, 103
  early boomers, 100
  executive and self-identified, 99
  financial difficulties, 106–107
  the GI Bill, 100
  heterogeneity of generational
    cohorts, 100
  institutions and medical technology, 107
  late boomers, 100
  older adults, 99
  older patients/clients, 108
  social isolation, 104
  social revolution, 101
  substance use, 104–105
  and suicide risk in late life, 104–107
  the United States, 100
  youth and aging, 101–102
Baconian project, 191
Beck Hopelessness Scale (BHS), 138
Borderline, 40

C
Capacity
  decision-making, 53–55
  patients with refractory medical
    disorders, 45
Catechism of the Catholic Church, 191
Cattell's review, 27

Printed in the United States
By Bookmasters